*Current and Historical
Perspectives on the
Borderline Patient*

Library of Congress Cataloging-in-Publication Data

Current and historical perspectives on the borderline patient / edited
  by Reuben Fine.
      p.   cm. — (Current issues in psychoanalytic practice)
    Bibliography: p.
    ISBN 0-87630-506-0
    1. Borderline personality disorder.   2. Psychoanalysis.   I. Fine,
  Reuben. 1914–   . II. Series.
  RC569.5.B67C87   1989
  616.85'852—dc20   89-7312
                                                                   CIP

Copyright © 1989 by The Society for Psychoanalytic Training

Published by
BRUNNER/MAZEL, INC.
19 Union Square
New York, NY 10003

MANUFACTURED IN THE UNITED STATES OF AMERICA

10 9 8 7 6 5 4 3 2

Contents

Contributors vii

Acknowledgments xiii

Introduction 1
    Reuben Fine

Part 1. Background: the Treatment of Schizophrenics

Excerpt from One Hundred Years of Psychiatry (1917) 19
    Emil Kraepelin

The Modified Psychoanalytic Treatment of
Schizophrenia (1931) 24
    Harry Stack Sullivan

The Relation of Onset to Outcome in Schizophrenia (1931) 46
    Harry Stack Sullivan

My Sixty Years with Schizophrenics (1979) 55
    Manfred Bleuler

Parents and Schizophrenia (1981) 59
    Bertram P. Karon & Gary R. VandenBos

Part 2. Theoretical Perspectives

Psychoanalysis and Psychiatry (1929) 83
    Ernest Jones

Borderline States (1953) 96
    Robert P. Knight

The Family Background (1968) 109
    Roy R. Grinker, Sr., Beatrice Werble & Robert C. Drye

Differential Diagnosis and Treatment (1975) 123
    Otto F. Kernberg

Discriminating Features of Borderline Patients (1978) 149
    John G. Gunderson & Jonathan E. Kolb

Theoretical Perspectives (1984) 161
    W. W. Meissner

The Interface Between Borderline Personality Disorder and
Affective Disorder (1985) 198
    John G. Gunderson & Glen R. Elliott

The New Psychoanalysis and Psychoanalytic Revisionism:
Book Review Essay on *Borderline Conditions and
Pathological Narcissism* (1979) 222
    Victor Calef & Edward M. Weinshel

Schizotypal Symptoms in Patients with Borderline
Personality Disorders (1986) 242
    Anselm George & Paul H. Soloff

Chicago Medical School, the University of Illinois Medical School, and Northwestern University Medical School; author of numerous books and articles.

Gunderson, John G., M.D.
Assistant Professor, Department of Psychiatry, Harvard Medical School; affiliated with Department of Psychiatry, McLean Hospital, Belmont, Massachusetts; author of numerous books and articles.

Handley, Robert B., Ph.D.
Staff Psychologist, National Jewish Center for Immunological and Respitory Medicine, Denver; Assistant Professor of Psychology, Department of Psychiatry, University of Colorado Health Science Center.

Hull, James W., Ph.D.
Assistant Professor of Psychology in Psychiatry, Cornell University Medical College; he works on the long-term unit for severe personality disorders and is Assistant Director of Training in Psychology, New York Hospital-Cornell Medical Center, Westchester Division.

Jones, Ernest, M.D. (1879–1958)
Member of the Royal College of Physicians in 1904, Dr. Jones is generally credited with introducing Freudian psychoanalysis to the English-speaking nations. He was instrumental in developing a worldwide organization devoted to the advancement of psychoanalysis. He was the founder of the *International Journal of Psychoanalysis,* which he was editor of until 1939. Jones made many original contributions in theoretical and clinical areas. He was a founder and past president of the British Psychoanalytic Society.

Karon, Bertram P., Ph.D.
Michigan State University; Michigan State Psychotherapy Project; clinician, supervisor and researcher in the area of the treatment of schizophrenia; co-author of *Psychotherapy of Schizophrenia: The Treatment of Choice.*

Kernberg, Otto F., M.D.
Medical Director, New York Hospital-Cornell Medical Center/Westchester Division; Professor of Psychiatry, Cornell Medical College; Training and Supervising Analyst, Columbia University Center for Psychoanalytic Training and Research. Dr. Kernberg has written extensively on the topic of the borderline personality.

Knight, Robert P., M.D.
Affiliated with the Menninger Foundation until he joined the staff of Austin Riggs, Dr. Knight has made many important theoretical and clinical contributions. He is most widely known for contributions regarding paranoia and borderline states.

Kolb, Jonathan E., M.D.
Instructor in Psychiatry, Harvard Medical School; Assistant Psychiatrist, McLean Hospital, Belmont, Massachusetts.

Kraepelin, Emil, M.D. (1856–1926)
Professor of Psychiatry and Director of the Psychiatric Clinic (Munich). Best known for his classification system of mental disorders, particularly the psychosis.

Lane, Robert C., Ph.D.
Clinical Professor of Psychology and Supervisor, Postdoctural Training Programs, Adelphi and Nova Universities; Training and Control Analyst and Director, Long Island Division of the New York Center for Psychoanalytic Training; past president, Division of Psychoanalysis, American Psychological Association and The Society for Psychoanalytic Training.

Levenson, Hanna, Ph.D.
Mental Hygiene Clinic, San Francisco Veterans Administration Medical Center, California.

McGlashan, Thomas H., M.D.
Director of Research, Chestnut Lodge; Research Professor of Psychiatry, University of Maryland School of Medicine; Instructor, Washington Psychoanalytic Institute; and a practicing psychotherapist and psychoanalyst.

Meissner, W. W., M.D.
Clinical Professor of Psychiatry, Harvard Medical School; author of numerous articles and books on many subjects including *The Paranoid Process* and *The Borderline Spectrum*.

Muth, Deborah Y., M.S.W.
Program Manager, The Therapeutic Community, Sacramento, California.

Acknowledgments

We wish to acknowledge for their kind permission to reprint:

Citadel Press for an excerpt from Emil Kraepelin's *One Hundred Years of Psychiatry,* 1917.

The Association for Research in Nervous and Mental Disease for Harry Stack Sullivan's "The Relation of Onset to Outcome in Schizophrenia," 1931.

Basic Books for Manfred Bleuler's "My Sixty Years with Schizophrenics," 1979; and Roy R. Grinker, Sr., Beatrice Werble and Robert C. Drye's "The Family Background," 1968.

Jason Aronson for Bertram P. Karon and Gary R. VandenBos's "Parents and Schizophrenia," 1981; Otto F. Kernberg's "Differential Diagnosis and Treatment," 1975; and W. W. Meissner's "Theoretical Perspectives," 1984.

Baillière Tindall for Ernest Jones's "Psychoanalysis and Psychiatry," 1929.

The *Bulletin of the Menninger Clinic* for Robert P. Knight's "Borderline States," 1953.

The American Journal of Psychiatry for John G. Gunderson and Jonathan E. Kolb's "Discriminating Features of Borderline Patients," 1978; John G. Gunderson and Glen R. Elliott's "The Interface Between Borderline Personality Disorder and Affective Disorder," 1985; Anselm George and Paul H. Soloff's "Schizotypal Symptoms in Patients with Borderline Personality Disorders," 1986; and David E. Reiser and Hanna Levenson's "Abuses of the Borderline Diagnosis: A Clinical Problem with Teaching Opportunities," 1984.

The Psychoanalytic Quarterly for Victor Calef and Edward M. Weinshel's "The New Psychoanalysis and Psychoanalytic Revisionism: Book Review Essay on *Borderline Conditions and Pathological Narcissism,*" 1979.

Human Sciences Press for Joseph Palombo's "Critical Review of the Concept of the Borderline Child," 1982.

Greenwood Press for Michael H. Stone's "Disturbances in Sex and Love in Borderline Patients," 1985.

The American Psychiatric Association for excerpts from Thomas H. McGlashan's "The Prediction of Outcome in Borderline Personality Disorder: Part V of the Chestnut Lodge Follow-up Study," 1985.

The Guilford Press for Les R. Greene, Judith Rosenkrantz, and Deborah Y. Muth's "Borderline Defenses and Countertransference: Research Findings and Implications," 1986.

*Current and Historical
Perspectives on the
Borderline Patient*

The reaction of the psychiatric world was not enthusiastic about Sullivan's results. Many doubted them; many called Sullivan himself "schizophrenic" and the like. Gradually, however, especially in the United States after World War II, when psychiatry began to develop more rapidly, psychiatrists began to develop more hope about the ultimate outcome for the schizophrenic patient. The facts are of course still very much in dispute. According to Kolb and Brodie (1982, p. 388), about one-third of those patients who are hospitalized during the first year of their illness make a fairly complete recovery; one-third improve but remain damaged; the remaining one-third will require indefinite care.

> The introduction of the modern pharmaceutical therapies has not brought about a reduction in the number of schizophrenic patients requiring hospital care whose illness pursues a chronic course. (p. 388)

Thus, in spite of the improvements brought about by drug therapy, theoretically for many psychiatrists the situation remained much the same as in Kraepelin's day: psychosis on one side, neurosis on the other, and never the twain could meet. The problem for them was to establish a clear-cut diagnosis; after that everything would fall into place.

But for a large number of other psychiatrists, more attuned to the findings of psychoanalysis, this attitude was unsatisfactory. They saw some schizophrenics get better, saw others have transient psychotic episodes remit without any therapeutic effort. The old saw that schizophrenics "have no anxiety" held on but eventually disappeared. A new type of classification was needed.

For the analysts the problem was much more simple. Freud had always believed in a continuum theory of a gradual transition from the normal to the psychotic. In fact, in his 1937 paper, "Analysis Terminable and Interminable," he made the remarkable statement:

> Every normal person, in fact, is only normal on the average. His ego approximates to that part of the *psychotic* in some part or other and to a greater or lesser extent. (p. 235, italics added)

In other words, as a consequence of analytic investigation, the differences among psychotics, neurotics and normals were considerably blurred. The problem arose, as never before, of clarifying the essential differences among them. Perhaps the clearest statement of the continuum theory was given by Ernest Jones in 1929 in his address at the opening of the Columbia University Psychiatric Institute:

> All mental morbidity is, therefore, a state of schizophre-
> nia, although Professor Bleuler has proposed to reserve
> this term for the most striking of its forms. What we meet
> with clinically as mental disorder represents the endless
> variety of the ways in which the threatened ego struggles
> for its self-preservation. In the nature of things, therefore,
> our conception of it can be cast only in terms of active
> dynamic strivings. (p. 372)

It is a mistake to believe that Sullivan's work stands alone. Prior to Word War I, hospital psychiatrists were not analytically oriented, which left them virtually resourceless in the management of the schizophrenic. Once analytic ideas began to come through, after the war, hospital psychiatrists applied them and found to their agreeable surprise that schizophrenics were by no means as narcissistic as had been supposed (Fine, 1979). In the 1920s many favorable results were reported with the psychotherapy of schizophrenia. August Staercke (1921), Paul Federn (1934) and many others communicated encouraging experiences with hospitalized psychotics, even though it was generally agreed that the results were not as good as those with neurotics.

Most interesting is a paper by Robert Waelder (1924), which has, so far as I can discover, the first use of the term "borderline."

> The subject of the present paper is in the first place an
> hypothesis concerning the conditioning factors by which
> a psychosis comes about or is avoided in those *border-line*
> characters in whom the phenomena of transition to a
> psychosis are so readily observed. The considerations
> which I shall bring forward should strengthen our hope of
> being able in the future to cure certain of the psychoses,
> for we shall convince ourselves that, in psychosis just as
> in neurosis, the distinction between "normal" and patho-
> logical is by no means a basic distinction in the psychic
> realm. (p. 260, italics in original)

It may also be noted in passing that while Freud had proposed a fundamental distinction between the narcissistic neuroses (pre-

American Psychoanalytical Association in 1979 was devoted to the question of technique, again with wide differences of opinion. A recent book by Wallerstein (1986) comes closer than any other work to clarifying analytic technique, but here too wide variations are noted, and long-held shibboleths, such as that analysis four times a week is more effective than once a week, have had to go by the board. In spite of the fact that no one could successfully define what a proper analysis should be, all the schools insisted on their particular version. Almost by definition a schizophrenic could not be analyzed, as far as most practitioners were concerned, so if he turned up improved or analyzed, something must be wrong with the diagnosis. A picture of widespread confusion resulted from the many personal and political battles that were fought after Word War II. Most recently, Otto Kernberg, who could certainly not be regarded as a rebel in any sense, has severely criticized the system of analytic education:

> I believe that psychoanalytic education is suffering from serious disturbances, which by analogy, might be examined as an illness affecting the educational structures of psychoanalytic institutes and societies. (1986, p. 799)

All of these historical observations are relevant to the current disputes about the nature, criteria and treatability of the borderline patient.

In the 1940s, when psychiatry first began to absorb the basic tenets of psychoanalytic theory, psychiatrists did note the inaccuracies inherent in the traditional Kraepelinian system but did not know what to do about them. The first solution was to suggest a wide variety of diagnostic categories into which they could fit the patients who, while obviously disturbed, were not classically either neurotic or psychotic. A variety of diagnostic labels were offered to characterize these patients: latent schizophrenia, pseudoneurotic schizophrenia, schizo-affective psychosis, psychotic character, incipient schizophrenia, socially recovered schizophrenia. None of these lasted very long before Adolph Stern suggested the term "borderline" in 1938, which was reinforced in a famous paper by Robert Knight, then president of the American Psychoanalytic Association, in 1953.

> The term borderline case is not recommended as a diagnostic term, for a much more precise diagnosis should be

made which identifies the type and degree of psychotic pathology. Far more important, however, than arriving at a diagnostic label is the achievement of a comprehensive psychodynamic appraisal of the balance in each patient between the ego's defensive and adaptive measures on the one hand, and the pathogenic instinctual and ego-disintegrating forces on the other, so that therapy can be planned and conducted for the purpose of conserving, strengthening, and improving the defensive and adaptive functions of the ego. (p. 172)

Although the term "borderline" was used by Adolph Stern in 1938, it was not until Knight's 1953 paper that it came into general use, even though he himself, as seen above, did not recommend it. Diagnostically, the numerous categories listed in the 1940s soon disappeared and were all generally replaced by the term "borderline." Some used it in the sense of "borderline psychosis," others in the sense of "borderline neurosis." Still others used it simply in the sense of severe personality disturbances (a term Kernberg himself uses in his latest book, 1984), with the implication that the further one gets toward the periphery of emotional disturbance (Stone, 1954) the harder it becomes to treat, yet there is no single category which is completely untreatable, if the therapist is willing to devote the time and the effort (cf. Searles, 1965).

In a widely quoted paper, Leo Stone (1954) confirmed the traditional continuum theory of psychoanalytic nosology and the general feeling of therapeutic optimism that existed among analysts:

The scope of psychoanalytic therapy has widened from the transference psychoneurosis, to include practically all nosological categories . . . While the difficulties increase and the expectations of success diminish in a general way as the nosological periphery is approached, there is no absolute barrier; and it is to be borne in mind that both extranosological factors and the therapist's personal tendencies may profoundly influence the indications and prognosis. Furthermore, from my point of view, psychoanalysis remains as yet the most powerful of all psychotherapeutic instruments, the "fire and iron" as Freud called it. (p. 593)

Within this general theory, however, the term "borderline," which, as Grinker et al. put it in 1968 (p. 172), had been in use for

substructures and functions, then analyzing the specific structural derivatives of internalized object relationships, which are relevant to this form of psychopathology. Under this heading he includes:

1) Nonspecific manifestations of ego weakness
2) Shift toward primary-process thinking
3) Specific defensive operations at the level of borderline personality organization. The most important of these defensive operations are:

   (a) splitting
   (b) primitive idealization
   (c) early forms of projection and, especially, projective identification
   (d) denial
   (e) omnipotence and devaluation

4) Pathology of internalized object relationships

Genetic Dynamic Analysis

The primary aspect is pregenital aggression, especially oral aggression. A frequent finding is a history of extreme frustration and intense aggression (secondary or primary) during the first few years of life. Excessive pregenital and particularly oral aggression tends to be projected and causes a paranoid distortion of the early parental images, especially of the mother. In both sexes, excessive development of pregenital, especially oral, aggression tends to induce a premature development of oedipal strivings, and as a consequence of a particular pathological condensation between pregenital and genital aims under the overriding influence of aggressive needs. All of these pathological solutions are unsuccessful attempts to deal with the aggressiveness of genital trends and the general infiltration of all instinctual needs by aggression.

Neither in 1968 nor in 1984 does Kernberg commit himself to any etiological formula. We are left in the dark about whether this kind of pathology is due to nature or nurture.

With regard to therapy, Kernberg has recently modified his views to recommend modified psychoanalytic psychotherapy:

> Although most borderline patients . . . do best with modified psychoanalytic psychotherapy, there are some who

can be analyzed without modifications of technique, and I have recently become more optimistic in this regard. (1984, p. 165)

Kernberg's work has in the past 20 years created a virtual "Kernbergian" revolution. Yet he is, of course, not without his critics, some of them quite severe. One article after another appears on the borderline, so, evidently, even the most essential questions have not been definitively answered by his formulations.

The first extensive critique of Kernberg's position was by Victor Calef and Edward Weinshel (1979). Their main conclusions are:

1) The borderline personality organization concept has blurred the already unclear distinction between psychoanalysis and psychotherapy. What emerges from his writings is a greater confusion of what constitutes the essence of psychoanalysis.
2) There has been a retreat from an emphasis on the vicissitudes of sexuality, the derivatives of libido, and the centrality of the oedipal conflict.
3) More and more, "psychological" conflict is seen in terms of conflict with the external world and its representatives rather than in terms of intrapsychic conflict.
4) Related to this shift in the arena of the "real" is a clear indication that the tripartite structural theory with all of its derivatives and implications is being replaced by the putative theories of object relations.
5) Kernberg introduces a shift, diagnostically, from the emphasis on understanding, on the recognition of continual and at least tacit acknowledgment that diagnostic labels are artificial and abstract. "We view this tendency as regressive, harking back to a sort of Kraepelinian taxonomy" (p. 489).
6) There is a significant tendency to depart from the very basic technical precepts of "free association," the rule of abstinence, the principle of the analyst's freely suspended attention, and the priority given to the admonition to respect "where the patient is now."
7) A bandwagon effect has been created which makes it virtually impossible to find a case which cannot be suspected and/or considered to fall within the borderline personality organization orbit. To make anything a virtually universal diagnosis, as is now being done with the borderline, is highly suspect.

As Calef and Weinshel (1979) have noted, everything seems to have been thrown into the pot, so that it becomes virtually impossible to find a patient who does not have some borderline traits. Further, the DSM III specifies that no "single feature is invariably present" (APA, 1980, p. 321).

Thus, we are brought back to the original continuum approach: normal-neurotic-psychotic, with now considerable clarification of the dynamics of all three. "Borderline" could replace neurotic on the current scene, but it seems to be just as varied as the definitions of neurosis were in the past.

Since borderline is so protean, covering such a wide range of pathology, there seems to be little justification for insisting that it is a definite pathological entity. Most studies have not been able to find that uniformity that Kernberg seems to desire. And even Kernberg, in his latest book, refers to *The Severe Personality Disorders* (1984).

Thus, it would seem to be simpler to say of a borderline that we are dealing with a very disturbed person, with a variety of pathological manifestations, who is nevertheless not psychotic, though transient psychotic symptoms may appear and/or disappear. With regard to treatability and the best mode of treatment, the best answer would seem to be provided by the exhaustive Wallerstein (1986) study. It made little difference there whether patients were diagnosed as psychotic, borderline, or neurotic, or had some other designation. The outcome of treatment depended more on the clinical sagacity of the therapist than on any standard diagnosis. In other words, whatever you call the patient, what is most vital is that the therapist has to treat the patient in an appropriate manner.

Inevitably, the diagnosis of borderline brings up the question of the treatability of the schizophrenic. The term "borderline" after all was originally devised to delineate those patients who could respond to treatment to some extent because they were not as far gone as full-blown psychotics.

In this respect, opinions again vary all over the lot. Some (perhaps the majority of organic psychiatrists) still assert unequivocally that schizophrenics cannot be analyzed, and cannot even be properly treated without medication. Others insist that the alleged untreatability of the schizophrenic is due more to the attitude of the therapist than to the severity of the illness, pointing to the numerous analysts such as Sullivan, Fromm-Reichmann, Searles, Karon and VandenBos, Bleuler and innumerable others who have reported reasonable results with the psychotherapy of schizophrenia.

In part, the question rests on the level of regression in the patient. Many call "borderline" today would have been called "schizophrenic" in the past. Many called "schizophrenic" are relatively mild and respond rather well to kindly care and understanding, as in the "moral treatment" of the early 1800s. Again, however, the emphasis is placed too squarely on the patient rather than on the interaction between patient and therapist. Herbert Strean (1988) has commented that the best therapist for the schizophrenic is a first year social work student. There is much to this apparently cynical comment, since the first year social work student can do little beside giving a little love and care, while the full-fledged psychiatrist is so full of complex jargon that he does not see the patient.

The example of the Belgian city of Gheel is still before us. There for centuries (since at least the twelfth century) schizophrenic patients have been lodged with the members of the local community, who have learned to live and get along with them.

Another event, from modern times, is the startling Italian decree of 1978, which at one sweep abolished all mental hospitals (Mosher, 1982). Patients were to be treated in small community installations, where they could be given close care and therapy, as well as whatever else they needed. It is too soon to tell how this experiment will work out, but it is in line with basic psychoanalytic understanding. The point is again that the emphasis must be placed not on the "diagnosis" but on the way in which the patient is treated, including the personality of the treating person.

Conclusion

This whole discussion, as well as the other papers contained in this monograph, stress two points. First of all, there is still no real agreement about whether borderline is a clear-cut diagnostic entity. Since it includes so much, the chances are that it is not, but only time and further research will tell.

Second, the training of the therapist is more significant than the diagnosis. It is in this sense that Kernberg's recent (1986) blast at the analytic educational system must be understood. Like Sullivan, he has evidently been disillusioned by the countertransferences of the average physician who undertakes psychotherapeutic treatment. Sullivan (1962) once commented that it takes the average physician on the staff of a mental hospital 12 to 18 months to "crack his crust" to such an effect that he can begin to learn what it is all about.

Thus, once more the topic of borderline personality leads back to the personal qualifications of the therapist, which turn out to be far more important than any textbook understanding of symptoms

Excerpt from

One Hundred Years of Psychiatry

Emil Kraepelin
(1917)

The revolution that occurred during the course of a century shows up clearly in the development of psychiatric methods in Munich. The old "lunatic cells" with their rings and chains in the first hospital were replaced in 1801 by 25 rooms in the asylum built by Griesinger. The asylum was soon notorious and so overcrowded that patients could not even be segregated according to sex. These conditions led in 1859 to the erection of a district asylum, later enlarged several times, which on April 1, 1860 accommodated 166 patients. The asylum was first directed by Solbrig, then by Gudden. Each of the four sections of the barracks-type structure was enclosed by a square garden. By 1877, the number of usable rooms had surpassed 500. When it too became overcrowded, the construction of the colonial-type Gabersee institution was undertaken. The old institution was finally abandoned altogether. It was replaced in 1905 by Eglfing's large rural asylum, to which the Haar institution was annexed in 1912. On January 1, 1917 the three institutions in Upper Bavaria and the psychiatric clinic erected in 1904 accommodated a grand total of 2,751 patients. This represents an increase of 1,657% over a period of 57 years.

The final topic in our survey of the evolution of psychiatry is family nursing, or the accommodation of selected patients in their own homes or in the homes of strangers under professional supervision. The pattern for family nursing was set by the Belgian village of Gheel. For centuries Gheel had been the mecca of mental patients in search of a cure. That is how a number of patients came to find lodging in private homes. In spite of many drawbacks, this type of treatment had so many good features that it was later imitated elsewhere. In Germany it was first adopted, more than a century ago, in Rockwinckel. It was not widely adopted in Germany, however, until the last few decades. Nowadays it is practiced with varying degrees of success in many different localities. Wherever the local population is suited to the practice, it is doubtlessly much better to entrust the care of the patient to a family rather than to place him in an institution. With the family he can enjoy full freedom of movement, worthy employment and familiar surroundings. Patients must be carefully selected, however, and placed under the constant supervision of a physician.

But today concern for the welfare of our patients does not end when they are discharged by the physician. The last several decades have witnessed the formation of benevolent associations in many places to help discharged patients. Most of them have been patterned after the one founded in Heppenheim by Ludwig. Their task is to facilitate the return of patients who have recovered or improved to a normal pattern of living, to help them with their problems, and by so doing, to preserve and fortify the good results achieved through institutional treatment. Equally important is the fact that these benevolent associations through their activities have narrowed the gap between institutional doctors and laymen, gradually weakened deep-rooted prejudices against asylums, and brought to the attention of a wider audience our obligations to our fellow men who suffer from mental disease. The same effects have resulted from greater accessibility to institutions for the insane on the part of the outside world; contributory factors have been the disappearance of surrounding walls, the performance of ordinary farm tasks by patients, provisions for greater freedom of movement, and cordiality toward visitors.

If we compare the situation of mental patients today with the circumstances that prevailed a century ago, the revolution that has been accomplished comes into clear focus. The words penned by Nostiz in 1829 ring true: "If we weigh objectively the accomplishments of the last half century and try to determine how far we are in theory, word and deed from our goal, then we may reasonably conclude that the progress now being made in psychiatry and the uses to which it is now being put in our institutions will result in its complete transformation before the end of the present century." One by one prejudices have been overcome, abuses and cruel practices eliminated, new means found to alleviate mental diseases. Spearheading this advance was the growing body of scientific knowledge relating to the nature and etiology of insanity and deriving from study of data in different fields of investigation and from the overall progress of the science of medicine. Unrelenting effort on the part of a large number of alienists gradually transformed the sad lot of the mentally ill, with the result that today we are actually nearing the end of our struggle. To be sure there are still many defects to be remedied and improvements to be made, but we are not being presumptuous in stating that we have discovered the approach to be followed henceforth in psychiatry.

Our satisfaction over the progress already made is tinged with regret. When we consider the extraordinary sacrifices made by those responsible for the evolution of psychiatry, we are constrained to lament the fact that all the hopes tied to it can never be fulfilled. We must openly admit that the vast majority of the patients placed in our institutions are according to what we know forever lost, that even the best of care can never restore them to perfect health. Our treatment probably makes life endurable for a vast number of mental cripples whose plight would otherwise be intolerable, but only rarely does it effect a cure. A study made at the request of Vocke showed that out of 1,183 patients in Eglfing on January 1, 1917, no less than 826, or 70%, were considered incurable. This should come as no surprise to anyone with psychiatric experience. Also to be considered is the fact that patients who recovered were always discharged while incurable patients accumulated; thus it is obvious that by itself even the best psychiatric therapy can not eradicate the scourge of mental disease.

We must therefore ask if there are other, more promising, approaches. The answer is a resounding yes. Most promising is the prevention of insanity, though this is possible today only to the extent that we are acquainted with the causes of the affliction and are capable of combating it. We know the basic causes of three major diseases: hereditary defects, alcoholism, and syphilis. They constitute, according to the most conservative estimates, at least one third of all mental disorders treated in our clinic. Then comes addiction to morphine and cocaine. Traumatic neuroses can also be prevented. An autocrat in possession of our present knowledge would be able, if he showed no consideration for the lifelong habits of men, to effect a significant reduction in the incidence of insanity within a few decades. We can entertain even higher hopes. The nature of most mental disorders is now obscured. But no one will deny that further research will uncover new facts in so young a science as ours; in this respect the diseases produced by syphilis are an object lesson. It is logical to assume that we shall succeed in uncovering the causes of many other types of insanity that can be prevented—perhaps even cured—though at present we have not the slightest clue; a case in point was cretinism before the discovery of the thyroid treatment.

Only scientific research can bring about the realization of such advances. In the past it has spearheaded medical advances, and on it will depend our success in the future. It is not, as might be assumed, the favorite pastime of a few enlightened minds but the basis for all further progress. The great war in which we are now engaged has compelled us to recognize the fact that science could forge for us a host of effective weapons for use against a hostile world. Should it be otherwise if we are fighting an internal enemy seeking to destroy the very fabric of our existence? Hardenberg said in his decree of February 16, 1805: "The state must concern itself with all institutions for those with damaged minds, both for the betterment of the unfortunates and for the advancement of science. In this important and difficult field of medicine only unrelenting efforts will enable us to carve out advances for the good of suffering mankind. Perfection can be achieved only in such institutions; here are found all the conditions necessary for conducting experiments to test basic theories and for using the results of such experimentation for the advancement of science."

Anyone familiar with the present state of our science will see that further advancement will require measures not now in use. The nature of psychiatry is such that questions which are constantly being formulated can be answered only on the basis of evidence supplied by a number of auxiliary disciplines; clinical observation must be supplemented by thorough examination of healthy and diseased brains, neurology, the study of heredity and degenerative diseases, the chemistry of metabolism, and serology. Only exceptionally well-trained specialists possess competency in each particular field; their ranks are thin and, because of unfavorable external conditions, they now have only a limited opportunity to exercise their skills. These observations clearly show that only a well-planned and comprehensive program of research can bring us closer to the goal which we are striving to attain. We ought therefore to note with pride and satisfaction that it was possible for us in Germany in the middle of a raging war to take the first step toward establishing a research institute for the purpose of determining the nature of mental diseases and of discovering techniques for effecting their prevention, alleviation and cure. All those who have contributed to the success of this great undertaking, especially His Majesty our King and the worthy authors of the program, merit our most cordial thanks. A far greater recompense than anything which we might be able to say today, however, is the hope that ground has already been broken for new approaches that will enable us to win a victory over the direst afflictions that can beset man.

But we have taken only the fist step toward our goal. Even under the most favorable conditions, the fruits of scientific labor generally ripen very slowly, and in our field quick, dazzling results are unthinkable; quite apart from these considerations, providing funds for the elaboration of a unified program of research poses a challenge still to be faced. We believe that we can face it with confidence. The cost of providing psychiatric care is staggering; efforts to lower costs, if promising, should receive unqualified support. According to figures supplied by Vocke, a large research institute could be operated on an annual budget of 200,000 marks, or one-tenth of one per cent of the total funds now required for the operation of our institutions. If each year the research institute succeeded only in preventing mental disease in one of 1,000 cases or in helping one out of 1,000 inmates to regain his freedom, it follows that the expense of the institute would soon be recovered. Can we ignore such important considerations? It seems to me that we should recall here the words used by Müller in 1824 to reject the notion that attempts to better the situation of the insane might be impeded by the impossibility of raising the necessary funds. "In this wide world," he said, "there are still many unmarried and childless men whose coffers have been richly blessed and whose sense of charity, which is not dead but merely dormant, needs to be awakened and guided toward this beautiful, sacred goal. And what goal could be more sacred than that of caring for a brother in distress, especially when the affliction is distinctly human and therefore more obvious than others, and when it respects neither reason nor rank nor riches?"

The Modified Psychoanalytic Treatment of Schizophrenia

Harry Stack Sullivan, M.D.
(1931)

In this presentation, an attempt will be made to contribute some factual material bearing on the nature of the schizophrenic mental disorders, and on their treatment by a procedure rather intimately related to the psychoanalytic method of Sigmund Freud. No argument will be offered as to the propriety of the use of "psychoanalytic" in referring to a definite variation from Dr. Freud's technique, nor will a review of the orthodox Freudian contributions to the schizophrenia problem be undertaken. The former cannot but remain a matter of personal opinion. For the latter we may await a presently forthcoming study by Dr. William V. Silverberg. Since a session of our current meeting has been devoted to the subject of schizophrenia, and since some of the views expressed therein are doubtless not consonant with those of the present writer, some attention must also be devoted to the meaning of schizophrenia as hereinafter used. No importance is attached, however, to the magnificent expression of my personal prejudices in these matters.[1]

Reprinted from *American Journal of Psychiatry, 88;* 519–540, 1931–1932. Read in abstract at the eighty-seventh meeting of the American Psychiatric Association, Toronto, June 5, 1931.

[In the process of examining early in the paper the whole concept of "prediction" in medicine and psychiatry, Sullivan gives, somewhat facetiously, the historical and professional setting for the paper and its predictability. — Helen Swick Perry]

24

Firstly, it is held that if there is any difference between the "schizoid" and "schizophrenic" mental disturbances, the difference is wholly one of degree, and not one of kind. The writer is no more entertained by "thobbing" about an essential organic disorder in schizophrenia, than is he by tedious speculation as to the relations of organic anomaly or defect to particular psychoses with mental deficiency. In contradistinction, for example, to Schilder's contribution at the earlier session [1931–32], this paper is intended to deal with consensually valid information about actual patients and actual procedures of therapy, rather than with ingenuity of thinking about hypotheses concerning possibilities of an unknown order of probability. It must follow the tedious scientific rather than the spectacular philosophic road, and its verbiage must be so carefully organized and so adequately elucidated as to provide the psychiatric reader with a formulation useful to himself and his patients. It does not set up any new frame of reference by use of which one can achieve a high percentage of "hits" at the game of prognostic prophecy: to the writer, the future of any particular person is a highly contingent matter, unless the subject-person be psychobiologically an adult— and in the latter case, unless also he be approaching the *senium,* the degree of contingency of his future is *distinct* if not still *high.* Had we persisted for many generations in an agrarian culture, and had this, improbably, been accompanied by extensive, well-integrated psychobiological research, so that we came to know a great deal about the living of our people, then, perchance, we would have come to a fair acquaintance with the actualities of *human probability.* Translated, however, in a few generations from such a culture to the unprecedented industrial situation, we are now in a state of almost complete ignorance of these facts of living, and therefore without any basis for prophecy as to the outcome of this or that poorly envisaged complex of more or less important but partly unrecognized factors. The future of each physico-chemical organism may subsist in some reality underlying our hypothetical time-dimension, but the future of each *person* must be recognized as a function of the eternally changing configuration of the cultural-social present. Conceivably, the identical germ plasm evolving in monozygotic twins may be representative in the present of a path in the future such that the twins shall arrive synchronously at a physico-chemical fiasco in the shape of appendicial inflammation. Conceivably, it was in some ultimately comprehensible fashion ordained at the moment of the writer's conception that he shall cease to live owing to rupture of the middle meningeal artery at the age of 57 years, 3 months and 5 days, plus or minus less than 100 hours.* But that the present fact of his contemning what Dr. Gregory Stragnell has so aptly dubbed the scholasticism of certain psychoanalytically inclined psychiatrists— in this particular case Paul Schilder about real and pseudo- schizophrenia—that this activity was determined more remotely than the occasion of the last meeting of the Association for Research in Nervous and Mental Diseases, is not true.[2]

No one could conceivably demonstrate any preordination of the effect on the protagonist's future of this situation, prior to the date first named. That which at least two people cannot demonstrate cannot be utilized in scientific procedure. It seems therefore fairly proven that the effects of the current interpersonal situation on the future of Dr. Paul Schilder, arise de novo from the configuration of the present; this in turn, in so far as it is focused in the writer, arising from configurations *actually existing* at particular moments on certain dates in the recent past; these, in further turn, arising from streams of events so complex in themselves, and so complex in their interrelations, that any prophecy of the current situation, on a date more distant than six months ago, would have been fantastic in the extreme.[3]

To return now to the crux of this point: *either no one* of the acutely schizophrenic young men received by the research service of the Sheppard and Enoch Pratt Hospital in the past two years was in fact schizophrenic but instead all were "schizoid"—in which case we might perhaps assume that schizophrenia *the* disease is not shown by native-born males before the age of 25—*or* there is no great importance to be attached to the organic substratum of personality in young acute schizophrenics, but rather great stress to be laid on the socio-psychiatric treatment to which they are exposed, in our studying of the factors relevant to outcome. It is my opinion that a consensus of qualified observers can be secured in support of the latter conclusion. The question of an "organic disorder" is therefore irrelevant to this consideration of schizophrenia.[4]

Secondly, in further delimitation of the term, schizophrenia, it is held that these disorders have not been defined psychoanalytically. It is necessary, before adumbrating the original communication herein attempted, to discountenance any conclusion that the writer's study of schizophrenia has "proven" or "disproven" psycho-

---

*Sullivan was born on February 21, 1892. He died of a cerebral hemorrhage on January 14, 1949, aged 56 years, 10 months, 24 days. — H. S. P.

analytic theory, or any part or parcel thereof, other than the doctrine of narcissistic neurosis. The psychoanalytic terms hereinafter utilized are terms as to the meaning of which, in the writer's opinion, a consensus of competent observers could be obtained. That these consensually defined meanings would be identical with or quite different from the most orthodox Freudian definitions, is unknown. Psychoanalytic formulations are extremely individualistic, in the sense that they are largely Prof. Freud's opinions about his experience with his patients, in the formation of which opinions—as in the great part of all psychiatric opinions—the social and cultural aspects of the thinker's opinion-formation have mostly been ignored. There could not be a meaningful use of the term schizophrenia in regard of a man who had grown from birth into adolescence in utter detachment from any person or personally organized culture. Again, it is possible so to organize a society that the living of its persons, normal to each other, would be regarded as schizophrenic by psychiatrists who studied any one of its members in sufficiently alien surroundings. In brief, schizophrenia is meaningful only in an *interpersonal context*; its characteristics can only be established by a study of the interrelation of the schizophrenic with schizophrenic, less schizophrenic, and nonschizophrenic others. A "socially recovered" schizophrenic is often still psychotic, but is certainly *less* schizophrenic than is a patient requiring active institutional supervision. To isolate the *non*-schizophrenic individual, however, is no small problem. It implies criteria of presence or absence of these processes, of which criteria there seems to be a marked dearth. One might use the following as a fundamental basis for classification: the non-schizophrenic individual, in his interaction with other persons, behaves and thinks in complete consonance with their mutual cultural make-up. Then, to the extent that one's behavior and thought in dealing with another diverges from the mutual culture— traditions, conventions, fashions—to that extent he would be schizophrenic. This seems to be a good working hypothesis, but it has not yet ensued in much consensually valid information. There is, as yet, no measuring of mutual culture; we know that being exposed to culture does not necessarily imply its incorporation in a personality; we know that there are certain personality differentials that greatly affect the incorporation of cultural entities; but we have not paid much attention to evolving techniques for distinguishing the cultural aspects of individual personalities.[5]

There is, however, an indirect approach to this problem—one, moreover, that has seemed to be of practical application. We know that the dream-life of the individual is to a very great degree, purely personal. This consideration applies to a lesser extent to the waking fantasy-life. While there is probably very little indeed of the waking fantasy that is uninfluenced by environing persons or personal entities not wholly of the self, we can assume that certain "primitive" dreams are almost entirely without external reference. We therefore conclude that the more like the dream of deep sleep a given content is, the more purely of the self it is. We can then surmise that a rough approximation to our basis for division into the schizophrenic and the nonschizophrenic can be hypothecated on the consideration of the more purely personal versus the consensually valid appercep-tion of a given interpersonal situation. If the "contact" with external reality is wholly unintelligible per se to the presumably fairly sane observer, then the subject-individual manifests a content indistin-guishable from a dream, and is either in a state of serious disorder of the integrating systems, or is schizophrenic. An individual manifest-ing behavior when not fully awake would thus be clearly schizo-phrenic. An individual suffering the disorder of interest manifested in severe fatigue would likewise come under this rubric.

A psychiatrist's initial reaction to this formulation can scarcely be one of instant acceptance. He knows of people who "awaken" in nightmares and have trouble in throwing off the content of the dream. He knows that most of these folk are comparatively normal, in their daily life. He is not ready to identify their transitory disturbance of consciousness on occasional nights with the mental disorder shown 18 hours or so per day, day in and day out by the "dementia praecox" patients in the wards of the mental hospital. It is the writer's opinion that neither phenomenologically nor dynami-cally can a distinction be shown between the two situations. Schizophrenics, in the first hours or days of the frank illness, show just as abrupt transitions among distinguishable states as does our troubled dreamer. The dream-state in their case tends to become habitual, or at least frequently recurrent, and whenever this occurs, the individual is definitely schizophrenic.[6]

The questions that would seem to require answer before acceptance of this formulation of schizophrenia are somewhat as follows: How does it happen that most of us are able to sort out our dreams and our waking experience with a very high degree of success, while the schizophrenic fails in this? Why do only some of those who have night-terror or nightmares progress into chronic schizophrenic states? And, from the organicist, why, if this definition is approximately correct, should not a treatment by alternation of rest and the use of a powerful cerebral stimulant like caffeine bring about at least a suspension of the schizophrenic state? As to the first of these questions, the actual sorting out of *some little* of our dream-life from waking experience is a difficult or impossible task. The little that is "hard to locate" as to whether dream or "reality" is often quite transparently related to important but none too well recognized tendency systems within the personality concerned. We come thus to the answer of questions one and two: To the extent that important tendency systems of the personality *have* to discharge themselves in sleep, to that extent the dream-processes tend to exaggerated personal importance, and to augmented "reality value." That which permits tendency systems no direct manifestation except during sleep and other states of altered consciousness is their condition of *dissociation* by other tendency systems of the personality—systems apparently invariably represented in the self. At this point, a digression must be made anent a fairly popular psychoanalytic "thob" about the "strength" versus "weakness" of the ego. We learn that the superego is "weak" in the schizophrenic; also, that it is "strong" in the schizophrenic; that the ego and the ideal of ego are weak or strong; that the feeble ego is ground between the powerful id of instinctual cravings and the superego; and so forth. Leaving aside the fact that there is plenty of clinical material to be observed by anyone seriously interested in *finding out* what this is all about— there being at least 250,000 patients diagnosed as schizophrenic in the hospitals of the United States—the writer would point out that no night-terror, nightmare, or schizophrenic disorder *can occur* unless there is a waking dissociation of some one powerful tendency system by another powerful tendency system. And, by direct implication of the formula, a continued dream-state, schizophrenia, cannot occur unless there is continued an approximation to a dynamic balance between the tendency system manifesting in the conscious self and the one dissociated from such manifestation.[7] As to the chemotherapeutic employment of agents to provide rest alternating with cerebral stimulants of the caffeine group, it may be noted that this very program, applied during the first hours of schizophrenic collapse, does delay the disaster. The cerebrum and the other areas responding to caffeine stimulation, however, are not solely the province of the conscious self, and the raised threshold of function is not solely at the service of the *dissociating* system. This topic, together with that of delirifacient drugs and of ethyl alcohol, has been discussed by the writer, elsewhere.

It appears, then, that no well-integrated personality—in whom there is no dissociation of an important tendency system—can show schizophrenic processes of more than momentary duration; and that any personality in whom there is a chronic dissociation of a powerful tendency system may show persisting schizophrenia after any event that destroys the balance by strengthening the dissociated tendency system, or by enfeebling the dissociating system. Physiological maturation and toxic-exhaustive states are frequent factors in this connection.

The partition of time to the schizophrenic processes—whether they occupy but moments during the time ordinarily devoted to sleep, or instead persist days on end in active psychosis—is determined by the balance between the dissociated and the dissociating systems. The "healing" process that ordinarily occurs in night-terror and nightmare is the source of an important insight into this matter. One "recovers" from the failing dissociation manifesting more or less lucidly in the nightmare, by reintegrating one's consciousness of circumambient reality, including one's "place," status, etc. If the pressure of the dissociated system is great, one "knows better" than to return to sleep until one has strengthened the dissociating system by a readjustment of interest and attention to one's waking world. In night-terror, the healing process is less conscious, but usually more directly *interpersonal.* In any case, in the writer's opinion, the restoration of balance in favor of the dissociating system is achieved by some *adjustment of interpersonal relations.* On the other hand, a persisting dream-state represents a failure of interpersonal adjustment, such that the tendency system previously dissociated is now as powerful in integrating interpersonal situations as is the previously successful dissociating system. The augmentation of the one may alternate somewhat with that of the other; the *degree* of consciousness may vary, but conflict and a consciously perceived threat of eruption of the dissociated system is sustained. It is evident that these dynamics may lead to the phenomena delineated in the paper of Dr. Mary O'Malley earlier in the program. It is equally clear that the "retreat" from the personal realities of others, the "seclusiveness" and the inaccessibility to easy personal contacts that are so classically schizophrenic are but the avoidance of accentuated conflict between the tendency systems, which integrate or "strive" to integrate the sufferer into mutually incongruous interpersonal relations, with the appearance of most distressing interests and attention.

We may proceed from this theoretic formulation of the facts of schizophrenia to consideration of the treatment of these disorders. It is to be noted that the basic formula of all psychotherapy is that of interpersonal relations, and their effects on the further growth of tendency systems within the patient-personality. Observation of the processes shown in improvements and aggravations of personality disorder is clearly in line with this formulation. One sees that there is no *essential* difference between psychotherapeutic achievement and achievements in other forms of education. There is, in each, an alteration in the cultural-social part of the affected personality, to a state of better adaptation to the physico-chemical, social, and cultural environment. No essential difference exists between the better integration of a personality to be achieved by way of psychoanalytic personality study, and the better integration to be achieved by an enlightened teacher of physics in demonstrating to his student the properties of matter. There are several differences in the technique required, but these are superficial rather than fundamental, and are to be regarded as determined by actual early training of the patient, in the end reducible to the common denominator of *experience incorporated into the self.* The principal factors responsible for the apparent gap between the ordinary good educative techniques and the orthodox psychoanalytic procedures are to be found in the peculiar characteristics of very early experience—viz., that of the first 18 to 30 months of extrauterine life.[8] Since the characteristics of this material are discussed in various psychoanalytic contributions—including that of Dr. Gregory Zilboorg in this session—and since the purpose of this paper is to present the necessary steps preliminary to dealing with the infantile and early childhood experience, we shall proceed immediately to a consideration of the *interpersonal requirements* for the successful therapy of the schizophrenic.

Psychotherapy, like all experience, functions by promoting personality growth, *with or without* improvement of personality integration. Pure suggestion therapy, if such there be, merely adds experience to one or more of the important tendency systems of the personality, thereby perhaps altering the dynamic summation manifested in behavior and thought. Even such a therapy could perhaps be useful in preschizophrenic personalities and, conceivably, even in acute psychosis. A purely rational therapy would be directed to the better integration of the personality systems, as well as to the provision of additional experience. Since it could apply only at the level of verbal communication, it should scarcely be expected to produce great affect in the field of extra-conscious processes. Hortatory therapy would generally be directed to the augmentation of the superego aspects of personality. This includes persuasion and the all too prevalent "bucking up" treatment. None of these procedures is in line with the information which we have secured as to the growth and function of personality.

Treatment in states of reduced consciousness, notably under hypnosis, could be more nearly adjusted to the total personality. Unfortunately, however, the integration of the treatment situation implied by the occurrence of the hypnotic or even the hypnoid states imposes a great responsibility on the physician. Unless he is expert indeed in dealing with the earlier experience incorporated in each personality, the net result of the treatment is sadly disappointing. Either there is little more achieved than could have been secured by a fairly rational exhortation, or there is disturbance of the superego functions and an increased severity of conflict. The integration of the hypnosis situation in the incipient or acute schizophrenic is difficult in extreme. This manipulation of the personality is therefore for us chiefly of theoretic importance. The attempt at hypnotizing distressed preschizophrenics should perhaps be emphatically discouraged, as the mandatory—even if self-determined—submission to the other personality is almost certain to cause a severe emotional upheaval, with the hypnotist thereafter in an unenviable role as chief personification of the goal of the dissociated system.

The only tools that have shown results that justify any enthusiasm in regard of the treatment of schizophrenia are the *psychoanalytic* procedures and the *socio-psychiatric* program which the writer has evolved from them. Before taking up these procedures, however, it may be well to note that the process of benefit by psychoanalysis seems none too clearly envisaged by many of its practitioners. One might be led to assume from the literature that a "cure" is achieved by a releasing of the libido from its "point of the fixation" existing somewhere in the past of the individual. A steadily increasing complexity of the map of possible fixation points is leading some of the outstanding thinkers in this field to doubt the importance of the doctrine of fixation. The writer has long since indicated his inability to discover anything corresponding to a point of fixation in schizophrenia, and has come to believe that "releasing the libido from its fixations" is but a figure of speech for something that occurs in recovery under analysis. Observation shows that psychoanalytic therapy consists of two major processes, the combination of which leads to growth and improved integration of personality. These are, firstly, a retrospective survey of the experiential basis of tendencies that conflict with the simple adaptation of the person to others with resulting growth to a more adult character;

and secondly, the provision of experience that facilitates the reorganization of the undeveloped or warped tendencies such that adaptation becomes more successful. The achievement of this double process requires the establishment between the physician and patient of the situation called by Freud the "transference."

There has been a good deal written about "transference," and many peculiarities of technique have been originated with view to its cultivation and management. There seems to the writer to be nothing other than *the purpose* of the interpersonal situation which distinguishes the psychoanalytic transference relation from other situations of interpersonal intimacy. In other words, it seems to be a special case of interpersonal adaptation, distinguished chiefly by the rôle of subordination to an enlightened physician skilled in penetrating the self-deceptions to which man is uniquely susceptible, with a mutually accepted purpose of securing the patient an increased skill in living. Like almost all other situations tending towards intimacy the early states of the psychoanalytic situation include a great body of fantasy processes that are not directly helpful to the achievement of the goal of the physician. Like all other interpersonal relations, this one includes a good deal of intercommunication by channels other than that of spoken propositions. As it is ordinarily applied, the psychoanalytic situation involves a patient the organization of whose self is not satisfactory, and whose self-regard is inadequate. This is very much the case in preschizophrenic and incipiently and acutely (catatonic) schizophrenic patients. By reason of the extreme distress caused by any threatened (or fantasied) reduction of the already distressingly small self-regard of these patients, and also by reason of specific painful experience with all previously significant persons, these patients are extremely uneasy about any situation in which the favorable cooperation of another is required for its resolution. The appearance of strong positive tendency towards the physician is thus attended by an extraordinary augmentation of attention for unfavorable signs, and very slight provocation may lead to a reversal of the tendency—from positive to negative, love to hate.

Before proceeding to develop the implications of these facts for the actual management of these patients, reemphasis must be made of the writer's distinction of schizophrenia from hebephrenic deterioration and from paranoid maladjustments. In brief, the patients to whom therapy may be applied with high probability of success are, firstly, patients in whom there has been a rather rapid change from a state of partial adjustment, to one of apparent psychosis, a matter of weeks, not months or years—this transition being the incipient schizophrenic state; secondly, patients who have not progressed into that regression of interests to early childhood or late infancy levels, to which we refer as the hebephrenic; and thirdly, patients who have not made a partial recovery by massive projection and transfer of blame, the "paranoid schizophrenic," or paranoid state with more or less of residual schizophrenic phenomena. The case of the chronic catatonic state is of potentially good outcome, this seeming to be but a chronic continuation of the purely schizophrenic state, but the actual duration in illness is a factor that is not to be ignored.

The procedure of treatment begins with removing the patient from the situation in which he is developing difficulty, to a situation in which he is encouraged to renew efforts at adjustment with others. This might well be elsewhere than to an institution dealing with a cross-section of the psychotic population; certainly, it should not be to a large ward of mental patients of all sorts and ages. The sub-professional personnel with whom the patient is in contact must be aware of the principal difficulty—viz., the extreme sensitivity underlying whatever camouflage the patient may use. They must be activated by a well-integrated purpose of helping in the re-development or development de novo of self-esteem as an individual *attractive* to others. They must possess sufficient insight into their own personality organization to be able to avoid masked or unconscious sadism, jealousies, and morbid expectations of results. They must be free from the more commonplace ethical delusions and superstitions. Admittedly, this is no small order, and the creation of this sort of situation is scarcely to be expected either from chance or from the efforts of a commonplace administrative agent.

Given the therapeutic environment, the first stage of therapy by the physician takes the form of providing an orienting experience. After the initial, fairly searching, interview, the patient is introduced to the new situation in a matter-of-fact fashion, with emphasis on the personal elements. In other words, he is made to feel that he is now one of a group, composed partly of sick persons—the other patients—and partly of well folk—the physician and all the others concerned. Emphasis is laid on the fact that something is the matter with the patient, and—once this is at least clearly understood to be the physician's view—that regardless of the patient's occasional or habitual surmise to the contrary, everyone who is well enough to be a help will from thenceforth be occupied in giving him a chance to get well. From the start, he is treated as a *person among persons.*

There is never to be either an acceptance of his disordered thought and behavior as *outré* or "crazy," or a "never-mind" technique that ignores the obvious. Everyone is to regard the outpouring of thought or the doing of acts as at least *valid* for the patient, and to be considered seriously as something that at least he should understand. The individualism of the patient's performances is neither to be discouraged nor encouraged, but instead, when they seem clearly morbid, to be noted and perhaps questioned. The questioning must not arise from ethical grounds, nor from considerations of mere convenience, but from a desire to center the patient's attention on the discovery of the factors concerned. If there is violence, it is to be discouraged, *unemotionally,* and in the clearly expressed interest of the general or special good. If, as is often the case, violence arises from panic, the situation must be dealt with by the physician. If, however, the patient seems obviously to increase in comfort without professional attention after the introduction to care, the physician can profitably await developments. A considerable proportion of these patients proceed in this really human environment to the degree of social recovery that permits analysis, without much contact with the supervising physician. Moreover, in the process, they become aware of their need for insight into their previous difficulties, and somewhat cognizant of the nature of the procedures to be used to that end. They become not only ready but prepared for treatment.

If the patient does not respond in so gratifying a fashion to the special environment, the physician must discover the difficulty. In some cases, the previously dissociated tendency system is integrating personal situations that precipitate panic or panicky states. This requires reassurance by a technique of realistic acceptance of the underlying tendencies, a bringing out into the open of the cause for the fear experienced by the self, with the resulting beneficent effects of a new feeling of group solidarity in that the harsh appraisal of the tendency incorporated in the patient's personality is temporarily suspended or enfeebled, by acquaintance with people to whom the situation is a commonplace of life. In all too many cases, the ideal-organization is such that the appearance of this solidarity-reaction is judged by the self to be ominous, and the attempt to diminish the violence of reaction to the previously dissociated tendency system fails. It is necessary, however, that the conflict be abated, otherwise the development of interpersonal security that is absolutely necessary for a social recovery cannot be achieved. In such cases, recourse is had to chemotherapeutic agencies, notably ethyl alcohol, which impair the highly discriminative action of the more lately acquired tendency systems, and permit the at least rudimentary functioning of the more primitive, without much stress. After from three to 10 days of continuous mild intoxication, almost all such patients, in the writer's experience, have effected a considerable readjustment. The modus operandi may be indicated roughly by remarking that these patients discover by actual experience that the personal environment is not noxious, and, having discovered this, have great difficulty in subsequently elaborating convictions of menace, plots, fell purposes, etc. It is the rule to have several interviews with the patient during the period of intoxication, and in them to carry out the reassuring technique above indicated.

Occasionally, an acute schizophrenic, showing a marked tendency to paranoid maladjustment, proceeds all the more rapidly in this direction under the type of care thus far outlined. Several devices have been used in combating the process, but the results are not yet satisfactory. It has become clear that this eventuality requires an extraordinary intervention, if the patient is to be saved; and some pioneering work has been done in this connection. The principle involved, however, is one sufficiently startling to justify hesitancy in reporting but two patients. For the present, it must suffice that patients who show progressively deepening paranoid developments or those who are received in florid paranoid states should not remain with the group under active treatment.

As the patient improves, and as his acceptance of the need for help grows, the efforts of the physician become more direct in their application. Energy is expended chiefly in *reconstructing the actual chronology of the psychosis.* All tendencies to "smooth over" the events are discouraged, and free-associational technique is introduced at intervals to fill in "failures of memory." The role of significant persons and their doings is emphasized, the patient being constantly under the influence of the formulation above set forth— viz., that however mysteriously the phenomena originated, everything that has befallen him is related to his actual living among a relatively small number of significant people, in a relatively simple course of events. Psychotic phenomena recalled from the more disturbed periods are subjected to study as to their relation to these people. Dreams are studied under this guide. During this phase of the work, the patient may or may not grasp the dynamics of his difficulty as they become apparent to the physician. Interpretations are never to be forced on him, and preferably none are offered excepting as statistical findings. In other words, if the patient's actual insight seems to be progressing at a considerable pace, it can *occasionally* be offered that thus-and-so has, in some patients, been found to be the result of this-and-that, with a request for his associations to this comment.

One of perhaps three situations now develops. Firstly, if the patient is doing very well, the family insist on taking him home, and generally ignore advice as to further treatment. Secondly, the chronology of the course of recent events running into the psychosis is rather well recorded, and the patient is found to have great difficulty in coming to insight. He is then discharged into regular treatment at the hands of a suitable psychoanalyst, experienced in the psychiatry of schizophrenia—and not too rigid in devotion to technique. Thirdly, the stage of chronology-perfecting is accompanied by so much growth of insight that it is shifted gradually to a close approximation to regular analytic sessions that follow a liberal variant of the orthodox technique.

In the writer's experience, covering some 11 years, there have been regrettable events to be charged off to precipitate and to rigid techniques of psychotherapy. From these mistakes and from the singular opportunities provided by patients themselves, the socio-psychiatric technique above indicated has finally evolved. When physical facilities were made available, it was tried out rather thoroughly. The condition of no patient was aggravated by its use, and the social and real recovery rates obtained were extremely gratifying. It would seem that, for the group as defined above, schizophrenia is an illness of excellent prognosis. The treatment required, however, is obviously far from widely available, and the schizophrenia problem therefore continues to be very urgently one of prevention.

Certain considerations bearing on the professional personnel for working with schizophrenics may not be amiss. In the first place, it seems quite clearly demonstrated in the Sheppard experience that the therapeutic situations must be integrated between individuals of the same sex. Two male patients treated by woman physicians did remarkably badly, while "cooperating" much better than the average. A number of women, treated by the writer, also "cooperated" nicely, as they progressed into deterioration or paranoid maladjustments. Male patients treated by the writer are not as comfortable in the treatment situation as were these women. But they are correspondingly more successful in achieving actual rather than fantastic results.

In the second place, the unanalyzed psychiatrist and the psychiatrist filled with the holy light of his recent analysis are in general not to be considered for this work. The former have generally a rigid system of taboos and compromises which are rather obvious to the schizophrenic intuition, so that the patient comes early to be treating the physician, and to be fearing him. The analytic zealot knows so many things that are not so that the patient never makes a beginning.

Thirdly, the philosophical type of person is a poor candidate for success as a therapist of schizophrenics; they too love philosophizing—it is so much safer to "think" than to go through the mill of observation and understanding. Also, most of these people get systematized so early that they are blind to experience less than a personal psychosis.

Fourthly, those elsewhere identified as the "resistant homosexual types" are poor material for schizophrenia therapists; they are too busy finding "homosexual components" in everyone to note the facts flowing past them.

Fifthly, the reformer element, who "know" how life should be lived, and what is good and bad, if they must do psychiatric work, should keep far from the schizophrenic. Perhaps the manic-depressive psychosis is their ideal field.

Sixthly, perhaps of all the people least fitted for this work are those that are psychiatrists because it gives them powers and principalities over their fellows; to them should go the obsessional neurotics.

Lastly, sadly enough, those to whom life has brought but a pleasant flood of trifling problems without any spectacular disturbances, who have grown up in quiet backwashes far from the industrial revolution, within the tinted half-lights of the passing times—these are afield in undertaking the schizophrenia problem. It is one up to the last minute in its ramifications, and can but bring them a useless gloom and pessimism about youth and the times. There are some ecclesiasts who find joy in tinkering with the mild mental disorders, in Church Healing Missions and the like. These folk might learn much from, for example, the Rev. Anton Boisen, Chaplain of the Worcester State Hospital, who has come by the tedious and often deeply disturbing road of observation and experimentation to a sane grasp of the relations of religious thoughts and techniques to the schizophrenia problem.*

In conclusion, it may be restated that, at least in the case of the male, fairly young schizophrenic patients whose divorcement from fairly conventional behavior and thought has been rather abrupt, when received under care before they have progressed either into hebephrenic dilapidation or durable paranoid maladjustments, are

---

[* A description of this experience is found in Anton T. Boisen. . . 1936. H. S. P.]

to be regarded as of good outlook for recovery and improvement of personality, if they can be treated firstly to the end of socialization, and thereafter by more fundamental reorganization of personality.

Discussion

Dr. Silverberg (Washington, DC). I have no doubt that one of the objections that will be raised to Dr. Sullivan's paper is that the method and the organization which he has described may work very well in the hands of Dr. Sullivan, who has peculiar means of dealing with schizophrenics, but in the hands of another individual, even with a reasonably good medical and psychiatric training, the method would not work. I most emphatically refute this objection. I was Dr. Sullivan's successor at Sheppard and inherited, so to speak, the organization which he had perfected there. During the year that I was at Sheppard, I made no essential changes in the organization that Dr. Sullivan had created there. During that time I dealt with 16 schizophrenics in the special six-bed ward that he used, and had rather good results. Of these 16 patients, 12 either recovered or improved. Of the 12 cases that had been cured or improved, nine were discharged and three remained under care at the end of the period. Of the four unimproved cases, three were discharged, and one remained under care. Of the three unimproved, discharged cases, two turned out to be patients who had been ill for some time, without its being known by their families. They had been paranoid for at least two years before coming to the hospital.

On the basis of these statistics, one sees that 75% of the cases going through this organization have been either recovered or improved. If one omits the two chronic cases for whom, as Dr. Sullivan has already said, such a method of treatment or any method of treatment seems to be of no great value, it will be seen that about 85% of these 14 cases have been either recovered or improved.

Another objection that might be made to this plan is: What is going to happen to those patients when they leave a situation of this sort, which is perhaps from a superficial point of view rather artificial? Will they not, in coming up against the world of reality again, have a return of their symptoms? I should say that this objection is rather more theoretical than real. The same question occurred to my mind when I first took over the ward. The patients, however, passed from this ward to the parole ward and from the parole ward out into the world without any significant difficulties.

I might also say that this particular method of treatment seems to be of greater value for the cases predominantly catatonic and schizophrenic than those predominantly paranoid in symptoms. I hope that the figures which I am able to present will be rather impressive and that the formation of similar organizations elsewhere will be encouraged.

Dr. Gregory Zilboorg (White Plains, New York). I think this is the first encounter between Dr. Sullivan and myself on the floor of the American Psychiatric Association, but in various other meetings we have had many pleasant opportunities to thresh out certain differences which I believe are more superficial than actual.

The fundamental contentions of Dr. Sullivan's paper could be briefly summarized as follows:

First, the schizophrenic presents no special difficulties as regards transference reactions. I think that this point at least, made by himself, will make it possible for him to agree that the psychoanalytic technique which I have used in schizophrenics is probably workable since it led me to the same conclusions.

Second, the point of view of fixation borrowed from the general theory of neuroses is not entirely justified in our work with schizophrenics, for the schizophrenic process presents a number of definite clinical features, the origin of which is not dependent upon any definite fixation; hence the essential features of our therapy in schizophrenia are not so much the release from the point of fixation as the reconstruction of the whole personality. So far so good. However, certain contentions of Dr. Sullivan's paper ought to be approached with at least some doubt. On the basis of my clinical experience I feel compelled to believe that one is not justified in viewing the problem of technique too casually; this technique permits us to enter into the deepest layers of the human personality and should not be discarded with that ease which permits Dr. Sullivan to say: "Send them to an analyst who is psychiatrically trained but who is not too orthodox with regard to psychoanalysis." My contention is: send the patient to an analyst who is very well trained but beware of the analyst who has had poor psychiatric training. The great difficulty of the situation lies in the fact that the psychiatrist looks with suspicion at the analyst because he knows no analysis, while the analyst is just as suspicious of the psychiatrist because the analyst knows no psychiatry. This attitude, covered with a mask of mutual admiration at public meetings, is based on the deep unconscious feeling: "I know something that thou dost not comprehend." This attitude does very little for the progress of therapy in general and that of therapy of schizophrenias in particular.

Dr. Sullivan's emphasis on the socialization of the personality of the schizophrenic is of extreme importance, and I believe that the so-called socio-psychiatric methods are those which are covered by the term "reality testing" which to me is a part of every scientific psychoanalysis of a schizophrenic. That is the reason why I consider Dr. Sullivan's method nothing more than a series of preliminary measures which do not reach deep enough.

The remark that the paranoid schizophrenic is much better off than a healthy individual cannot obviously be taken seriously. Any psychotic prefers his psychosis to being well; otherwise he would not have embarked upon a psychotic path. If this were to serve as an impulse for and criterion of our therapeutic measures, we should refuse to treat a manic because he is so much happier than when he was well.

I have already talked more than I should have, and said less than I wanted to. I shall therefore conclude by emphasizing that in psychiatry, as in medicine, we cannot and should not concentrate on treating symptoms rather than diseases; that the subjective alleviation of symptoms, particularly in schizophrenics, is of no therapeutic significance; and that social recovery is not a recovery in the real sense of the word, since a patient may make a complete social recovery and continue to remain psychotic.

Chairman Brill. I would like to have this discussion continued, but I regret very much that we have not much time. As Chairman, I will use my prerogative to say a few words about the subject.

I have been interested in this problem from the beginning of my existence as a psychiatrist, and I have treated schizophrenics psychotherapeutically, I might say analytically, for a long time. In fact, I have in mind patients who were treated by me psychoanalytically 18 or 19 years ago. When I reported here some of these cases about two years ago, I entitled my paper "Psychotherapy of Schizophrenia" because I did not use *lege artis* analyses because I found that I had to change my analytic technique to suit my cases. The reason I did not use such definite terms as were given here by the speakers is because I really do not believe that we have reached the stage of definite formulations. One thing I am sure of, and that is that by using as much of psychoanalysis as the patient can digest and by resorting to the techniques mentioned by both speakers, modifying them to suit the occasion, I have been able to accomplish results. I did not do exactly what Dr. Sullivan recommends. Thus, some of my greatest successes have been with female patients. Nor have I done everything that Dr. Zilboorg describes. But, listening to them, I do know that I have done everything that they recommend and have deviated as much as they did to suit the particular patients.

The patients I have in mind I did not have to send to any hospital. They were all cared for at home. With such cases I had the best results.

What impressed me in Dr. Sullivan's paper is the hopefulness that it inspires. It is very pleasant to hear such papers and such discussions as were given by Dr. Zilboorg and the others. The therapeutic future of schizophrenia looks quite hopeful.

I know perfectly well there are many others who would like to discuss, but owing to the late hour, I regret that I have to ask Dr. Sullivan to close the discussion.

Dr. Sullivan.   Many important things have come up in the discussion. I can only express my gratitude to Dr. Silverberg for the report on what has been going on at Sheppard, and take this opportunity of emphasizing again the great prognostic importance of *insidious onset* where the individual has very gradually gotten eccentric and become far different from his previous personality, before conspicuous phenomena pointed to his being psychotic. That patient, so far as I know, is in a very bad way, and not apt to profit from the sort of effort I have been talking about.

The urgency of the early socialization is one of the points I am most anxious to carry over to you. Every disappointment the patient undergoes is another obstacle to his recovery.

As to the possible institutional results, there Dr. Silverberg and Dr. Zilboorg were superficially at difference; Dr. Silverberg remarked that the social recovery, which is accomplished in this process, is a definite growth in personality, and Dr. Zilboorg made the statement, which may have been the result of limitations on his time, that social recovery does not mean any sort of recovery. It seems beyond argument that there is an improvement in personality if one changes from obvious psychosis to a considerable measure of ability to live in one's environment. The fact that the patient can be carried to the point where he knows how to keep out of trouble is at least economically and pragmatically useful. It seems a century or two too early for enforcing perfection in this one field of human welfare work.

I have heard a good deal about the "choice of psychosis" and the difficulty of "curing" schizophrenics because they were "so much better off" in the psychosis than were they previously. I think that this interpretation is only one of several possible interpretations; I have seen a good many schizophrenics, and it does seems to me that they have passed from the frying pan into a very active fire by becoming schizophrenic. I do not think we are laying a sound foundation for therapeutics by holding that the patient prefers being psychotic to being well. That this is a superficial statement of the view, I quite realize. It is fairly close, however, to the discoverable content of those who talk this way. If some profound truth is concealed in it, so much the worse for those who cannot express it more adequately—and for those who might profit from understanding it.

The paranoid maladjustment, by which others are found to blame for one's difficulties, does contribute a certain measure of self-respect, and these patients require that you will guarantee them more self-respect before they will give up their paranoid adaptation. That is apparently a difficult achievement, at least for me. That is what I meant when I said they had something much better than at least can be our first offers to them in socialization.

I am grateful to Dr. Brill for his comment. I do not regard the conceptions I am presenting as wholly revolutionary or original. I am most emphatically in accord with his remark on the feasibility of non-institutional care for early schizophrenics; a work to which I am now devoting myself. His comment supports my thesis; namely, that the general adoption of this orientation in the treatment of incipient schizophrenia and of all younger patients of acute onset—with the creation of convalescent camps and open institutions to which these patients can be sent—should be regarded neither as a hope of the distant future nor a particularly expensive procedure. It seems to me that this addition to the modern state hospital service will pay far larger dividends on the taxpayers' money, than does the current type of custodial care and accidental treatment of schizophrenics, and that it would give the youth of today something like a fair chance of surviving at least the first episode of schizophrenic disorder.

Notes

1. The reader is respectfully referred to the perhaps redundant but no less relevant "Thobbing" of Henshaw Ward (1926). To *thob* is to *th*ink out

something, which opinion is glorified as an extravasation of one's personality, and most vigorously believed and "defended," thereafter.

2. The most significant determining factors in this particular situation, *so far as the writer is chiefly concerned,* may be "dated" as follows: March 12, 1931, psychiatric meeting at which the protagonist "presented" a case illustrating the alleged relations of the organic and the functional; March 18, 1931, dinner discussion; April 10, 1931, psychiatric meeting, as previous; April 24, 1931, psychiatric meeting, as previous; April 28, 1931, protagonist's discussion of "The Pathogenesis of Schizophrenia" by Dr. Gregory Zilboorg, New York Psychoanalytic Society; May 13, 1931, reading of summary of protagonist's paper in the program of the current meeting; May 17, 1931, realization that someone must be made a "goat" for illustrating pseudopsychiatric contributions; May 21, 1931, conclusion that the ends justified the risk of this sort of illustration before so kindly and democratic an audience as the present one.

    The *situation* under discussion is *interpersonal*; involving, as major nexus, (a) the writer variously expanded, (b) his "impersonal" hearers and readers, (c) the person, Paul Schilder as protagonist, auditor, reader, and reactor, and secondarily those who "side" with him in the alleged "controversy" which many conceive all psychiatric criticism to be, (d) the body of valid and other information that is the psychiatry of schizophrenia; and so forth.

3. The best that could have been ventured is something as follows: The present writer, being deeply interested in schizophrenia, and having amassed consensually valid information which he interprets as evidence convincing to any intelligent observer to the effect that *no such illness of acute onset is apt to manifest a dependable sign of bad outcome regardless of treatment,* being moreover activated by a drive to insure the active attention of all concerned to the importance of early care in determining the outcome of schizophrenic disorders, being also interested in the growth of psychiatric knowledge and its refinement from fantasy, *will to a considerable probability,* sooner or later, subject the views of the protagonist to more or less effective criticism. If suitable occasion arise, this will doubtless occur in the course of a psychiatric meeting. Since the writer will be activated to reach the largest audience, it will probably occur at a meeting of The American Psychiatric Association. After reading the program of the current meeting—a prophecy the more probable in that it is but a few weeks "ahead of" the events—an astute prognostician might have said, "It is *quite probable* that this situation will arise on June 3 or 5, 1931." Even if, on May 27, he had read this paper, he would have had clearly in mind the fact that the occurrence of the present situation *continued to be contingent* on many actually unpredictable factors.

4. The acuteness or insidiousness of *onset of the observed psychosis,* however, may finally give the question of underlying organic state new relevance. It is quite *possible,* in the writer's opinion, that an ultimately measurable something of great prognostic significance may be found to underlie these insidious disintegrations of personality attended by more or less of schizophrenic phenomena, that are now lumped with disorders of acute *observed onset.* Statistics of the Sheppard experience

indicate so great a difference in course of the two groups, that one cannot but wish that effort might be directed to the comparative study of individuals of acute versus insidious observed onset.

5. The development of this topic—*viz.,* the cultural entities built into and going to make up the individual personality—is to be found in the writer's forthcoming text, "The Sickness of The Modern Mind: The Psychopathology of Interpersonal Relations" [probably *Personal Psychopathology*].

6. That this conception of schizophrenia is broad enough to include the clinical entity, *hysteria,* has not escaped the writer. This is not the occasion on which to develop the implications of a classification of levels of consciousness, nor of the dynamics underlying major and minor dissociations.

7. Since it is not the present purpose to discuss the strength or weakness of the ego and so forth, no comment will be made on, for example, the highly relevant data provided by psychopathic personalities.

8. Consideration of these factors is not directly relevant to the contribution herein attempted, and has been outlined elsewhere [*Personal Psychopathology*].

The Relation of Onset to Outcome in Schizophrenia

Harry Stack Sullivan, M.D.
(1931)

Introduction

The writer will assume that the concept of schizophrenia has been stripped of an implication of inevitable chronicity and deterioration. He will not accept recovery as "remission" or "arrest," but instead will hold that an individual who has undergone a schizophrenic illness, ceased to show schizophrenic processes, and resumed social living with a gradual expansion of life-interests, has in fact to the limit of the meaning of such terms actually *recovered* from the schizophrenic illness. Having noted that such recoveries are by no means infrequent, he will then offer some tentative notions bearing upon crude observational factors seemingly sequents of the favorable outcome, and useful to the psychiatrist who cannot engage in any detailed study of his patients.

Review of Cases

In the seven years during which the research staff of the Sheppard and Enoch Pratt Hospital has been occupied with the

Reprinted from *Schizophrenia [Dementia Praecox]: An Investigation of the Most Recent Advances, 10*, 111–118; Baltimore: Williams & Wilkins, 1931, with permission from the Association for Research in Nervous and Mental Disease, Inc., New York.

problem of schizophrenia in males, about 250 patients have been subjected to more or less elaborate investigation. To simplify this orientation, the discussion will be limited to the first hundred, of whom fairly dependable correlations of the crude (nonstatistical) sort can be made. This hundred occur in the first 155 serial admissions. Fifty-five patients were eliminated from this study for the following reasons: (a) defective information coupled with failure of the physician to establish satisfactory contact with the patient, 30 patients; (b) mentally defective patients coupled with defective information, 11 patients; (c) schizophrenic nature of the illness questioned (often in earlier admission elsewhere), 14 patients. In other words, there is useful data in 64.5% of the consecutive male schizophrenic admissions. This higher percentage results in part from such factors as the hospital's policy and prestige, so that the patient-material cannot be held to be a representative cross-section of the general schizophrenic population. Many of the notions derived from this study, therefore, may or may not be of general application. The positive conclusions, however, which are the subject of this paper, must be accepted as only very modestly related to defects of the clinical sample, and as generally valid.

Of the 100 cases on which comment is made herein, the onset of mental illness was insidious in 22. In other words, in each of these 22 individuals, there was a life-course in which the patient underwent no dramatic separation from ordinary living, but instead became gradually more and more peculiar until finally, by reason of some more or less spectacular occurrence, his mental illness was recognized. In no one of these was the prolonged phase of insidious divorcement from approximate mental health a matter that was overlooked because of the indifference or stupidity of the persons making up the environment. The insidious characteristic of the change may be accepted as genuine.

Of these patients, a liberal figure for those improved is seven. That is, less than 32% of these patients showed marked modification of the processes towards that state of approximate mental health. Of the seven, two patients are in perhaps as good mental health as is the general population, three are definitely paranoid states, one is a defective without psychosis, and one is decidedly reduced in the interest and activity range.

Of the basic 100 patients, the onset of schizophrenic mental illness was acute in 78 cases. In other words, in each of these 78 individuals, there was a life-course in which the patient underwent a rather abrupt change in behavior and expressed thought such that the personal environment was emphatically impressed by his transition from a state of approximate mental health to one of mental disorder. Of these, 48, or somewhat over 61%, have shown marked improvement; in a considerable number, the change has amounted to a recovery from the mental disorder.

Of the 30 patients in whom the onset of grave illness was acute, but improvement did not follow, the following data may be of interest: four are dead, two having killed themselves; four are defectives, two of whom improved greatly under care, but relapsed to grave disorder under social pressure after discharge. In two instances, the illness appeared late in life; these are now both in chronic paranoid states. Nine younger patients have progressed into chronic paranoid states from which recovery is not to be expected, since the disorder is preferable to the real situations to which the patient might hope to return. In five hebephrenic cases, deteriorating processes are evident—one at least as a result of errors in the psychiatric handling of the patient. Another one progressed swiftly into a dilapidated paranoid state, but continued subacutely ill for some years, killed a bystander while on parole, and was in turn killed by a policeman. This was the fifth death in the group. Of the remaining five, one has had recurrent waves of psychosis over a period of about 11 years, and is rather badly disintegrated; one has been in a subacute catatonic state with great hostility to the personal environment—a form of paranoid state, according to a descriptive psychiatrist—for about four years; one slipped into the acute psychosis owing to the extraordinary fragility of his personality, which had been held to some semblance of integration only by a quite bizarre disregard for ordinary standards, coupled with a wife willing to co-operate in his extraordinarily perverse modus vivendi; another is a subacute catatonic of several years duration, tending strongly to paranoid maladjustment, also the result of poor therapy on the part of the writer; the fifth is a man singularly handicapped by physical factors, who stumbled along until about 36 years of age before failure, and has little indeed to recover to—he is progressing into a paranoid state.

Impervious barriers generally keep one from establishing rudimentary interpersonal relations with the unfavorable patient of insidious onset. This is probably a direct result to be expected from consideration of the environmental personal situation in which the personalities had their development. In the seven cases of improvement after the insidious onset, to which reference is made above, a rather good superficial contact was established with six of them. One proved to be of extraordinary intellectual equipment, who had had only a small number of truly schizophrenic processes in the course of an insidious deviation from conventional life, towards a life of extreme radicalism. He underwent partial psychoanalysis and is now studying medicine. Another was of decidedly superior intellectual equipment, had very few schizophrenic processes, but early retired from active social life and efforts towards achievement. He has been gainfully employed for two years or so. Another is a seriously defective boy *in whom the onset had been acute,* but in the course of such chronic maladjusted living that the change did not impress the personal environment. He made a "transference cure" of low grade and has been working for about a year. He thus comes to belong among those cases of acute onset, but is reported here because of the *apparently* insidious onset.

The Significance of the Type of Onset

In brief, an insidious onset of schizophrenic processes is of much more grave omen as to outcome than is an abrupt onset. Two theoretical considerations may be advanced in this connection. Either the insidious disorder is *different from* the acute, or the personality distortion underlying the insidious onset is more severe, although of similar nature to the distortion underlying the acute onset. Moore [1929–30] has presented some evidence derived from statistical operations with tetrad differences, pointing to the existence of a syndrome of "cognitive defect" positively related to so-called praecox conditions. This author finds that "cognitive defect" has positive correlation with "what are probably two phases of dementia praecox: the uninhibited and the catatonic." This is taken to move the "praecox disorders off into the realm of neurologically founded maladies. It is easy to divide the material under consideration into "praecox" illnesses based on organic pathology and "schizophrenic" illnesses based on functional pathology. The division, however, is irrational and unprofitable, for some of the former cases recorded a good measure of mental health just as did most of the latter. In other words, in frankly defective patients, undergoing severe and relatively typical schizophrenic processes,[1] nothing fully distinctive from extraordinarily talented individuals suffering schizophrenia has appeared in this investigation.

Moore's syndrome includes the "shut-in" personality factor. This inclusion results from mathematical operations, and not directly from descriptive psychiatric procedures. How does the material under discussion bear on the "shut-in" factor? Taking the 48 patients in whom the onset was acute and recovery considerable, there are, roughly, 36 clearly negative and 12 more or less positive. Taking the 30 of acute onset without material recovery, there are, again roughly, 10 showing what might be described as a "shut-in personality." Of the 78 acute onsets, then, 56 did not impress the writer as occurring in personalities to be placed under the rubric of "shut-in." The question arises as to those showing insidious onset. Of the 22, there were 14 distinctly "shut-in"; these did not include any of those that actually improved markedly.[2]

Comment

Very briefly, quite in keeping with the work of Edward J. Kempf and with the other findings of the Sheppard study, a crude correlative study such as that any hurried psychiatrist might make, indicates that an acute dramatic divorcement from more or less commonplace living is of good prognostic omen in schizophrenic illnesses. This sort of psychotic onset implies a personality that has *grown farther* towards adulthood than is the case with insidious illnesses. In this is the factor of promise. The acute onset means that one is dealing with a personality integration that has gone on a long distance in spite of the dissociated homosexual cravings or the masturbation conflict from which the illness has finally taken origin. It, therefore, includes a good deal that can be re-integrated into a "going concern." The insidious onset means that the growth of the personality has failed long before the hospital admission, and that there is relatively much less that is useful for a re-integration of anything like an average life-situation. Disregarding all the factual material which can be elicited in psychopathological study of individual patients, one is justified in prognosticating on the actuteness of the divorcement from reality in the schizophrenic illness, and may give a heavy favorable weighing to the dramatic outcropping of the psychosis. The chances for "recovery or remission from dementia praecox" are alleged to be in the neighborhood of one in four or five of the younger patient. This may be amplified by saying that the chances for recovery are twice as good in the patient of acute onset as in the one insidiously separated from reality.

Discussion

The following questions submitted to Dr. Sullivan before the Commission, together with the answers to them, are here reported verbatim.

Dr. Strecker. In Dr. Sullivan's excellent presentation, I was particularly interested in the fact—and I take it this is the point of the paper—that what has been designated as an acute stormy onset is a relatively favorable prognostic sign. It is an old observation and one which I think is well borne out in clinical practice.

The other point is that I do not think we should be too much disturbed about what might be called the criteria of restitution. I wonder if some of our disturbed frame of mind about the matter is not due to the fact that we tend to lean over backwards in regard to the possibility of favorable outcomes. In discussing my presentation at the meeting of the Association when this subject was previously presented [Strecker & Wiley, 1925], Dr. Jelliffe put it very well when he said that every one of us, not only these restituted patients but every one of us found it necessary to carry a mental potato with which to get on in life. By that he meant (referring to the old Irish superstition of carrying a potato to ward off rheumatism) that we all needed perhaps a crutch or two. Now, when we ourselves need that sort of help, which we extract from our environment as best we can to meet our individual needs, it seems hardly fair that we should expect the ex-schizophrenic patient to get on without anything at all. Therefore, I should like to point out that we should not be too rigid in our definition of what constitutes restitution.

Dr. Sullivan. Dr. Strecker's comment, stating the point, if any, of my talk, requires reply. I shall also amplify my presentation, although I had intended nothing more than a crude prognostic indication for general use. As to the prevailing notion regarding the type of onset and outcome, not only does an acute stormy outlook indicate a relatively good prognosis, but an acute stormy onset is frequently overlooked or unrecognized by members of the patient's family. It is the character of the onset as it actually occurred in the patient that bears on the outcome. Sometimes the outcropping of schizophrenic phenomena is very clearly reproduced by the patient and shows an abrupt appearance of the abnormal content. This may have occurred when his behavior was not observed to be seriously disordered. The prognosis in such cases is good. The consideration of the sufficiency of the exciting situation seems to me to be practically of very little value to the institutional psychiatrist. I have attempted in other studies to show that the sufficiency of the exciting situation is an almost irrelevant consideration—certainly one on which I would accept the patient's opinion rather than that of the investigating psychiatrist. Since the insidious onset does not arise out of an "exciting situation," this consideration is wholly irrelevant, in every sense, to the group of patients in whom, in my opinion, the prognosis is most gloomy.

As long as I am led to touch upon the dynamics of the schizophrenic break, I feel that I should mention certain considerations which have appeared to me to be valid and which I presented at a recent meeting of the New York Neurological Society. Study of the life history of a considerable number of people, including those patients mentioned in the present paper, has convinced me that the onset of schizophrenia can frequently be divided into two states. A considerable number of people experience the first step towards schizophrenic phenomena a considerable time before the psychosis makes its appearance. The interval between the initial *stadium* and the appearance of psychotic experience may be a matter of moments or the matter of a lifetime. I call the first stage the collapse of the individual world synthesis.

Individuals come to a certain age with a body of what I suppose one might describe as implicit assumptions about themselves and the universe. We all depend upon a large number of things that we are really not justified in depending upon, but we have never had any reason to suspect them. The sun rises pretty regularly and our alarm clocks work if we give them a chance, and so on and so forth. A great body of assumptions is the foundation upon which our life processes rest. In a remarkable number of adolescents, however, there comes a time when their faith in this background of implicit assumptions about their own abilities or about the consistency of the universe, and so on, is abruptly shattered. Then, instead of building the rationalizations as we do when someone points out that we have been an ass, these individuals go on feeling terribly upset about things. From that time on, instead of building the sort of rationalizations with which we heal the wounds to our self-respect and all that sort of thing, these people are different from what they were before. Perhaps I might mention three or four groups. In one case the individual becomes a superficial individual from then on; he deals with social contracts in what we call a sort of hysterical fashion; he has all sorts of enthusiasms and distresses and what-not, but acquaintance with him shows that this is just a sort of surface play. In another instance the individual becomes retiring, secretive, he seeks a much more restricted environment and avoids all social contacts. As a third case I might perhaps mention the resort to a wild compensatory program, this often leading to schizophrenia.

I belive we can isolate by further study a type of situation which I will call the first stage of schizophrenia (because it is so very frequently associated with the second or definite schizophrenia), in which there is a rapid loss of faith in the self and the universe, without the remedial maladjustments or actual remedial processes which go on with most of us when we receive a severe bump in life. Such situations are not, however, in any necessary close association with the gradual separation of the individual from reality, of which I have spoken.

Briefly, the second stage of schizophrenia, as it has become formulated in my mind, is somewhat as follows. The individual, with serious impairment of the dependability of his self and the universe progresses into a situation in which the dissociated parts of his personality are the effective integrating agencies. The factors which he experiences are then of two varieties. He lives the sort of life to which he is accustomed; this under the domination of the accepted egoistic structure. And he has from momentary to extended intervals during which the experience the experience which he is having is dominated by the dissociated systems. The result is a condition which I cannot distinguish by any important characteristic from that undergone by an individual in attempting to orient himself on awakening in the midst of a vivid nightmare. To all of this condition I apply the term incipient schizophrenia. If it goes on, the clinical picture becomes that of catatonic illness. So far as I can see, an individual may remain in this state of difficulty almost indefinitely. On the other hand, he may, as a result of appropriate experience, undergo one of three changes—this at any time in the course of a catatonic illness of any duration. An integration may begin between the dissociated and the dissociating systems of his personality—in which case all proceeds toward recovery. A massive transference of blame may occur, as a result of which he progresses into a chronic paranoid state, the particular type of which is related in a simple fashion to the conflicting systems. Or there may be a dilapidation of the dissociating system and a regression of interest and impulses to an early childhood or infantile level—in which case we see what is called hebephrenic dilapidation.

You will notice that my considerations imply that a gradual detachment from reality, occurring rather early in the evolution of personality, follows an ominous course quite distinct from that of the more dramatic type to which I have invited your attention. Further, that in the latter connection, it has appeared to me from study of the problem, that so-called hebephrenic and paranoid praecox illnesses are separate processes from the essential schizophrenia, incipient or catatonic.

Notes

1. In other words, not typical "psychoses with mental deficiency." [See American Psychiatric Association, 1918.]
2. If all defectives are to be accepted as, by definition, "shut-in," then these figures are subject to revision, for several of the mentally defective patients did not impress the writer as having shown a "shut-in" personality.

My Sixty Years with Schizophrenics

Manfred Bleuler, M.D.
(1979)

I was born and spent my entire childhood in a psychiatric hospital of which my father was the director. Altogether I have lived with schizophrenics for 60 years. After graduation from medical school I spent 10 years as a resident physician. Eventually I served as the director of a psychiatric hospital, Burghölzli, in Zurich, Switzerland, for 27 years. The remainder of my time was spent either in general hospitals or in general practice. These many years of day-to-day contact with schizophrenics have contributed to the development of the following views regarding this pathology.

The obvious symptomatology is but one level of the schizophrenic's personality. A healthy life exists buried beneath this confusion. Somewhere deep within himself the schizophrenic is in touch with reality despite his hallucinations. He has common sense in spite of his delusions and confused thinking. He hides a warm and human heart behind his sometimes shocking affective behavior. We must know how to approach the schizophrenic. We must enter and feel with him his vision of reality. We must never relinquish this endeavor. With perseverance there will come a time when the schizophrenic is as we are, when there is mutual understanding and sharing of feelings and mood. This short but invaluable moment might well result in a lasting improvement or even in recovery.

I began my work with schizophrenics before the introduction of insulin, electroshock therapy (EST), and neuroleptics into the field. Consequently I was able to observe the effects of various physical,

From the Foreword, by Manfred Bleuler, M.D., to *Disorders of the Schizophrenic Syndrome,* edited by Leopold Bellak, M.D. Copyright © 1979 by C.P.S., Inc. Reprinted by permission of Basic Books, Inc.

psychotherapeutic, and analytic treatments. I have come to the following formulations regarding the essentials in the treatment of schizophrenics. There must be an active communion with the patient, a communion founded upon the patient-therapist relationship. This relationship is necessary but not sufficient. A community, whether it be in a hospital or in a family, is of paramount importance. In this community the schizophrenic must reach a state of equilibrium between an optimal amount of activity which stimulates him, and an optimal amount of routine and order which helps to calm and control him. When ready, the patient needs to be confronted with new situations and responsibilities which encourage him to mobilize his vital forces. During certain phases of his illness he will require a calming agent such as psychotherapy or drugs. The success of a therapy is contingent upon the organization of an active community, opportunities for the patient to become involved, and possibilities for tranquilization. A social environment, and the ability to deal effectively with stress at times and to relax at other times, are of unparalleled importance in the development and formation of our personality from birth to old age. It is precisely the control of these elements which permits the healthy individual to inhibit his prelogical, unrealistic, and disordered mental life from overflowing.

Schizophrenic thinking is a part of every human being's life. It occurs in our everyday functioning as daydreams, dreams, art, fantasy, and fanatic thinking, among other phenomena. In a normal person this type of thinking prevails in a small part of life and is under control; in a schizophrenic it has become the predominant way of dealing with life and of communicating with oneself and with others. Furthermore, we now recognize that certain types of brain damage can elicit a psychosis similar to schizophrenia. Intoxications, infections, tumors, and temporal epilepsy have been known to produce schizophrenialike symptoms.

Over the years I have asked myself if schizophrenic patients were physical patients, and vice versa. The answer is clearly that the overwhelming majority of schizophrenics are physically, and particularly endocrinologically, healthy, and that the overwhelming majority of physical and endocrine patients are not schizophrenic. To this day a physical process in the etiology of schizophrenia has not been discovered; but we should definitely not discount the possibility of a future discovery in this area. We are at a loss to give a physical interpretation of human intelligence, of human genius, of the understanding of beauty and of the sublime, and of human love and goodness. Biology has contributed to an understanding of the physical basis of human life but not to the human mind in its complexity or to schizophrenic life.

I have always been impressed by the degree of suffering experienced by my schizophrenic patients, as seen through their family and personal history. The schizophrenic female has suffered predominantly from her relationships with parents, siblings, other children, and beloved ones. The schizophrenic male has suffered most frequently from competition with other men. The mental suffering of future schizophrenics is, however, not essentially different from the suffering of future normals. For this reason among others, the development of a schizophrenic psychosis cannot be explained without postulating an inherited disposition. Nevertheless I have found no proof that such a disposition might be accounted for by a single error of metabolism or by some other single inherited defect. The following assumption seems much more probable: the inherited traits for the personal disposition of a future schizophrenic are not in harmony with each other. Such a disharmony, coupled with the disharmony of the social environment, is conducive to loss of a peaceful inner life and an integrated ego at the beginning of psychosis.

I have worked with the families of many schizophrenic patients. In most cases, I was touched by the parents' love and care for their schizophrenic child, and by the child's love for his parents. Assuredly there are schizophrenics who have suffered from their relatives' hate, rejection, aggression, and cruelty. However, this is the exception rather than the rule. Communication within the families of both the parents of the schizophrenic and of the schizophrenic himself is bizarre and idiosyncratic. Furthermore, the nonpsychotic family member's negative attitude toward the development of the schizophrenic member affects the schizophrenic and the other family members. Conversely, the nonpsychotic member develops peculiar attitudes or even neurotic problems as a result of his contact with the future schizophrenic.

In considering schizophrenics, we are dealing essentially with the same problems facing us all regarding heredity, environmental factors, and psychopathology. The schizophrenic is involved in the same struggle each of us is: the struggle to be an integrated person with the ability to adapt one's inner drives and desires to reality. Because of this similarity we must understand the schizophrenic and be hopeful. We must never lose faith. There is no doubt that some cases will be cruel disappointments. On the other hand, 50% of our schizophrenic patients are completely or socially recovered some years after the onset of psychosis, and a substantive percentage of the rest are at least improved.

In conclusion, it is realistic to be hopeful in working with schizophrenics; and our faith is an ingredient immensely helpful to the patient in his treatment. In this volume the editor and the many expert contributors present our latest knowledge of the many-faceted disorders of schizophrenia.

Parents and Schizophrenia

Bertram P. Karon, Ph.D., and
Gary R. VandenBos, Ph.D.
(1981)

In our society, there is a general belief that parents have an enormous impact on children, which to a large extent is obviously true. No one in our society really knows what the ideal way is to raise a child, however. Even the so-called experts disagree, as can readily be ascertained by going to the child-care section of any bookstore or library. Radically different advice for handling almost any situation is given by professionals with apparently solid credentials.

There are some areas of child rearing about which we know a great deal, but they are only islands of knowledge. We generally know more about how to produce pathologic conditions than health. Good mental health professionals could probably tell you one or more ways to raise your child to ensure that they would develop any particular symptom. It is the other question—what is the reasonable way to raise normal children—about which there is disagreement. If this is true for the mental health professionals, it is true for parents as well.

All parents make mistakes. Luckily, human beings are very rugged. What seems to destroy a child is not a single mistake, but parents who seem dedicated to that mistake, who make the same mistake over and over again and act as if they were determined never

Reprinted with permission from *Psychotherapy of Schizophrenia: The Treatment of Choice,* by Bertram P. Karon and Gary R. VandenBos, Chapter 5. Copyright © 1981 by Jason Aronson, Inc.

to discover or permit the child to discover that the parents might have made a mistake. Obviously, such unfortunate consistency should be thought of as a symptom, with unconscious dynamics, motivated by anxiety, as are most symptoms.

Parents of Schizophrenics Are Not Criminals

It cannot be said too many times that parents of schizophrenics are not evil people. In some psychologic discussions, the parent of a schizophrenic is described in a way that would make you think the author was referring to a criminal. Fortunately, most professionals are not that simple-minded.

But the parent who talks to a professional saying, "You are accusing me of destroying my child," is as much dealing with self-accusation as with any perceived accusation from the professional, and the wise professional will deal with this guilt feeling. Moreover, the parent has usually raised the child to the best of his or her knowledge or capacity.

Most parents dealing with the awful problem of living with a severely disturbed child, even a grown-up severely disturbed child, who seek help and try to understand how this could happen, do feel like criminals. Because of their own self-rebukes, they hear any implication that they are in some way involved in their child's pathologic condition as meaning that they are really criminals. The disturbance of the child is so massive that the parents feel there is no way they could be involved, unless what they had done was itself massive, and they are not consciously aware of anything they have done that could be that destructive.

Of course, the confusion arises from the fact that the destructive pressures from the parents in the majority of schizophrenic cases lie in the parents' unconscious. The destructive pressures on the child are a symptom of the parents—a symptom for which the parents are no more to blame than the hysterical patient is for having a paralyzed arm, or the obsessive patient for needing to carry out a ritual, or the schizophrenic patient for hallucinating. This symptom, however, arouses more guilt if it is recognized, because it directly affects another person, indeed, a loved one, and affects him or her in a severely destructive way.

The parents are engaged in a struggle, to live with and provide for a very sick, puzzling, and difficult child. The treatment of the child often means intense personal and psychologic discomfort for the parents, because it means changing techniques of adaptation that have worked for them; yet parents will go to extraordinary lengths to see that their child gets help, and to do what has to be done for the child's best interest. This is realistically admirable.

It is nonetheless understandable that some therapists feel hostile toward the parents of schizophrenic offspring. The therapist sees the parents through the eyes of the patient, sees the terribly devastated life and the pain and sees how the reactions of the parents over a lifetime have helped to produce this devastation. The therapist empathizes with the rage and pain of the patient. That is why it is often easier to have a different staff member work with the parents, if continuing therapy of the parents is undertaken, since the other staff member does not have the same immediate emotional identification with the pain of the child and can more readily see the parents as themselves victims, coping as best they can with the problems of their own childhood and with their responsibilities as adults.

It is important to remember that in most cases whatever part of the parents is involved in and needs the symptoms of the child is unconscious, and no one is responsible for his or her unconscious, since no one can control anything until after it becomes conscious. The conscious rational part of the parents does not want and does not understand the patient's symptoms. The parents may be less anxious at the thought that it is the child and not the parent who is sick. Accepting the child's healthy development, like normal mastur- bation, independence, need for privacy, etc., may have required accepting things in the child which would have created enormous anxieties in the parents, but all of these conflicts are unconscious. Part of the help a professional can give is to bring these matters tactfully into conscious awareness, and hence conscious control, but this requires adept handling. It is easy to traumatize the parents. It is even easier to irritate them so that they become the therapist's enemies rather than the therapist's allies. Changing the destructive part of the parents' interaction with the child means changing a symptom; consequently, unconsciously motivated resistance is to be expected.

For example, one mother of a schizophrenic child, knowing that I (Karon) felt there was parental involvement in the vulnerability to schizophrenic symptoms, said, "Parents of schizophrenics should be shot." The woman seemed to be almost shaking with anger.

"No, parents of schizophrenics should be given counseling." She relaxed and smiled. She had expressed the intense hostility she thought I felt toward her and was relieved when she was offered help. While it is difficult enough to get the schizophrenic patient to accept you as being on his or her side, it is even more difficult for the family to get the feeling that you are on their side, particularly after the therapy begins.

Parents of schizophrenic children vary in how amenable they are to help. Ordinarily, when, as a professional, one suggests, "It is very difficult to be a good mother, and I'd like to be of help," most mothers are relieved.

But one mother of eight, four of whom had been hospitalized as schizophrenic, smiled when she was offered help, "Oh no, Doctor. You don't understand. It's very easy to be a good mother."

She was very resistant to any kind of therapeutic assistance. We had just begun to talk when she immediately perceived what the problem might be. She said, even though I (Karon) had never raised the issue of her relationship to her parents, "You are trying to make me hate my mother, and I won't do it." She correctly perceived that her difficulties in being an adequate mother were related to the inadequate mothering she had herself received, but that was a relationship that she was not ready or willing to explore. It was easier for her simply to act out the trauma by repeating it again and again with her own children, this time with herself as the active rather than passive member of the pair. The result was tragic.

Difficulties in Assessing Specific Dynamics

In trying to understand the familial pressures that predispose a child to serious psychopathology, the clinician and researcher alike are struck by the fact that some families seem obviously pathologic, and it is not surprising that the children develop severe symptoms. If a schizophrenic child is raised by parents who feel there is nothing strange about burning a young child with matches to teach him the danger of fire, because the parent was treated that way himself as a child, the child's susceptibility to terror is not surprising. The majority of parents in our society would consider this grossly unreasonable and cruel. Similarly, some schizophrenic individuals come from families in which thought patterns and the ways in which the family deals with each other are clearly bizarre. Such families literally teach the pathology.

But there are families in which some of the members seem normal and others pathologic. Occasionally, a seemingly "good parent" has a schizophrenic child, and only one child in the family is schizophrenic. The symptoms of the child seem surprising because of the apparent health of the family. Moreover, there are even families that seem pathologic, but the children survive and are psychologically healthy. One is tempted to dismiss the problem with "innate biologic susceptibility." Such a glib explanation would make careful examination unnecessary, but it does not seem plausible when the family interactions are given careful scrutiny. Close screening reveals subtle isolated "family-syncratic" thought disorder shared by the "normal" members of the family of a schizophrenic child, with the symptomatic child playing a special role in the familial interactions.

In such seemingly "good" families, the parents will often report that their house is a stable middle-class home and that they have provided materially for the child and been concerned about him or her. The patient, too, will tell you that he or she has had a good home and good parents. A routine social history frequently may not reveal anything that will explain the disorder. In some cases, the pathologic pressures become obvious only when the patient is treated or observed over a period of time. The key may occasionally be obtained in detailed interviews which review all of the events in the family, not just events the family presents as pertinent.

One set of parents brought their adult schizophrenic son for evaluation. They were proud of their "good middle-class way of life" and the material benefits they had given him. They could not understand why he was catatonic. When the three of them were interviewed together, the son sat rigidly and said nothing. The parents talked about him in the third person as if he were not there. Each member of the family was then interviewed alone. As soon as the parents were absent, the apparently catatonic man talked freely and responsively. As soon as the parents entered the room again, he relapsed into his stonelike appearance and unresponsive posture. This dramatic difference in symptoms clearly indicated the relationship that existed between his family and him. None of us, even if we had a sick child, would refer to him in the third person if he were there. We would try to bring him into the conversation; we would acknowledge that he ought to speak for himself and be included in any discussion of him. These parents habitually dealt with him on this level, because at some level there was a part of them that wished he were as inactive as a stone and as little trouble.

Lidz (1973), whose studies of the families of schizophrenic individuals reveal pathology-producing patterns of interaction in every such family, reports that many of the families were referred to his project because the referring psychiatrist felt the referred family was so healthy that they could not have played any significant role in producing the designated patient's pathologic condition.

The schizophrenic person may hold a special meaning or position with the family, e.g., the oldest child or the youngest child, the only boy, or the only girl, or the first boy, or the first girl. The special significance of the individual to the family may come from events that were happening at the time of birth. The patient may be the child the mother had at the time the father was having an affair. A not uncommon pattern is that the child was born in close proximity to the death of a grandparent, about whom there were ambivalent feelings. The parents may act out these feeling in relationship to the child.

The family members may confuse therapists (or researchers) because they know more than they acknowledge. Sometimes they suppress what they know because they believe it to be irrelevant, or too shameful. Adelaide Johnson and her co-workers (Beckett et al., 1956) conducted an interesting investigation. Each member of families of schizophrenic patients was taken into therapy with a different therapist. The therapists for a given family compared notes. If traumatic events were mentioned by one member of the family, each of the therapists then probed their patients and were able either to confirm or not confirm its actuality. In each family, there were disturbing events that every member of the family knew about, but these were not disclosed initially to either the patient's therapist or anyone on the treatment team.

Interestingly enough, if the designated patient mentioned the traumas, they were most likely to mention them as delusions, misinterpretations, or false memories. "This didn't really happen, but I keep thinking it happened." These workers found that after verification, it was extremely useful to bring the patient back into touch with reality: "Improbable as it may seem, this really did happen to you."

Sometimes the family may have rational reasons for withholding information. Patients who are lower on the socioeconomic ladder have good reason to be distrustful of authorities with respect to information that could get them into legal difficulties. Patients from any socioeconomic class may be fearful of their reputation in the community. One family with a 19-year-old schizophrenic daughter did not reveal that the stepfather had seduced her, that the mother was training her to be a prostitute, and that the patient and her sister had had an ongoing homosexual relationship for many years. All of these were legally defined crimes, and understandably no member of the family wanted to go to jail. But it was difficult to understand the daughter's symptoms until this information came to light in therapy.

Positive statements by a schizophrenic patient about how good a parent he or she has had cannot be taken at face value. The child has had no one outside the family to compare. The parent has always said, "I am a good parent, and think how awful it would be if you had a bad one." The patient, for security, has maintained this fantasy and tries to maintain it with desperation.

Probably no parent treats all of his children in the same way. The child who becomes schizophrenic, with nonschizophrenic siblings, has not been treated exactly the same as the other children. Paradoxically, the mother will often report in private that the schizophrenic child is or was her favorite. She may even say she had to be careful not to show her favoritism too much. An objective account of the handling of the patient as compared to other children readily reveals differences in what actually occurred that would hardly be called favors. The reason the "favorite" is the sick individual is that the mother has unconsciously used this particular child psychologically to maintain her own adjustment; that is, without the mother's being aware of it, this child has reduced some of the mother's important anxieties. Therefore the child is her favorite, but what that means is an intimate psychologic intertwining in which the child's needs do not determine how they interact.

In one case, the mother had toilet-trained her "favorite" harshly, and, without being aware of his feelings, terrorized him into compliance by 6 months of age. The "less favored" child was treated more gently; as late as 5 years of age, he was not beaten for "accidents." This information was at no point volunteered by the mother. She nonetheless confirmed it in answer to specific questions, after it had been reconstructed in her "favorite's" therapy. While she had gone to great lengths to cooperate with treatment, the initial and continuing social history data only included information in which the "favorite" had been treated at least as well or better than his nonschizophrenic brother. It is not unusual that parents of schizophrenic children will "gloss over" major differences in the handling of two children in general terms as being "similar" or both having been handled "well."

Sometimes a mother may relate psychologically to the child in such a manner that she becomes worthwhile on the basis of the child's achievement, but the child does not become worthwhile on the basis of his own achievement. This process is illustrated by a family in which there were two sons, one of whom became a businessman and made a lot of money, and the other became a college professor and also did very well. When talking separately to the parents, the businessman heard only about his brother's brilliance, and the college professor heard only about how much money his brother made and was asked why he earned so little. Both of them felt worthless; both of them eventually had psychotic breaks. Meanwhile, the mother, who was neither able to be an intellectual nor to earn a lot of money, was able to maintain her self-esteem at the cost of her children's self-esteem. She did not know she was being destructive. She probably was not even aware that she was defending her own self-esteem, fending off her own feelings of her inadequacy compared to the achievements of her sons.

Another example of this is a patient with artistic ability whose mother took his paintings, from childhood on, even though he begged her permission to keep them. She showed them to her friends, rationalized to herself and to her son that she was only trying to show how proud she was of him. She derived the satisfaction of the attention and praise the paintings received. Her son's achievement tended to make her feel good about herself. At another level, however, it still touched off her envious rivalry. The son, however, got no direct gratification and believed that people admired his work solely because of his mother. Before intensive therapy, he had developed no realistic view of his talent. As he said to his therapist, "If it wasn't for my mother, nobody would think I was worthwhile." The mother, in her need to feel worthwhile, also bragged about nonexistent achievements of her son, so that the therapist was surprised to find out that his art was really extraordinarily good.

An adult catatonic patient was the second of a family of 11 children of whom he was the only reportedly sick individual. He made bizarre gestures, involving among other things his neck and face: he habitually turned to one side and bent his neck. When the family was interviewed, they said that he had never made unusual gestures before he came into the hospital. After several weeks of psychotherapy, the patient seemed in pretty good shape, and the relatives visited him in the hospital. The therapist observed them from across the room and noted that as the patient talked with his family, he began to relapse into his dramatic gestures and posturings. As the parents were leaving, the therapist stopped them and asked, "How did your son seem today."

"Very good," they said.

"Did he seem sick?"

"Not at all," they said.

"Did he make any peculiar signs or gestures?"

"Oh no, he's like he always is—very healthy."

The therapist then asked about his neck postures and imitated the patient.

The mother said, "Oh well, he's done that a lot. We thought he did that because he sleeps on a couch that is too short for him"

The patient, who was in his mid-20s, had been removed from school at the age of 16, that is, as soon as it was legal to do so. His parents had taken him directly to the employment office of an automobile factory. He had worked on the assembly line ever since. His entire salary was turned over to the mother, and neither the mother nor the father held a full-time job. The largest salary in the household was that of the patient. His oldest brother had been allowed to keep the money he made, however, and eventually to leave the household. The younger children derived some security from the patient. As long as he went to work, brought the money home, gave it to his mother to help support the household (keeping only a small allowance), and, despite working very hard at an arduous job, was content to sleep on a couch which was too short for him, he was considered healthy; that is, he met the needs of the family as a system. Indeed, he met the needs of everybody except himself.

It was only when he refused to go to work that he was brought to the hospital. As in many poor families, clothes were highly valued. The patient had bought some new clothes out of his small allowance and he cherished them. His older brother, who was not required to turn his income over to the family and was bigger than he, borrowed them and, of course, split them. The patient was told by his mother that he must not complain and that it was all right. This was the point at which he stopped going to work. The posturing of his neck was his physical way of complaining about the fact that he had no adequate place to sleep, but such complaints were just as ignored as more realistic verbal complaints would have been; at least he was not punished.

Traumatic events are frequently seemingly little things that are continued over a lifetime. The woman who got angry every time she fed her son is a good example. This destructive pressure was not something of which she was aware. All she knew was she had had a quarrel that day with her son, and she had felt annoyed with him that day. No one of these quarrels would in itself have had any permanent effect. It is the fact that from infancy to adulthood, whenever she fed him, anger was communicated either by the way she had handled him as an infant or by her quarreling with him as a child and later as an adult. This persisting inevitable pattern of hostility under specific circumstances produced in the son the persisting symptomatic feeling that all food was poisoned.

In schizophrenia, it is important to remember that this pervasive quality of the interpersonal pressure is central to the development of severe symptoms. A specific single traumatic incident is usually an intense and dramatic presentation of a chronic problem. Part of the confusion about the nature of traumatic events and pressures arises from the fact that the one major difference between what is reconstructed in a careful psychoanalytic therapy and what really happened is that what is remembered as a single event is always a summary of many events with similar meaning. There is increasing acknowledgment of this with neurotic patients, as well as with schizophrenic patients.

As noted earlier, Freud's discovery that the repressed seduction fantasies of conversion-hysteric female patients in the Victorian era were most often fantasies, led us astray. Later analysts have interpreted this as if he said in all cases, hysteric or not, you are dealing with a fantasy. In schizophrenic persons, the fantasies of seduction, of rape, and of torture most often turn out to be based upon an interpretation of real events. The way the patient first tells about it may not be realistic, but after he has discussed it with the therapist a number of times, what will be reconstructed will turn out to be real events, or misunderstanding of real events. Schizophrenia is a much more serious disorder than conversion-hysteria, and big effects do not result from little causes.

Some of our psychoanalytic colleagues, when we have discussed the families of schizophrenic patients, have objected and said that they have seen neurotic patients whose families were every bit as destructive in their impact as those described; however, there is a critical difference. For these neurotic patients, there is always one or more people outside the family who provide much of what the parents have not provided, but, as mentioned previously, the families of individuals who ultimately become schizophrenic systematically discourage contacts with people outside the family—that is, they discourage the identification with and the learning from peers and adults outside the family.

Parental Determinants of Disordered Behavior

The specific symptoms of schizophrenia are exceedingly varied and the people called schizophrenic are an exceedingly varied group of people. Since this is so, the particular parental pressures that have led to such disordered behavior would also be expected to be exceedingly varied. This is, in fact, the case. One parent may beat a patient unmercifully to teach him an important lesson. Another parent may teach a grossly distorted view of the outside world, because the parent believes it. Another parent may starve a patient to teach the child not to be greedy, and still another intrusively stuff a patient with food to reassure themselves that they care about the child. Indeed, the various specific behaviors of parents that are destructive are almost endless.

The parental pressures that tend to produce schizophrenia are not themselves necessarily schizophrenic symptoms. This distinction has not been understood by genetic researchers. They tend to look for schizophrenia in the parent as being the cause of schizophrenia in the offspring, even when they are supposedly investigating psychologic pressures, not genes. It is true that schizophrenic individuals are very difficult to live with and consequently may produce a higher rate of psychologic disorder in their children. It is also true that their children identify with them, as all children identify to some extent with their parents. But the specific pressures that lead to schizophrenia are different from schizophrenic pathology itself. There exist people whose functioning in other contexts is healthy, who are nonetheless "pathogenic" parents. There also exist severely schizophrenic individuals whose parenting is surprisingly unaffected by their pathologic condition. Admittedly, as with any complex task, the sicker one is, the harder it is not to be destructive in the complex interaction of parenting.

We have tried to conceptualize, at a very general level, what it is that produces schizophrenia. While some parents of schizophrenic offspring are obviously unpleasant people, most parents of schizophrenics are not consciously destructive and would not harm their child if they had conscious control of the process. The parent whose offspring tends to become schizophrenic has used that child to solve his own psychologic problems. Therefore, we conceptualize it as follows: to what degree does the parent act in terms of the child's needs or his own when the two sets of needs conflict?

To measure this tendency, the unconscious functioning of the individual should be investigated. Therefore to examine this process, we defined a score for the TAT. The stories could be scored when there was a potential conflict between the needs of the dominant person and the needs of the dependent person. The degree to which the dominant person takes the dependent person's needs into account is scored: "pathogenic" (the dominant person does *not* take the dependent person's needs into account), "benign" (the dominant person *does* take the dependent person's needs into account), or "unscorable." A pathogenesis score is derived by the formula: number of pathogenic stories divided by the total number of scorable stories, that is, stories scored either pathogenic or benign.

In a series of studies, blindly scored TATs differentiated parents of schizophrenic children from parents of normal children. In the original study, Meyer and Karon (1967) had found almost no overlap between the mothers of schizophrenic children and the mothers of normal children in this psychologic trait. This was replicated by Mitchell (1968). In a further study, Mitchell (1969) scored TATs gathered by Singer and Wynne (1965a, 1965b) and found that both fathers and mothers of schizophrenic children were more "pathogenic" than parents of normal children.

In another study, on adult schizophrenic individuals, the degree of maternal pathogenesis correlated with the severity of patient pathology (Nichols, 1970). This was a very stringent test. Since all the patients were schizophrenic, the range of variation was small. Statistically, a reduced range of variation tends to make all correlation coefficients smaller.

Interestingly enough, Mitchell (1969) found that on the average the mothers were more pathogenic than the fathers. Here we see a congruence between clinical work and research when appropriately carried out. From the early days of psychotherapy with schizophrenic persons onward, those psychotherapists who have done intensive work have talked about the role the mother has played in producing the pathologic condition. This has been doubted by people who felt that it was unfair to mothers, and by people who felt that childhood could not be that important, and by people who preferred to believe that schizophrenia was a mystery. The research evidence is that, for schizophrenic individuals from intact families, not only are the mothers more important because mothers are more important for both healthy and unhealthy development than fathers for most children in our way of organizing the family, but also because, on the average, the mothers of schizophrenic children do tend to be somewhat more destructive in their impact than the fathers of schizophrenic children, even though these fathers may be more destructive than normal fathers.

An interesting sidelight on this is that Mitchell found the reverse to be true for delinquents, namely that the fathers tended to be more "pathogenic" in this specific sense that the mothers, who were more nearly like the mothers of "normals." A male delinquent from an intact family tends to have a sense of identity (which one would expect with a better relationship with the mother), but to have trouble with social controls (which one would expect with an impaired relationship with the father). This latter finding has been replicated.

Pathogenesis has also been found to differentiate child-abusive mothers from normal mothers, and child-abusive fathers from normal fathers, in both black and white populations (Melnick & Hurley, 1969; Evans, 1976).

In our studies of psychotherapy, as described in Chapter 10, pathogenesis has been used to examine the TATs of therapists, where it was found that "pathogenesis" differentiated ineffective from effective therapists. This should not be surprising. Therapy, like being a parent, is a situation in which one person has a dominant role in determining what happens, but what occurs is supposedly for the benefit of the dependent person. If the therapist is meeting his or her own needs unconsciously and not the needs of the patient, not much therapy is likely to be accomplished.

Do Children Teach Parents to Be Destructive?

In every case in our experience the schizophrenic individual's life has been such as to make his or her pathologic condition inevitable, and in most cases that means that the parents have been unconsciously "pathogenic." If even one parent is both strong and "benign," a schizophrenic outcome is improbable. As the evidence for unusual dynamics in the families of schizophrenic persons has accumulated, two alternative explanations of these data have emerged. One is genetic: schizophrenia, sometimes in mild form, leads to schizophrenia. But "pathogenesis" as we have defined it, and "parental communication deviance," as Wynne and Singer (1963) have described it, have been found to be more closely and consistently related to schizophrenia in the offspring than specifically schizophrenic traits, whether observed behaviorally or measured in psychologic tests.

The second alternative explanation is that the deviant child elicits deviant behavior from the parent. There is, of course, a certain amount of truth to this. Living with a very sick person is frustrating and may well exhaust a parent's tolerance and capacity to cope rationally.

Nonetheless, if one examines the specifics of the parent-child interaction, the specifically destructive interactions are usually such that no child could have taught them to the parent. The research problem is that the specifically destructive behavior varies from family to family.

Thus, no child teaches a mother to hold his hand in a flame for a minor offense, or to toilet-train the child by 6 months of age with severe measures, or from infancy on to get angry whenever she feeds him.

The one prospective study of the impact of family deviance to date (Doane et al., 1980) reports on the families of maladjusted but not psychotic adolescents. They measured Singer and Wynne's (1965a, 1965b) schizophrenia-producing communication deviance from the parent's TATs and so-called expressed emotionality (i.e., intrusive hostility) of the parents, a variable reported (Vaughn & Leff, 1976) to be characteristic of parents whose schizophrenic offspring tend to be rehospitalized early. If both of these parental measures were in the schizophrenia-producing direction, all the offspring were, 5 years later, diagnosed as schizophrenic or borderline. If neither variable was in the schizophrenia-producing direction, none of the offspring was schizophrenic or borderline. If the parental measures were not both in the same direction, there was an intermediate frequency of severe pathologic conditions.

Some Aspects of Family Dynamics

The views of Lidz (1973) are so cogent that they are worth briefly summarizing. We human beings depend upon our families to provide positive support and pressure to make it possible to grow up as independent human beings. When the family fails to provide the proper nurturance, support, identifications, and acculturation, we do not develop the strengths and abilities to make an adult individuated adaptation. The family that produces schizophrenic patients, according to Lidz, consists of disturbing and, sometimes, disturbed people. That is not to say that they are consciously malevolent people; on the contrary, they are typically very upset by the patient's illness.

All of us depend on our families to teach us cognitive categories similar to those used by other people in our culture. Lidz finds that families of schizophrenic offspring tend to teach cognitive categories which differ in meaning from those of people outside the family. Lidz describes two types of schizophrenia-producing families, which he terms the "skewed" and "schismatic." The skewed family is oriented around the needs of one of the parents, usually the mother. A distorted view of the world, of family life, and of how children should be raised is accepted by the other spouse and by the children. These distortions are needed by the dominant parent to maintain the parent's own psychologic survival. The parent does not differentiate the child from the self in any clear way. Usually the schizophrenic child is a boy in such families.

The schismatic family involves two parents, each of whom attempts to impose his own distorted view of the world, family life, and of the proper way to raise children upon the family. No consensus is arrived at by the parents, and the child internalizes two conflicting parental introjects. Usually the schizophrenic child in such a family is female.

In both types of families, the differences between parents and children, between male and female roles, and between the self and the other are blurred and confused. In the skewed family, the overidentification of the mother with her son, who is among other things the man she could not be, is very common. In this schismatic family, the identification of the daughter with the mother is made difficult by the mother's own derogation of her sex role, plus the father's derogation of the mother. These may account for the apparent sex-specific destructive effects.

The schizophrenic thought disorder, Lidz points out, is central to the pathology, and is clearly not like any organic thought disorder. He characterizes it as "egocentric overinclusiveness." By this he means the belief that everything that happens is related to one's self, and the belief that one can influence all sorts of outside events over which one has no realistic control.

In the so-called schizophrenic state, the patient's thoughts are thoroughly dominated by this egocentric overinclusiveness. But this is an adaptation to which the patient has been sensitized by a family that itself shares the same kind of thought disorder, but to an attenuated degree and usually restricted to intrafamilial transactions. The patient for most of his life is not so much egocentric as "parent-centric" in his or her functioning; that is, the patient's deficits are those required to make up the deficits in parental functioning. Such functioning on the part of the patient, however, appears to be egocentric from the standpoint of the rest of the world, particularly when it become so severe that it is no longer a viable way of life.

Lidz differentiates schizophrenic people into developmental versus regressive disorders in that some patients never have developed capacities, while others attain more mature functioning and then, under stress, regress to a prior level of more primitive intellectual functioning. What for a potentially schizophrenic individual might comprise an intolerable stress, however, may be no more than the normal stresses of human life for people with a different life history: the problems of independence and separation from one's family at adolescence, the need to be able to relate to people outside the family, the need to develop closeness and sexuality with other human beings, and/or the need to find a career and an adult way of life in the outside world.

Some Common Patterns of Bad Parenting

Frequently, there is a reversal of roles in families of schizophrenic individuals, so that the child feels as if he or she ought to be able to parent the parents, and that the parent should be able to enjoy the psychologic status of a child, and, if not, the parent is being unjustly used.

With male schizophrenic patients, the unconscious need of the "pathogenic" mother is usually to maintain control of her boy so that he never becomes independent of her. He may be allowed to become competent in some ways, but not to the point where it would lead him to separate and depart. Even his competence is used as a necessary addition to her fulfilling her own narcissistic needs.

This frequent pattern of destructive mothering is paralleled by a different pattern of "pathogenic" fathering. The father is generally not troubled about separation; in fact, in many cases, the father would just as soon the son did not bother him. The father's need is to set up competitions in the areas in which he feel inadequate. The role of the son is to lose that competition. If the father is unsure of his masculinity, the son is to be feminine or a homosexual. If the father is unsure of his intellectual competence, the son is to be "dumb." If the father is not sure of his ability to hold a job, the son is to be occupationally inadequate. The son's inadequacy reassures the father and makes the child necessary for the father's adjustment.

The fathers of schizophrenic children of either sex often express their "pathogenesis" by emotional absence, thus not providing an alternative relationship or model for the child. They do not interfere with even obviously hurtful practices of the mother, either because of "weakness," or because "one shouldn't argue in front of the children." Projective examinations generally reveal that, dynamically, such a father is just as "pathogenic" as the mother, allowing her to act out the destructiveness he might otherwise act out himself.

In our experience with female schizophrenic patients, this sex-role typing of the pernicious interaction does not seem as clear-cut. As in so many other issues of developmental psychology, the pressures involved in the development of schizophrenia in females are not as clearly patterned and tend to be more confusing. Mothers do seem to have more conflict about psychologic separation (that is, of identity), but both the fathers and mothers may equally generate problems with independence. The fathers may, however, be physically or emotionally absent. Competition in areas of anxiety may occur with either parent. A mother may reject the daughter as a child, but exploit her as a caretaker for younger siblings, or even for her. Sexuality is even more of a conflict than it is for males. The fathers either become seductive, or more frequently, emotionally withdrawn from the girl, for fear of their own sexual fantasies. The little girl almost never understands why she has been rejected.

Advising the Parents

Parents of schizophrenic children, whether being seen in treatment for themselves or in consultation regarding their child, may ask if they have caused their child's problems. They feel guilty. Like all patients, parents project onto the therapist the condemning superego based on the punitive part of their own parents. It is well known that in therapy every interpretation is twisted into an accusation; likewise, every bit of advice we give to parents is frequently twisted into an accusation.

But "In what way have I been culpable?" is not a fruitful question. Rather, we want to focus the parents on "What should I do now, given what has happened, and what I now want to happen?" It is important to help them talk about how frustrated they are dealing with a child whom they see as headstrong, out of touch with reality, and demanding totally unrealistic things. There is generally considerable truth in their complaints.

There are clinicians who intentionally intensify the guilt in order to get cooperation (or a high fee), but cooperation elicited through guilt is not recommended here, any more than in other relationships. Inevitably, it leads to anger, denial, and sabotage of the therapy. There are other clinicians who bolster the parents' self-esteem by telling them they have nothing to do with the child's problem, even if the clinician believes otherwise. This makes it difficult to investigate and change current parental practices later.

In most cases in which the parents initially cooperated, but later disrupted therapy, either the parents and the therapist colluded to avoid the issue, or the therapist blatantly lied to the parents about their involvement.

In our opinion, the proper approach, when parents ask about their role in the child's problems and it is too early to know, is to say: "I don't know. It may take us a long time to know exactly what caused your child's symptoms; however, it is our job to find out. Even if your child had no symptoms, being a parent is very difficult. When your child has problems, it is even more difficult, and I would like to be of use to you." It is helpful simply to add: "I don't know yet, but what do you think?"

The therapist thus is honest about how much he specifically knows, and yet he is not denying the possibility of some involvement by the parents. After all, the degree and nature of parental involvement will not be clearly understood until a good deal of work has been accomplished. Moreover, there are some cases of unusually severe life circumstances in which parental involvement is minimal. This honesty and uncertainty leave the door open for the parents to raise specific concerns later, and makes it easier for the therapist to raise such issues at a later point in therapy, if it would be useful. Obviously, there is more need for the therapist to have contact with the parents if the patient lives with them, and with a severely disturbed younger child living at home the concomitant treatment of the parents is an absolute necessity.

Over time, the schizophrenic offspring and their parents have developed a complex relationship. By the time a therapist typically sees them, the child's behavior confirms the parents' conscious experience of the child as crazy and unrealistic. The child's symptoms and other interactions with the parents express a mixture of hostility and compliance which is very frustrating. Indeed, a superficial evaluation of the parent-child interaction would lead to the conclusion that the parents were simply being victimized. The therapist must help the parents to handle their frustration with their difficult child. As he talks with them about what they are doing, he clarifies what is appropriate or inappropriate and helps them move to doing things with the child in different, more positive ways. Alleviating their realistic discomfort provides the leverage for the therapist to have an impact.

But when the child begins to change, the parents frequently panic. They now confront the anxiety and guilt they have been avoiding through their previous handling of the child. The therapist must take the lead in discussing what the child's changing behavior and the parents' reactions do and do not mean, consciously and unconsciously. The therapist needs to have prepared for this by having begun the relationship in a way that allows such discussions. The therapist also needs to function as a benign parent figure for the parents, providing emotional support during this difficult transition.

The therapist's view of human nature and of normal development needs to be communicated to the parents, including the role of the unconscious. Particularly important for the parent as well as for the child is the differentiation between thoughts and actions, the harmlessness of all thoughts and feelings, and the evaluation of actions by the seriousness of consequences. The importance of privacy, the normality of anger, crying, sexual feelings and curiosity including masturbation, must be discussed, as relevant.

The therapeutic view of child rearing that long-run goals should outweigh short-term inconveniences should be communicated to the parents. Thus, for example, the mother who is afraid of being kind to her child ("too kind," according to her), because her relatives will disapprove and think she "spoils" him, should be enlightened about probable long-term effects, so her guilt over kindness can be alleviated. She needs to be told that the evidence (e.g., Levy, 1943) is that "spoiling" a child by overindulging or being too "kind" tends to produce a nuisance in the short run, but the problems are readily overcome in the long run, while excessive deprivation or severity tends to produce chronic problems. Therefore, when in doubt, err in the direction of kindness.

Of course, it is not kind to undercut independence. Parents need to be told that independence is best achieved from a position of security, that human beings want security and will accept control when they are afraid, and feel burdened by control when they feel safe and want independence. It is important that they understand children vacillate between wanting security and wanting independence. Ideally, the parent needs to provide security when the child wants dependence and freedom when the child wants independence.

Both preventing independence and not providing security are hurtful, and, of course, teaching the skills that make independence possible is essential, as well as having independence as an important value.

Most parents want their children to be well behaved. The role of discipline in the socialization process is troublesome to most parents. They often feel some guilt about physical discipline and yet feel they have no alternatives. Like all problems, these are more serious for the parents of schizophrenic children and they need concrete help. Consider the father who beats his child for swearing. Both the issue of swearing and the issue of beating need to be discussed. The father's concern about swearing can be refocused: "Do you know any grown-ups who don't swear?"

Father, surprised (as if it's a new idea): "No."

"Then the problem isn't to teach him not to swear. That's not possible. The problem is to teach him when to swear, and when not to swear." This a paradigm for discussing many issues (e.g., sex, cleanliness, card-playing, dancing, alcohol, etc.), namely, what is a reasonably socialized adult like, rather than an overconforming "perfect" child.

Beating is an issue in its own right. Serious physical injury is never to be tolerated. The parents must be told that it is possible to raise children without ever hitting them, usually a new idea to them, and that the therapist would like them to consider, with his help, other ways of handling specific problems. It is also important, however, to let them know that very few parents are capable of never hitting their children, despite their best intentions. Otherwise the parents hear the therapist condemning them, or as being unrealistic. The therapist's emphasis on long-term consequences permits the therapist to point out that physical punishment is the fastest way to stop an immediate problem but tends to make the general discipline problem worse. In dealing with parents, it is essential for the therapist to try not to be seen as the condemning superego, or as someone whose standards are impossible to live up to. He should, of course, deal with the most serious destructive situations first, and expect only gradual and imperfect compliance on the part of the parents with any suggestions.

Parents need to be told that all children want their parents to like them, no matter how much the children's behavior seems to belie that. This powerful lever is there, if the parents will make use of it constructively. Punishment frequently serves primarily as a communication about what the parent does and does not want.

Therefore, the parent can learn to communicate his or her wishes in other ways, often more direct and differentiated, as in verbal communication. Of course, inconsistent reactions or consistent unconsciously motivated reinforcements in the "undesired" direction will produce unwanted counter-reactions by the child.

We frequently tell parents that they can have any kind of specific improved behavior from the child they want if they will be absolutely consistent in their reaction for a minimum of 6 months. It is not unusual for them to say, "But it's not worth it," which immediately places the so-called major problem in perspective.

There is no single bit of advice more useful to most parents who are having difficulties with their children (or who are concerned about their children's difficulties) than to suggest that every week each parent separately make some time available to the child that the child can depend on. The time is best spent with each child alone, although with large families that may not be practical. The child should have the right to cancel, but not the parent. When this is done, the disappearance of apparently "serious and unsolvable" problems is often dramatic. In some schizophrenic cases, there is a nonexistent father-son relationship which both would like, but feel they ought not to have, and that the "other" would not want, and only the authority of the therapist can permit the relationship to develop (generally over the mother's objections). In other schizophrenic cases there is a mother or father who withdraws from the child because the parent feels he is emotionally hurtful and he is trying to save his child (cf. Searles, 1965), who can be helped in reestablishing a relationship. Such advice, however, is unnecessary for most of the parents of schizophrenic children because of the elaborate psychodynamic intertwining that already exists. Rather, the problem is encouraging the parents to allow meaningful contacts outside the family.

In advising parents, and in working with families of schizophrenic adults, one's primary goal must be to prepare the child (or adult patient) for the role of a healthy independent adult. The secondary, short-term goal is to produce a temporary living situation that is tolerable for all concerned. (Normal child rearing is, of course, a temporary situation, although it is not always conceptualized that way.)

Part 2

Theoretical Perspectives

Psychoanalysis and Psychiatry

Ernest Jones, M.D.
(1929)

Without wishing to make an invidious list of the many institutions in America devoted to psychiatry, I think it may be said that this is the third great institute of psychiatry* to be inaugurated in this country, the third of the institutes which, by the magnificence of their foundation and the searching spirit that informs them, are destined to arrest attention even beyond the world of psychiatry. It was my privilege, nearly 17 years ago, to participate in the opening exercises of the first of them, the since renowned Phipps Clinic. The honour I now feel at being invited to play a part on the present occasion moves me to unburden myself of some general reflections, but they are such as have a direct bearing on the proper theme of this address. On revisiting this country for the first time since that event at Baltimore, I cannot refrain from reviewing in my mind the changes that have taken place in that time in the world of American psychiatry, a world to which I once myself belonged.

It is not my duty here to comment on the important technical advances in knowledge that have taken place in these years, but it might be of interest if I related my impression of three important events that have occurred in the general position of psychiatry in America. The most outstanding of these, and one on which this country has every right to congratulate itself, is what might be called

Address delivered at the opening exercises of the Institute of Psychiatry, Columbia University, New York , December 4, 1929. Published in *The State Hospital Quarterly,* January, 1930, and in *Mental Hygiene,* 1930, vol. xiv. Reprinted with permission of Baillière Tindall, London.

the social consolidation of the profession of psychiatry. So much impressed is the outside observer by this that it does not seem unmerited to say that America has actually created a new profession. In a very important respect one can almost say that the profession of psychiatry does not exist in any other country in the world. You, and still more of my European colleagues, may be astonished at such a statement, but I make it because the respect in which it is true is in my judgement of far-reaching significance. It is this: If we consider for a moment the three great fields of the psychoses, of the psychoneuroses, and of so-called normal psychology, with its vast social implications, then one is bound to admit that the presence of a relationship between them is perceived much more widely in America than in Europe. You observe I say "more widely," not "more deeply," for the scientific study of this relationship has certainly been carried much further in Europe, even though only by a small group of workers. Still, the fact remains that in America both the medical profession and society at large have accorded a much more general recognition than elsewhere to the community of interests subsisting between these branches of study. In Europe, broadly speaking, the psychoses are the care of the psychiatrists; the psychoneuroses are vigorously claimed by both neurologists and asylum psychiatrists, the battle being complicated by the appearance of a small, but increasing, number of specialists in that department; and academic psychology—with minor exceptions, such as limited contributions to industrial psychology—remains as aloof from the concerns of mankind as it does in America.

The importance I attach to the observation just made is this: I am convinced that progress in any one of the three fields in question can be only very partial and limited until the relationship between them is fully explored. It is easy to pay lip service to the existence of this relationship, but it is quite another matter to take it seriously and investigate its deeper meaning. Yet only in this way can we come to understand that the normal, the neurotic, and the psychotic have reacted differently to the same fundamental difficulties of human development, and to penetrate into the exact nature of these difficulties. Parenthetically, I wish to express here my conviction that the strategic point in the relationship between the three fields is occupied by the psychoneuroses. So-called normality represents a much more devious and obscure way of dealing with fundamentals of life than the neuroses do, and it is correspondingly a much more difficult route to retrace. The psychoses, on the other hand, present solutions so recondite and remote that it is very hard for the observer to develop a truly empathic attitude towards them, and unless this can be done, any knowledge remains intellectualistic, external, and unfruitful. If a man's main interest is in the psychology of either the normal or the psychotic, it is fairly safe to predict that his understanding of the deeper layers of the mind will remain strictly limited. In America, however, thanks to the broad conception of psychiatry there prevailing, a psychiatrist is less exposed to these dangers. Society will see to it that he is chiefly occupied with the problems of the psychoneuroses, though his interest will extend along the mental-hygiene movement in the one direction and into the field of the psychoses in the other. The problems of social adaptation, or maladaptation, will therefore always stand in the foreground of his attention.

It would be tempting to inquire how this broad conception of psychiatry came to be developed only in America. It is definitely a matter of the last 20 years. I am not familiar enough with the details of growth in this period to venture a firm opinion on the point, but my impression is that the change has been brought about by a developing attitude on the part of society in general quite as much as by the influence of a few outstanding personalities. It appears, in fact, to be an expression of the American social conscience. It is easy for Europeans to wax satirical over this conscience, for assuredly the raw guilt out of which it is evolved has at times produced manifestations grotesque enough to warrant any satire. But to ignore this feature would be a venial error compared with the blunder it would be to ignore or underestimate the vast positive value of that social conscience. After all, perhaps the greater part of social progress emanates from an uneasy conscience, from dissatisfaction with a state of affairs unpleasant to our feelings or repugnant to our cultural sentiments. In the present case, for instance, the widespread social recognition that the psychiatrist's work—whether it is concerned with mental hygiene, with the therapy of the psychoneuroses, or with the care of the psychotic—constitutes an essential unity would seem to have proceeded in large measure from a dawning realisation that there exists in the community a vast amount of mental suffering to which attention needs to be directed.

The mention of the word "suffering" induces another reflection. It is noteworthy that, whatever pressure may have come from the side of society, the psychiatric movement in America to which I am now referring is essentially a medical one, is indeed an immense extension of the scope of the medical profession. It is not at first sight evident why this had to be so. A priori it might have seemed just as likely, and even more logical, if the increasing light thrown on mental problems had come from the side of the pure psychologist. Just as in physiology, where an accurate knowledge of the normal processes of bodily functions must precede the study of their derangements in disease, it might have been supposed that the proper order would have been for psychologists to obtain insight into the structure and development of the normal mind and then for this knowledge to be applied to the investigation of various departures from the normal. The reverse of this has happened. Almost all insight into the deeper structure and development of the mind has come from psychopathology, and it is only through this knowledge that we are beginning to understand something of the more obscure problems of the normal mind. It may sound paradoxical, but I venture to predict that in a not far distant future psychopathology, particularly of the psychoneuroses, will constitute the standard study of psychology, the basis from which the student will proceed later to the more obscure and difficult study of the so-called normal, and moreover I should not be altogether surprised if America achieved this consummation before any other country.

There are two objective grounds why this prediction is a very safe one to make. Investigation of the deeper layers of the mind has shown irrefragably that the basic elements out of which our minds are developed persist with the psychoneurotic—in the unconscious, it is true—in their original form to a much greater extent than they do with the normal, and further that they present themselves in a magnified and perspicuous aspect as if under a clear lens, so that from every point of view they are far more accessible to examination there than with the normal. Fundamental complexes and mechanisms, the effects of which radiate throughout the whole mind, can be very plainly demonstrated in the psychoneurotic when the same processes can often be only dimly inferred in the normal, and yet anyone who urges the objection that there is a qualitative difference between the two classes is merely displaying his omission to investigate the relationship between them.

The second ground on which the prediction can be based is even more interesting. We know nowadays that the reason why psychology has lagged so extraordinarily behind all other branches of science is because there exist in the mind—both, be it noted, of the subject and the object—the most formidable obstacles which interpose themselves in the path of any exploration designed to penetrate below the surface. Unlike any other man of science, therefore, the psychologist is from the beginning cut off from the object of his study—the human mind. So far as our present experience goes, there is only one motive strong enough to overcome these obstacles—that of wishing to be delivered of suffering; even the keenest scientific curiosity offers only a very partial substitute for this motive. Now in the history of the world the theme of suffering has been the special concern of three classes of men: of poets, of priests, and of physicians. Until recently it has been the first of these three, the poet, who has contributed most to our understanding of mental suffering, and we owe some of our most precious insight to his flashes of genius. But he is, after all, primarily concerned, not with the understanding of suffering, but with the transmuting of it into beauty or whatever else would raise it to another plane. Few have thought more profoundly about the function of poetry than Keats, and he tells us:

> . . . they shall be accounted poet kings
> Who simply tell the most heart-easing things.

The priest's interest, too, has been mainly therapeutic. Starting with a vested interest in a particular cure, he has been chiefly engaged in transmitting his cure to those in need. Nevertheless, the more profound theologians, having—so to speak—a scientific interest in their work, have also furnished us with much knowledge concerning the nature and sources of suffering. They have rightly laid especial stress in this connection on the importance of moral problems, notably on the problem of evil—nowadays called the problem of the sense of guilt. The physician likewise did not proceed very far so long as his attitude was a purely therapeutic one, showing once more how the passion for therapeutics—laudable as it is on humanitarian grounds—has often proved the bane of medicine and has blocked progress in real prevention and cure based on knowledge. Those over-anxious to heal cannot pause to find out how to do so. It is only when the desire to relieve suffering was infused by the scientific thirst for knowledge that we began to have serious insight, not only into the meaning of all this suffering, but—what is still more important—into the dynamic factors that move both the depths and the surface of our minds. In this achievement there is, in my opinion, one man's name that will be for ever preeminent, and that is the name of Freud, now so contemned, but in the future to be honoured above all his contemporaries.

This expansion of psychiatry into what were previously non-medical fields was either stimulated by or, at all events, responded to the special social sense of the American people. It is appropriate, however, in addressing the new Psychiatric Institute of the New York State Hospitals to remember that, although the names of workers elsewhere—such as Dr. White, of Washington, and Dr. Putnam and Dr. C. Macfie Campbell, of Boston—will not be forgotten in this connection, the main inspiration for the broadening and humanising of the conception of psychiatry in America emanated from the forerunner of this institute—namely, the Psychiatric Institute of the New York State Hospitals, situate on Ward's Island. That inspiration will always be associated with the names of Dr. Adolf Meyer and Dr. August Hoch, together with their brilliant pupils, Drs. A. A. Brill and George H. Kirby, who now, by their presence on the staff of Columbia University, link the two institutions that have co-operated in founding this impressive and promising institute. In saying this I would not have you think that I underestimate the important part played, particularly in the mental-hygiene movement, by lay co-operation. Although I think it desirable that the movement in question should always remain essentially a medical one, I am not one of those who think that laymen should be jealously excluded from psychiatric work, for I have ample experience of their value even on the therapeutic side itself.

The second event of the past few years to which I wished to make a short reference was the use American authorities made of psychopathology and psychology in the war. It is well known that this was more extensive and more enlightened in America than in any European country, and I mention it here only as an illustration to confirm the thesis just put forward of the remarkable extent to which psychiatry in America has become associated with the national life and has ceased to be regarded as a narrow speciality.

The third event is perhaps the most interesting of all and will bring me closer to the theme proper of this address. I mean the extent to which knowledge of psycho-analysis has permeated psychiatry itself in America. When I was last here, before the war, psycho-analysis had certainly established a foothold, particularly in New York, but they have extended this foothold only very slowly in the time that has elapsed since then. On the other hand, the extent to which a varying degree of knowledge of psycho-analysis has been accepted by American psychiatrists at large is truly noteworthy and is something for which there is no parallel in any country in Europe. Oddly enough, however, I think it could well be maintained that this open-mindedness on the part of American psychiatrists redounds less to their credit than might at first sight appear. For it looks sometimes as if they had purchased this open-mindedness by indulging in certain superficiality, in fact at the expense of their imagination. To put the matter cursorily, and therefore very partially, it might be said that European psychiatrists have been loath to accept psycho-analysis just because they realised it was a grim business, an affair of tremendous import from which they preferred to keep aloof; whereas American psychiatrists welcomed it as a novelty, but have failed to realise adequately its significance. This remark, like all such facile generalisations, is distinctly unfair, but what interests me is the modicum of truth it contains. If you find it over-sharply expressed, perhaps you will allow me to put the matter in a more objective way. What concerns us here is the precise relationship of psycho-analysis to psychiatry, the extent to which psychiatry can profit from psycho-analysis, and—last, but not least—the danger it is in of not securing this profit. I propose that we consider these questions in this order.

It has been said that the relationship of psycho-analysis to psychiatry resembles that of histology to anatomy. The point of similarity is evident; the one studies the finer details, the other the gross outlines. Let us see how far the analogy can carry us. It is hard for us nowadays to picture what anatomy was like before the discovery of the microscope, but we know enough to realise something of the revolution this instrument effected. It was not merely that far more became known about the actual anatomical structure of the various organs; more important than this was the contribution histology made to our knowledge of function and genesis. This is a matter too obvious to need stressing, but the point I am making here is that just the same is true of psycho-analysis. The addition to our knowledge through the detailed study of the finer content of various mental processes—i.e., the purely interpretative side of psycho-analysis, the revealing of the latent content of dreams, delusions, and so on—interesting as all this may be, is relatively unimportant in comparison with the illumination psycho-analysis has thrown on the more vital problems of motivation and psycho-genesis; in other words, it can explain, not only what has happened, but also why it happened. The exploration of the unconscious layers of the mind, made possible for the first time by psycho-analysis, has yielded knowledge of such inestimable value for psychiatry and psychology that it is hardly exaggerating to term it a revelation. We are in fact introduced to a new world, the world of the unconscious, where all the important events take place the results of which are simply documented in the consciousness.

Though it is of course impossible for me here to substantiate these extensive claims by citing any of the endless detail of which psycho-analytical work is composed, may I at least try to specify a little more definitely something of the nature of the contributions psycho-analysis has, in my judgement, made to the subject of psychiatry and to select for this purpose three particular considerations. It will be understood that I am using the word psychiatry here in the broad sense previously indicated and not merely as denoting the field of the psychoses. I am also speaking purely of its psychological aspects; of the relation of these to its organic aspects I shall say a word in conclusion. Well, to me the outstanding achievement of psycho-analysis in psychiatry is that it has given us for the first time a real comprehension of the meaning of mental morbidity. One may even go further and say it has taught us that mental morbidity has a meaning. Before the advent of psychoanalysis the prevailing view was that psychopathological symptoms had no psychological meaning; they were supposed to represent— from a psychological point of view—meaningless manifestations of a breakdown on the part of the mental apparatus. Various toxic and other organic influences were supposed to derange the brain, and the resulting symptoms were believed to be as meaningless as from a musical point of view the jangling sounds are meaningless that result from a clumsy weight crashing on to a piano. The infinitely detailed investigation of such symptoms by means of psycho-analysis has shown that they are full of meaning to their finest ramification, that they are throughout informed with purpose, with intent, and with aim. The achievement of imaginary gratification, the allaying of guiltiness and remorse, the protection against the most terrible dangers—all these are processes that we are as yet very far indeed from being able to express in any other than psychological terms.

One of the most startling discoveries psycho-analysis has made of a general nature is that most of the phenomena comprising a mental disorder are symptoms, not in the Greek sense of morbid casualties, but in the modern sense of indicators. But they are indicators, not so much of disease, except by implication, as of a healing process. This is a point of view that had hardly been suspected before psycho-analysis, and it is one that has important therapeutic as well as pathological bearings. It means not merely that the delusions of the paranoiac, the phobias of the hysteric, and the obsessions of the obsessional neurotic are not the disease, but signs of a disease—so much had been conjectured previously—but that they are the products of an attempt to heal the underlying trouble. Appreciation of this must radically affect our attitude toward such phenomena in our therapeutic endeavours. By merely thwarting them (e.g., by suggestion) an apparent success may be achieved that is purchased by a worsening of the disorder itself underlying them, one that may then manifest itself in more sinister ways.

In the second place, we know at last something—in fact, a great deal—about the nature of this underlying disorder, the disease itself, if we use the word in a broad and not too medical a sense. It may fairly be said that before psycho-analysis not even the site of the lesion was known, to say nothing of the nature of the lesion. This site is nothing more nor less than the unconscious mind, a region of the universe the very existence of which was only vaguely surmised before psycho-analysis explored and defined it, and yet one that is almost certainly of greater practical importance to humanity than consciousness itself. The disorder underlying all mental morbidity can be defined as a failure on the part of the ego to deal in any final manner with certain fundamental intra-psychical conflicts that are the inevitable lot of every human being. These conflicts arise from the difficulty in adjusting the claims of the sexual instinct in its earliest stages with those of other psychical forces. The integrity of the ego needs on the one hand secure possession of certain sexual impulses, or their derivatives, and on the other a secure relation to external reality. It is threatened if the conflict in question is not solved, and the ultimate danger menacing it is paralysis of mental functioning, a hypothetical condition to which I have given the name aphanisis, one to which some approximation is found in the dementia of psychotics and the inhibitions of psycho-neurotics. All mental morbidity is, therefore, a state of schizophrenia, although Professor Bleuler has proposed to reserve this term for the most striking of its forms. What we meet with clinically as mental disorder represents the endless variety of the ways in which the threatened ego struggles for its self-preservation. In the nature of things, therefore, our conception of it can be cast only in terms of active dynamic strivings.

The third psycho-analytical contribution to psychiatry I would cite is its extension of psychopathology into the realm of ætiology. It has long been surmised that certain psychoses were due to errors in development—indeed, with idiocy it is obvious—but the investigations of psycho-analysis have been able to establish this as a general proposition. What is termed "fixation," with the closely allied "regression," is a fundamental concept in psycho-analysis, and from this point of view it may fairly be said that all mental morbidity signifies an arrest in development. A potential neurotic or psychotic is someone who still carries about with him a conflict that is normally solved in infancy; he is someone who has never successfully passed a given stage of infantile development. Various precipitating factors decide whether this state of affairs will come to expression in the form of symptoms early or late in life. The relation between the arrest in ontogenetic development and particular difficulties in the phylogenetic history of humanity opens up a fascinating chapter, to which psycho-analysis has already made promising contribution. To sum up the three considerations just advanced, psycho-analysis has provided psychiatry with an interpretative, a dynamic, and a genetic point of view.

We may now profitably compare what I have said about American psychiatry and about psycho-analysis respectively. American psychiatry has the distinctive feature of breadth. It has already absorbed the psycho-neuroses in its scope and is making serious encroachments into normal psychology. The three fields have to be united, and American psychiatry and psycho-analysis are the two movements that are most alive to this truth. It was dimly perceived many years ago by Hughlings Jackson when he made his famous remark: "Find out about dreams and you will find out about insanity." It was Freud who found out about dreams and applied his findings to insanity, but it is to be noted that he found out about dreams by applying a psychopathological method derived from the study of the neuroses, thus uniting the three fields. If one takes the trouble to appreciate at their full value the three psycho-analytical points of view I have just sketched, it must be evident that psycho-analysis, while coinciding with its aims in the psychiatric ones we considered earlier, is still broader in its scope. Any attempt, therefore, to dismiss psycho-analysis to a corner of a chapter on the therapeutics of psychiatry, as if it were an alternative to hydrotherapy or a subvariety of suggestion, is simply to exhibit ignorance of its meaning and significance. When the doctrine of evolution made its appearance, it had either to be denied in toto or else to fertilise the whole of biology, to cause natural history, embryology, and comparative anatomy to be viewed afresh in a flood of light; even its bitterest opponents, to do them justice, realised that to have regarded it merely as a contribution of detail would have been simply foolish. Yet there is to-day a real risk of a corresponding blunder being committed with psycho-analysis. The forces of repression that veil first the existence and then the significance of the unconscious are hard to overestimate in their strength and subtlety; to accept a discovery with lip service and subsequently to discount the importance of it is only one, though a potent one, of its workings. To my mind there has never been any likelihood of psycho-analysis being stifled even by the most relentless opposition. But there is a very real danger, particularly in America, lest the gifts it can confer on psychiatry be put aside for long through complacent acceptance without proper appreciation of their value. This, in one word, is the message I make bold to bring from psycho-analysis to American psychiatry.

I have said something about the relation of psycho-analysis to the psychological aspects of psychiatry. What, now, is its relation to the organic aspects? I need not correct here the common misconception that psycho-analysis ignores the organic factors in mental disorder. Psycho-analysis has, it is true, to point out that attention has been too exclusively focused on them in the past, to the neglect of the psychological factors, and it has tried to restore a due proportion between the two sets. The same holds good for bodily disease in general, for it is probable that mental factors play a considerable, and possibly even an important, part in this field also. Into the vexed question of the connection between mind and body I do not propose to enter, my point of view here being purely clinical and empirical. But how is one to bring together the two indisputable facts that unconscious conflicts and bodily poisons may both operate in the production of mental disorder?

I hinted earlier that the ego, the kernel of the personality, on the integrity of which mental health depends, has two essential tasks to perform and two corresponding difficulties or dangers to cope with. It has to assimilate, and to respond adequately to, stimuli proceeding from two very different sources, from perceptions of the outer world and from stimuli arising in the inner world, respectively. It has not only to do this, but also to bring these two sets of stimuli into some sort of harmony with each other. Psycho-analysis finds that these tasks are much more formidable than is commonly thought, and that they are very rarely carried out with any degree of smoothness. It can point to endless imperfections in the performance of this task— for it is in essence a single task, the uniting of the inner with the outer world of the demands of the instincts with the demands of reality. When the imperfections are gross, mental morbidity will surely result. When they are less so, the issue, wavering in the balance, may be influence by changes in the forces with which the ego had to deal. Changes may occur in the demands on the part of reality, through the fluctuating circumstances of life and of human relationships, and changes may take place in the insistence of the inner needs, for example, at various times of life—puberty, climacteric, and so on. But not only may there be all these manifold variations in the task set the ego, but the capacity of the ego to perform it may also be affected by factors directly influencing it itself. By these I mean somatic factors, principally—so fair as we know—toxic ones. We are all familiar with the profound alterations in mental functioning that can be induced in this way, but the contribution psycho-analysis has been able to make is to indicate the nature of these alterations. They are the very same as those in the other case we considered previously, where the ego, without being weakened by any somatic influences, has proved unequal to its great task. The mental morbidity represents—in the organic just as in the psychogenic cases—the triumph of the imperfectly controlled unconscious impulses.

That this conception of mental morbidity can, thanks to recent researches, be seen to reign over the whole field, in both the psychogenic and the organic realm, is a scientific generalisation of supreme theoretical interest. The knowledge gained from it must enable us to direct our prophylactic and therapeutic efforts more intelligently than before. The immediate practical application of the knowledge is another matter. The work done by Ferenczi and Hollós on the psychology of dementia paralytica and by Tausk and Kielholz in respect of the alcoholic psychoses has shown that the mental manifestations of these disorders are in no way to be explained as a direct result of the toxins concerned; they are expressions of individual conflicts which can no longer be coped with by an ego weakened by the cerebral poisoning. Obviously this discovery has no immediate bearing on the necessity of dealing with the toxins, but nevertheless the suggestion that the more stable is the relation between consciousness and the unconscious the less liable is the mind to be disturbed by toxins may well prove to have important practical applications in the future. At the other end of the scale, there is no doubt that where the ego shows spontaneous failure to cope with this task, the approach can, at least at present, only be psychological. In the intermediate cases, where the ætiology is more mixed, the decision of which is the most suitable mode of attack will of course be a matter of judgement, and there will be some in which both are indicated. There is no contradiction whatever between the psychological and the organic point of view; they are of necessity interrelated.

We have not, however, exhausted this interrelationship by the consideration just advanced, which is concerned with only one way in which bodily factors can affect the mind. Quite apart from the direct influence of such factors in weakening the ego, we have to remember that the very existence of any bodily disturbance is in itself a psychological fact the importance of which to the mind may be very great and indeed momentous. On the other side, that the mind can affect the body is well recognised, though in my opinion the extent to which it can do so is still very much underestimated. It is not merely that psychogenic disorders—e.g., hysteria—often express themselves by disturbance of bodily function where the physical symptoms actually symbolise various mental processes. There are many other ways in which mental disorder—e.g., in the anxiety states—can affect somatic functioning more directly and can produce even structural changes with or without the co-operation of somatic factors. Finally, there remains what may perhaps prove to be the most important consideration of all. I refer to the probability that conceptions generated in the field of psychopathology—such as, for example, the connection between the pleasure principle and relief of tension—may in the future by applied to corresponding mechanisms in the somatic field and thus become established as biological principles of unconjecturable significance.

From all these considerations it will be evident that pathological psychiatry—i.e., that part concerned with somatic changes—forms an essential link between internal medicine on the one hand and psycho-analysis on the other, indeed, one might say between medicine and psychology in general. It will not be the only one—genetics or endocrinology, for example, may rival it in importance in the future—but it will surely remain an indispensable one. More novel, however, is the conclusion that psycho-analysis must become an increasingly important link between medicine and psychiatry on the one hand and the whole of society on the other. There are already a few feeble links of the kind, physical hygiene perhaps the most prominent. But when one reflects that there is no aspect of human endeavour that can long remain unaffected by psycho-analysis—from ethnology to politics, from education to sociology, from art to economics, from philosophy to religion; in short, the whole fabric of civilisation—then we must see that to-day we are witnessing the birth of an enormous widening of medical endeavour and of the significance of medicine in the body politic. And in this widening, psychiatry, as the chief link between psycho-analysis and medicine, will, I trust, play an honourable part.

Borderline States

Robert P. Knight, M.D.
(1953)

The term "borderline state" has achieved almost no official status in psychiatric nomenclature, and conveys no diagnostic illumination of a case other than the implication that the patient is quite sick but not frankly psychotic. In the few psychiatric textbooks where the term is to be found at all in the index, it is used in the text to apply to those cases in which the decision is difficult as to whether the patients in question are neurotic or psychotic, since both neurotic and psychotic phenomena are observed to be present. The reluctance to make a diagnosis of psychosis on the one hand, in such cases, is usually based on the clinical estimate that these patients have not yet "broken with reality"; on the other hand the psychiatrist feels that the severity of the maladjustment and the presence of ominous clinical signs preclude the diagnosis of a psychoneurosis. Thus the label "borderline state," when used as a diagnosis, conveys more information about the uncertainty and indecision of the psychiatrist than it does about the condition of the patient.

Indeed, the term and its equivalents have been frequently attacked in psychiatric and psychoanalytic literature. Rickman (1928) wrote: "It is not uncommon in the lax phraseology of a Mental O. P. Department to hear of a case in which a psychoneurosis 'masks' a psychosis; I have used the term myself, but with inward misgiving. There should be no talk of masks if a case is fully understood and certainly not if the case has not received a tireless examination—

Read at the joint session of the American Psychoanalytic Association and the Section on Psychoanalysis of the American Psychiatric Association, Atlantic City, May 12, 1952. Reprinted with permission from the *Bulletin of the Menninger Clinic, 17,* 1, 1–12, 1953.

except, of course, as a brief descriptive term comparable to 'shut-in' or 'apprehensive' which carry our understanding of the case no further." Similarly, Edward Glover (1932) wrote: "I find the terms 'borderline' or 'pre'-psychotic, as generally used, unsatisfactory. If a psychotic mechanism is present at all, it should be given a definite label. If we merely suspect the possibility of a breakdown of repression, this can be indicated in the term 'potential' psychotic (more accurately a 'potentially clinical' psychosis). As for larval psychoses, we are all larval psychotics and have been such since the age of two." Again, Zilboorg (1941) wrote: "The less advanced cases (of schizophrenia) have been noted, but not seriously considered. When of recent years such cases engaged the attention of the clinician, they were usually approached with the euphemistic labels of borderline cases, incipient schizophrenias, schizoid personalities, mixed manic-depressive psychoses, schizoid manics, or psychopathic personalities. Such an attitude is untenable either logically or clinically. . . ." Zilboorg goes on the declare that schizophrenia should be recognized and diagnosed when its characteristic psychopathology is present, and suggests the term "ambulatory schizophrenia" for that type of schizophrenia in which the individual is able, for the most part, to conceal his pathology from the general public.

I have no wish to defend the term "borderline state" as a diagnosis. I do wish, however, to discuss the clinical conditions usually connoted by this term, and especially to call attention to the diagnostic, psychopathological, and therapeutic problems involved in these conditions. I shall limit my discussion to the functional psychiatric conditions where the term is usually applied, and more particularly to those conditions which involve schizophrenic tendencies of some degree.

I believe it is the common experience of psychiatrists and psychoanalysts currently to see and treat, in open sanitaria or even in office practice, a rather high percentage of patients whom they regard, in a general sense, as borderline cases. Often these patients have been referred as cases of psychoneuroses of severe degree who have not responded to treatment according to the usual expectations associated with the supposed diagnosis. Most often, perhaps, they have been called severe obsessive-compulsive cases; sometimes an intractable phobia has been the outstanding symptom; occasionally an apparent major hysterical symptom or an anorexia nervosa dominates the clinical picture; and at times it is a question of the degree of depression, or of the extent and ominousness of paranoid trends, or of the severity of a character disorder.

The unsatisfactory state of our nosology contributes to our difficulties in classifying these patients diagnostically, and we legitimately wonder if a "touch of schizophrenia" is of the same order as a "touch of syphilis" or a "touch of pregnancy." So we fall back on such qualifying terms as latent or incipient (or ambulatory) schizophrenia, or emphasize that it is a *severe* obsessive-compulsive neurosis or depression, adding, for full coverage, "with paranoid trends" or "with schizoid manifestations." Certainly, for the most part, we are quite familiar with the necessity of recognizing the primary symptoms of schizophrenia and not waiting for the secondary ones of hallucinations, delusions, stupor, and the like.

Freud (1913) made us alert to the possibility of psychosis underlying a psychoneurotic picture in his warning: "Often enough, when one sees a case of neurosis with hysterical or obsessional symptoms, mild in character and of short duration (just the type of case, that is, which one would regard as suitable for the treatment) a doubt which must not be overlooked arises whether the case may not be one of incipient dementia praecox, so-called (schizophrenia, according to Bleuler; paraphrenia, as I prefer to call it), and may not sooner or later develop well marked signs of this disease." Many authors in recent years, among them Hoch and Polatin (1949), Stern (1945), Miller (1940), Pious (1950), Melitta Schmideberg (1947), Fenichel (1945), H. Deutsch (1942), Stengel (1945), and others, have called attention to types of cases which belong in the borderline band of the psychopathological spectrum, and have commented on the diagnostic and psychotherapeutic problems associated with these cases.

Some Diagnostic Considerations

In attempting to make the precise diagnosis in a borderline case there are three often used criteria, or frames of reference, which are apt to lead to errors if they are used exclusively or uncritically. One of these, which stems from traditional psychiatry, is the question of whether or not there has been a "break with reality"; the second is the assumption that neurosis is neurosis, psychosis is psychosis, and never the twain shall meet; a third, contributed by psychoanalysis, is the series of stages of development of the libido, with the conceptions of fixation, regression, and typical defense mechanisms for each stage.

No psychiatrist has any difficulty in diagnosing a psychosis when he finds definite evidence of falsification of reality in the form of hallucinations and delusions, or evidence of implicit loss of reality sense in the form of self-mutilation, mutism, stupor, stereotypies, flight of ideas, incoherence, homicidal mania, and the like. But these are all signs of advanced psychosis, and no present-day psychiatrist of standing would be unaware of the fact that each patient with one or more of these psychotic manifestations had carried on for some previous years as a supposedly normal individual, albeit with concealed potentialities for a psychotic outbreak, and that there must have been warning signs, various stages of development, and a gradually increasing degree of overtness of these gross expressions of psychotic illness. All science aims at the capacity to *predict,* and psychiatry will become a science the more it can detect the evidences of strain, the small premonitory sings of a psychotic process, so that it can then introduce the kinds of therapeutic measures which have the best chance of aborting the psychotic development. The break with reality, which is an ego alteration, must be thought of not as a sudden and unexpected snapping, as of a twig, but as the gradual bending as well, which preceded the snapping; and sound prognosis must inevitably take into account those ego factors which correspond to the tensile strength of the twig, as well as the kinds and degree of disruptive forces which are being applied.

A second conception which leads to misdiagnosis is that neurosis and psychosis are mutually exclusive, that neurosis never develops into psychosis, and that neurotics are "loyal to reality" while psychotics are "disloyal to reality." It is, to be sure, one of the contributions of psychoanalysis that neurotic mechanisms are different from psychotic mechanisms, and that psychosis is not simply a more severe degree of neurosis. However, it is quite possible for both psychotic and neurotic mechanisms to have developed in the same individual, and this is the crux of the problem in many borderline cases. Furthermore, there is a sense in which there is a loss of reality even in neurosis. As Freud (1924) pointed out: "The difference at the beginning comes to expression at the end in this way: in neurosis a part of reality is avoided by a sort of flight, but in psychosis it is remodeled. Or one may say that in psychosis, flight at the beginning is succeeded by an active phase of reconstruction, while in neurosis obedience at the beginning is followed by a subsequent attempt at flight. Or, to express it in yet another way, neurosis does not deny the existence of reality, it merely tries to ignore it; psychosis denies it and tries to substitute something else for it. A reaction which combines features of both these is the one we call normal or 'healthy'; it denies reality as little as neurosis, but then, like a psychosis, is concerned with effecting a change in it. This expedient normal attitude leads naturally to some active achievement in the outer world and is not content, like a psychosis, with establishing the alteration within itself; it is no longer *autoplastic* but *alloplastic.*" Again, on the point of gradations in loss of reality, Freud (1922) discussed normal jealousy, projected jealousy, and delusional jealousy, pointing out their transitions from one to the other, and describing how an individual may for a time maintain his critical judgment over paranoid ideas which are already present but do not yet have the strength of conviction of delusions.

Anna Freud (1936) describes how children can use the defense of denial—denial in fantasy and denial in word and act—in ways which represent temporary breaking with reality while retaining an unimpaired faculty of reality testing. However, if adolescents and adults persist in, or resume, this kind of denial after the normal development of ego synthesis has taken place "the relation to reality has been gravely disturbed and the foundation of reality-testing suspended." The varieties of channeling psychotic (usually paranoid) tendencies in eccentric or fanatical ways—even to the point of developing a following of many people—and the various degrees of inappropriate emotions seen in many individuals further highlight the vagueness of the criterion of reality testing, and of the distinction between neurotic and psychotic. Also, we are well aware that in these and other borderline conditions the *movement* in the case may be toward or away from further psychotic development.

The third frame of reference, that of the levels of psychosexual development—oral sucking, oral biting, anal expulsive, anal retentive, phallic, and genital—and of the attempts to build a classification of mental disorders by linking a certain clinical condition to each level of libidinal fixation, has presented a one-sided, libidinal theory of human functioning. This psychoanalytic contribution has been of major value, but it needs to be supplemented extensively with the findings of ego psychology which have not, as yet, been sufficiently integrated with the libido theory. Reliance on the "ladder" of psychosexual development, with the line of reality testing drawn between the two anal substages, has resulted in many blunders in diagnosis—especially in the failure to perceive the psychosis underlying a hysterical, phobic, or obsessive-compulsive clinical picture.

I believe it was Freud who used the metaphor of a retreating army to illuminate the mixed clinical picture in libidinal regression. I should like to borrow the metaphor and elaborate it for the purpose of illuminating ego-defensive operations. Various segments or detachments of the retreating army may make a stand and conduct holding or delaying operations at various points where the terrain lends itself to such operations, while the main retreating forces may have retired much farther to the rear. The defensive operations of the more forward detachments would, thus, actually protect the bulk of the army from disaster; but these forward detachments may not be able to hold their positions, and may have to retreat at any time in the face of superior might. On the other hand, the main army may be able to regroup itself, receive reinforcements or gain new leadership, and recapture its morale. In that event, the forward positions may hold long enough for the main forces to move forward to, or even well beyond, the stubbornly defended outposts.

I believe this metaphor conceptualizes in an important way the psychoeconomy and the indicated therapy in the borderline cases. The superficial clinical picture—hysteria, phobia, obsessions, compulsive rituals—may represent a holding operation in a forward position, while the major portion of the ego has regressed far behind this in varying degrees of disorder. For the sake of accurate diagnosis, realistic prognosis, and appropriate therapy, therefore, the clinician must be able to locate the position, movement, and possibilities of resynthesis of the main ego forces and functions, and not be misled by all the shooting in the forward holding point. An important corollary of this conception is that the therapy should not attempt to attack and demolish the forward defensive operations when to do so would mean disaster for the main ego operations. Some forward defensive operations are a matter of life and death.

Without defending the term "borderline state" as a diagnostic label, I have thus far developed the argument to show that there is a borderline strip in psychopathology where accurate diagnosis is difficult. I have tried to show the general characteristic of such borderline conditions, and to point out why the often used diagnostic criteria of break with reality, mutual exclusiveness of neurosis and psychosis, and the libido theory are insufficient and misleading in reaching accurate diagnosis, prognosis, and appropriate therapeutic recommendations for such cases. What, then, are the more reliable methods of evaluating these cases so that one will not have to be content with using as a diagnosis the unspecific term "borderline state"? The attempt to answer this question will involve a discussion of certain dynamic considerations as they relate to the diagnostic techniques available to us—the psychiatric interview, the free-association interview, and the use of psychological diagnostic tests.

Some Dynamic Considerations

We conceptualize the borderline case as one in which normal ego functions of secondary-process thinking, integration, realistic planning, adaptation to the environment, maintenance of object relationships, and defenses against primitive unconscious impulses are severely weakened. As a result of various combinations of the factors of constitutional tendencies, predisposition based on traumatic events and disturbed human relationships, and more recent precipitating stress, the ego of the borderline patient is laboring badly. Some ego functions have been severely impaired—especially, in most cases, integration, concept formation, judgment, realistic planning, and defending against eruption into conscious thinking of id impulses and their fantasy elaborations. Other ego functions, such as conventional (but superficial) adaptation to the environment and superficial maintenance of object relationships, may exhibit varying degrees of intactness. And still others, such as memory, calculation, and certain habitual performances, may seem unimpaired. Also, the clinical picture may be dominated by hysterical, phobic, obsessive-compulsive, or psychosomatic symptoms, to which neurotic disabilities and distress the patient attributes his inability to carry on the usual ego functions.

During the psychiatric interview the neurotic defenses and the relatively intact adaptive ego functions may enable the borderline patient to present a deceptive, superficially conventional, although neurotic, front, depending on how thoroughgoing and comprehensive the psychiatric investigation is with respect to the patient's *total* ego functioning. The face-to-face psychiatric interview provides a relatively structured situation in which the conventional protective devices of avoidance, evasion, denial, minimization, changing the subject, and other cover-up methods can be used—even by patients who are genuinely seeking help but who dare not yet communicate their awareness of lost affect, reality misinterpretations, autistic preoccupations, and the like.

Several interviews may be necessary to provide the psychiatrist with a sufficiently comprehensive appraisal of the total ego functioning, and to provide the patient with enough sense of security to permit him to verbalize his more disturbing self-observations. In spite of the patient's automatic attempts at concealment, the presence of pathology of psychotic degree will usually manifest itself to the experienced clinician. Occasional blocking, peculiarities of word usage, obliviousness to obvious implications, contaminations of idioms, arbitrary inferences, inappropriate affect, and suspicion-laden behavior and questions are a few possible examples of such unwitting betrayals of ego impairment of psychotic degree.

In regard to such manifestations the appraisal of total ego functioning can be more precise if the psychiatrist takes careful note of the degree of ego-syntonicity associated with them. Momentary halting, signs of embarrassment, and attempts at correction of the peculiarity of expression are evidences of a sufficient degree of ego intactness for such psychotic intrusions to be recognized and repudiated as ego-alien; whereas unnoticed and repeated peculiarities and contaminations provide evidence that the ego has been overwhelmed or pervaded by them and has lost its power to regard them as bizarre. Likewise the expression of suspicions accompanied by embarrassed apologies or joking indicates preservation of the ego's critical function with respect to paranoid mistrust; whereas unqualified suspiciousness indicates the loss of that important ego function. Sometimes this capacity for taking distance from these psychotic productions has to be tested by questions from the psychiatrist which call attention to the production and request comments from the patient about them. Obviously such confrontations should be made sparingly and supportively.

In addition to these microscopic evidences of ego weakness in respect to id eruptions in borderline cases, there are more macroscopic manifestations which may be either frankly stated by the patient or may be implicit in his attitudes and productions. Lack of concern about the realities of his life predicament, usually associated with low voltage wishes for help or grossly inappropriate treatment proposals of his own, is one such macroscopic sign. Others are the fact that the illness developed in the absence of observable precipitating stress, or under the relatively minor stress which was inevitable for the point where this patient was in his life course; the presence of multiple symptoms and disabilities, especially if these are regarded with an acceptance that seems ego-syntonic, or are viewed as being due to malevolent external influence; lack of achievement over a relatively long period, indicating a chronic and severe failure of the ego to channelize energies constructively, especially if this lack of achievement has been accompanied by some degree of disintegration of the ordinary routines of looking after one's self; vagueness or unrealism in planning for the future with respect to education, vocation, marriage, parenthood, and the like; and the relating of bizarre dreams, or evidence of insufficient contrast between dream content and attitudes on the one hand and waking activities and attitudes on the other. All of these macroscopic manifestations will be observable, if they are present, only if the psychiatrist keeps as his frame of reference the patient's total ego functioning, with appropriate allowances for the patient's age, endowment, cultural background, previous level of achievement, and the degree of severity of the recent or current life stresses.

The question of using the free-association interview, with the patient on the couch, frequently comes up with borderline cases. The associative anamnesis has been advocated by Felix Deutsch (1949) and many analysts use free-association interviews either as a limited diagnostic tool or as a more extended trial period of analytic therapy. This technique changes the fairly well-structured situation of the face-to-face psychiatric interview into a relatively unstructured one, so that the patient cannot rely on his usual defensive and conventionally adaptive devices to maintain his front. Borderline patients are then likely to show in bolder relief the various microscopic and macroscopic signs of schizophrenic illness. They may be unable to talk at all and may block completely, with evidence of mounting anxiety; or their verbalizations may show a high degree of autistic content, with many peculiarities of expression; or their inappropriate affect may become more obvious. The diagnosis is aided by the couch–free-association technique, but the experience may be definitely antitherapeutic for the patient. Definitive evidence of psychotic thinking may be produced at the expense of humiliating and disintegrating exposure of the patient's naked pathology. Clinical judgment must be used as to how far the psychiatrist should go in breaking through the defenses in his purpose of reaching an accurate diagnosis.

In the face-to-face psychiatric diagnostic interview the patient is in a fairly well-structured situation and is reacting to the interested listening and active questioning of a visible and supportive physician; in the couch–free-association interview the patient is in a relatively unstructured situation, more or less abandoned to his own fantasies, and relatively unsupported by the shadowy and largely silent listener. Diagnostic psychological tests combine the advantages of support from a visible and interested professional listener, as in the face-to-face psychiatric interview, and the diagnostically significant unstructured situation of the couch–free-association interview.

The various test stimuli are unusual and unconventional, and there are no "correct" answers, so that the patient does not know what he is revealing or concealing. The psychological tests also have one significant advantage over either of the two kinds of diagnostic interview. The tests have been standardized by trials on thousands of cases, so that objective scoring can be done and comparisons can be made of this patient's responses to typical responses of many other patients with all kinds of psychiatric illness, whereas even the experienced psychiatric interviewer must depend on impressions and comparisons of the patient's productions with those of other remembered patients in his particular experience. The psychologist can also determine the patient's capacity to take critical distance from his more pathological responses, and thus assess the degree of ego-alienness or ego-syntonicity of the pathological material, by asking questions which elicit comments from the patient about certain of the unusual responses.

As Rapaport et al. (1945 and 1946), Schafer (1948), and others have pointed out, the interpretation of diagnostic psychological test results is far from being a mere matter of mathematical scoring followed by comparisons with standard tables. There is also required a high degree of clinical acumen, and it is just in the field of the borderline cases that expert interpretation of the test results in essential. The Rorschach is probably the most sensitive test for autistic thinking, and the word association and sorting tests are most valuable for detecting the loosening of associations and disruption of concept formation. The Thematic Apperception Test is less sensitive to schizophrenic pathology but can give a sharply etched picture of the patient's projected image of himself and of the significant people in his life, while describing what the patient feels he and these significant people are doing to each other. The Bellevue-Wechsler intelligence test may, on the other hand, especially in borderline cases, show excellent preservation of intellectual functioning. The relatively clean and orderly responses of the Bellevue-Wechsler do not cancel out the contaminated and disorderly responses of the other tests and thus make the diagnosis doubtful. Instead, the former highlight the preservation of certain ego functions in the face of the impairment of other ego functions revealed by the latter, and thus provide a basis for critical appraisal of ego strengths in relation to threatening eruptions from the id. The Rorschach alone is often given as a test to check on possible schizophrenia, but only a balanced battery of tests can provide the range of responses which will permit accurate appraisal of total ego functioning.

In all of these diagnostic methods, then, the aim should be to take a complete inventory of ego functioning in order to discover the kind of equilibrium which exists between ego controls on the one hand and threatening impulses on the other, and to learn whether the *movement* in this patient is toward less ego control and poorer adaptation. The qualitative appraisal of ego functions is, if anything, even more important than the quantitative estimation of impulse-control balance. Even quite severely neurotic defenses may be capitalized, through therapy, and become reintegrating forces leading to a dynamic shift away, for example, from dereistic thinking to fairly well-organized compulsive striving, with marked improvement in both the defensive and adaptive aspects of ego functioning.

Some final comments are in order regarding the clinical picture in the borderline group of cases before turning to the therapeutic considerations. A useful distinction can be made between internalized or autoplastic illnesses, such as the schizophrenias, depressions, and clinical psychoneuroses, and the externalized or alloplastic illnesses, such as the neurotic and psychotic characters. In the autoplastic conditions, the ego, in various stages of enfeeblement, is attempting to hold out against a barrage of ego-alien impulses and their autistic elaborations; in the alloplastic conditions, or character disorders, the ego itself has been molded and distorted by the gradual infiltration of pathogenic impulses and defenses, and the invasion of id impulses appears much more ego-syntonic. In some respects the alloplastic conditions thus represent greater integration of the ego, but just because of this integrated infiltration of pathogenic impulses into the ego these cases are more difficult to influence therapeutically. On the other hand, the autoplastic conditions may appear more severely ill than the alloplastic ones but the prognosis for therapy may be more favorable. Both the psychiatric interview and the psychological test results can aid in establishing whether the structure of the illness is primarily autoplastic or alloplastic.

Some Therapeutic Considerations

The ego of the borderline patient is a feeble and unreliable ally in therapy. In the incipient schizophrenias the ego is in danger of being overwhelmed by the ego-alien pathogenic forces, and in the psychotic character disorders the ego is already warped by more or less ego-syntonic pervasion by the same pathogenic forces. Yet a few adaptive functions remain, and certain psychoneurotic defense measures may still be in operation, even though the impulse-defense balance is precarious. In an environment which maintains its overtaxing demands on such patients, further regression is likely. If these patients are left to their own devices, in relative isolation, whether at home or in closed hospital, they tend toward further intensification of autistic thinking. Similarly, if they are encouraged to free-associate in the relative isolation of recumbency on the analytic couch, the autistic development is encouraged, and the necessary supportive factor of positive transference to an active, visible, responding therapist is unavailable. Thus even though a trial analysis may bring forth misleading "rich" material, and the analyst can make correspondingly rich formulations and interpretations, the patient's ego often cannot make use of them, and they may only serve the purpose of stimulating further autistic elaborations. Psychoanalysis is, thus, contraindicated for the great majority of borderline cases, at least until after some months of successful analytic psychotherapy.

Psychotherapists can take their cue from the much better front these patients are able to present and maintain in face-to-face psychiatric interviews, where the structured situation and the visible, personal, active therapist per se provides an integrating force to stimulate the patient's surviving adaptive, integrative, and reality-testing capacities. Our therapeutic objective, then, would be the strengthening of the patient's ego controls over instinctual impulses and educating him in the employment of new controls and new adaptive methods, through a kind of psychotherapeutic lend-lease. With our analytic knowledge we can see how he defends himself, and what he defends himself against, but we do not attack those defenses except as we may modify them or educatively introduce better substitutes for them. Our formulations will be in terms of his ego operations rather than of his id content, and will be calculated to improve and strengthen the ego operations.

The psychoneurotic defenses and symptoms especially are not attacked, for just these ego operations protect the patient from further psychotic disorganization. Particularly the obsessive-compulsive defense line is left untouched, except as it can be modified educatively. To return for the moment to the metaphor of the retreating army, our therapy should bypass the outposts of neurotic defenses and symptom formation, and should act as a *rescue force* for the main army of ego functions to the rear, helping to regroup them, restore their morale, and provide leadership for them. Then we might hope to bring them forward to or beyond the neurotic outpost which we by-passed. We may even take our cues for morale building and leadership from the kind of neurotic outpost we observed. If it was primarily obsessive-compulsive we might strive therapeutically for a reintegration based on strengthened compulsive trends. If it was phobic we could attempt to build counterphobic defenses.

Not only do we try to consolidate the more neurotic defenses available, but we also attempt to convert autoplastic (self-crippling) defenses into alloplastic (externally adaptive) ones. This attempt will often require considerably more therapeutic impact than can be provided in an hour a day of modified analytic psychotherapy. Both the motivation and the specific opportunities for alloplastic adaptation can be provided through group dynamics measures—group discussions, group projects, and initiative-stimulating group and individual activities. In a comprehensive attempt at providing such a setting in which to conduct the individual psychotherapy of these borderline cases, we have discovered that many such patients can be carried on a voluntary basis and in an open hospital facility, thus avoiding the encouragement toward isolation, regression, and inertia which closed hospital care sometimes introduces.

Summary

Borderline cases have been discussed in their diagnostic, dynamic, and therapeutic aspects. The term borderline cases is not recommended as a diagnostic term, for a much more precise diagnosis should be made which identifies the type and degree of psychotic pathology. Far more important, however, than arriving at a diagnostic label is the achievement of a comprehensive psychodynamic and psychoeconomic appraisal of the balance in each patient between the ego's defensive and adaptive measures on the one hand, and the pathogenic instinctual and ego-disintegrating forces on the other, so that therapy can be planned and conducted for the purpose of conserving, strengthening, and improving the defensive and adaptive functions of the ego.

The Family Background

Roy R. Grinker, Sr., M.D., Beatrice Werble, Ph.D., and Robert C. Drye, M.D.
(1968)

The Trend Toward Family Studies

Since psychoanalytic theory demonstrated its heuristic value and psychoanalysis or some of its modifications became the American therapeutic method of choice in psychiatry, at least until recently, the focus of interest in etiology has been on deviance from the supposedly healthy path of development according to theoretical time-specific phases. This is the so-called genetic frame of reference. Experiences in early life focused especially on the mother-child relations to the point where some rejecting mothers were called "schizophrenogenic" and "Momism" was a perverted term publicly applied to a maternal attitude of overindulgence.

During the last decade, as a result of the pragmatic appeal for psychiatrists to do more for more people, community psychiatry has become a popular public health concept, group therapy is widely practiced, and focus on the individual is decreasing. In addition on sound theoretical grounds a few pioneers concerned with etiology began to study the families of psychiatric patients (Ackerman, 1958). With some exceptions these began with investigations of families in which one offspring was schizophrenic. According to Wynne and Singer (1963): "These studies have suggested that intrafamilial

communication and relationship patterns can be linked in considerable detail to forms of personality organization, including styles of
thinking, in offsprings who have grown up in these families."

The role of the family in furthering the development of the child
is summarized by Goldfarb (1955) who states that the presence of
family rewards and gratification are the source of the child's social
emotions. Deprivation of sensory and emotional stimuli is the
precursor of psychopathology. To quote a summarizing statement of
Lidz, Fleck and Cornelison (1965):

> Man's biological make-up requires that he grow up in a
> family or a reasonable substitute for it, not simply for
> protection and nurturance during his immaturity but in
> order to assimilate the techniques he needs for adaptation
> and survival. It requires that he grow into and internalize
> the institutions and instrumentalities of structured social
> systems as well as identify with persons who themselves
> have assimilated the culture. He acquires characteristics
> through identification but also by reactions to parental
> objects and through finding reciprocal roles with them.
> His integration is guided, in part, by the dynamic structure
> of the family in which he grows up, which channels his
> drives and guides into proper gender and generation
> roles, and provides a space relatively free from role
> conflict in which the immature child can develop and feel
> secure. His appreciation of the worth and meaning of both
> social roles and institutions is affected by the manner in
> which his parents fill their roles, relate maritally, and
> behave in other institutional contexts.

Theories on Family Pathology

Mischler and Waxler (1966) have recently written an analytic
essay on the theories of family interactional processes and schizophrenia proposed by the three groups headed by Bateson, Lidz and
Wynne. In brief the Bateson group proposes a theory based on
processes of communication, including the famous "double bind."
Bateson states, however, that this is really not a theory but more like
a new language. Lidz deals with content of interactions among
members of the family according to psychoanalytic theory. For
example, the male schizophrenic evolves from a dominant mother
("skewed" pattern) and the female from a seductive father ("schism"
pattern), and the entire family is seen as pathological. Wynne uses

sociological theory viewing the family as a unit whose roles are ambiguously structured under a façade of "pseudo-mutuality" and isolated from the extended social environment by "rubber fence" protective devices. These theories are in agreement that the family structure is a mode of defense, and that the schizophrenic member is a scapegoat whose illness is necessary for the family's stability.

In spite of defects in each of these theories, they focus on the family as a unit implicated in etiology, and are fruitful for the derivation of hypotheses that can be empirically assessed. In his discussion of the review Spiegel (1966) expresses our own views in somewhat different language. He states: "Little progress in theory-building can take place without better articulation of the paradigmatic models among themselves." This we have discussed under the title of Systems in Chapter 10.

The Borderline Family

Few references to the specific characteristics of the borderline family can be found in the literature. Singer and Wynne (1966) state:

Those patients who, in the global, over-all ratings, are classified as borderline schizophrenics have not been clearly psychotically disorganized, but may have a questionable history of a transient psychotic episode, and on examination may show similarities to schizophrenics in their styles of thinking. However, even when they are temporarily quite nebulous or fragmented in their thinking, when one follows these patients in the sequences of their thoughts and actions over a period of time, they are seen to "recover" point and meaning. Their thinking seems disjunctive only when observed in isolated portions of behavior. On over-all view—crucial to adequate evaluation—there is evidenced both to these patients, themselves, and to observers, an underlying connectedness and coherent, meaningful pattern in their thinking and in their lives. Such persons may be highly conflicted, disturbed, and disturbing, but they are not basically schizophrenic.

Singer and Wynne have some evidence:

Suggesting that clear-thinking fathers can reduce the impact of even very disturbing mothers. Sometimes the contribution of the less disturbed parent is not an active one, but rather a passive collusion and acquiescence with the style of the more disturbing parent.

Wolberg (1952), without specifying the number of her cases or the methods she used in her study, states that the borderline comes from a disorganized family. The mother is unable to plan and to conceive a functioning social unit for which she is responsible; or she thinks of her current family according to the culture and society of her own past. As a result the patient has no stable relations to any family member except accidentally to a member of the extended family. He finds the outside culture different and confusing. Wolberg classifies the mothers of the borderline patients as 1) obsessive, 2) narcissistic-masculine, 3) paranoid, and 4) passive-schizoid. Thus they may repudiate femininity, desert family responsibility for a career (the child becomes an obstructive monster), communicate distrust of the hostile world, or just "not be there" but withdrawn from the child into fantasy.

Beck's (1964) studies of the families of his six schizophrenics contrasted careful interviews by psychiatrists and social workers of the parents of sick children against similar interviews with parents of neurotic and healthy children as controls. From the 106 traits which he utilized, four categories each with three modes were used in the analyses. The parental attitudes elicited included rejecting, attacking, coercing, indifference and coldness. The parents of schizophrenic children showed considerable psychopathology with symptoms similar to their children. In general he states that the family as a unit moved a lot, was unstable, and that the father was weak and the mother dominant. Since this was really not a study of the family unit per se such as Wynne and Singer (1963) published, but of the parents, it was not unexpected that the families of neurotic children were not much different. On the other hand, the families of healthy children were not at all similar. These parents were ambitious for their children, often coercing, but they placed great emphasis on achievement which they rewarded.

There are other references to the families of the borderline patient in many individual case reports but they were not systematically studied. There seems to be no doubt that the family of the borderline is unhealthy but how specifically does it differ from the schizophrenic family or any other type is not known. Furthermore, many clinicians think that when they describe the mother or father they are focusing on the family. In truth, the family is a system which should be studied as a unit greater than its component parental parts (Zuk & Nagy, 1967).

The Families of the Research Patients

Our purpose in conducting this limited investigation of the families of our research patients was to describe in some manner their functioning as families, in other words, as a social system. The main question for investigation was, "At what level does the family function as a system over time?" It was our premise that the major functional task of the family—the nuturant care and enculturation or socialization of children—is a time-limited process. The family must maintain its integration through its allotted life-span. When the children are adults they should be ready to distribute themselves into new families, which initiates a process of disintegration of the family of origin.

The question of how the family functions was divided into four parts:

1. How does the family function in relation to the patient's illness and hospitalization as a family crisis?
2. How does the family maintain its integration?
3. How does the family resist the natural process of disintegration?
4. How does the family function in relation to other systems, for example, the community and the larger social system?

A *check list* of 69 family traits was organized in relation to questions 2, 3, and 4, and *narrative statements* were required for question 1. The major source material for completing the check list and the narrative statements was the record of information obtained in the course of usual practice by the social workers assigned to the Nursing Unit on which this study was conducted. A social evaluation of the patient and service to families are prime responsibilities of the ISPI Social Work Department. The department uses a standard format for recording the social evaluation. Included in the outline are: 1) the worker's assessment of the informant, usually a member of the family, which covers how the informant views the patient's problems and hospitalization and his attitude toward the patient and the illness; 2) background information which is basically a descriptive picture of the patient as he developed within his unique social, economic and cultural setting, covering the patient's pertinent experiences within the family and broader environment and the nature of interpersonal relations within the family. Supporting data from the psychiatric resident's summary were also used. We did not use any family data reported only by the patient. The data used were provided by one or more family members. . .

A psychiatric social worker on the staff of the Department of Social Work who had never worked on the unit on which this research was conducted completed the check lists for 47 families of origin of the sample of 51 patients; additionally separate check lists were completed for the few nuclear families of which the patient was a spouse in the sample. The worker had had no contact with the patients in the sample or with any other aspect of the research. Information about the family of origin was not available for four patients (two patients born illegitimately had no families, and two other families lived far from Chicago so that social service had no contact with them). The social worker was trained to use the check list by filling it out for 15 patients who were not in the sample of 51. She and one of the authors (B.W.) independently checked the lists for the 15 patients and compared and discussed the results. For the core sample the check list was filled out only by this one part-time staff worker, who had been trained to use the check list; further, the worker was required to write a brief statement of evidence, a sentence or two for every check representing the presence of a trait. This procedure insured that the factual basis for every check had been given consideration and thought.

Family Functioning in Relation to the Patient's Hospitalization

On entry into the hospital, more than half (27) of the patients (single, never married) had been living with their families of origin. Both parents were present in the majority of these homes; however, some patients (11) did come from homes where one parent, usually the father, was absent. Thirteen patients entered the hospital from intact nuclear families (either a husband or a wife was the patient), and a few patients came from broken nuclear-family homes. The remainder, including several separated or divorced and several single, never married, were living independently in the community. The heads of families were primarily in occupations classified as clerical, craftsman, operative and service, and a few were receiving public assistance.

The family's functioning in relation to the patient's illness and hospitalization was described by three variables: 1) the family's involvement on behalf of the patient, for example, keeping appointments, providing patient with needed articles such as clothes, and planning for discharge; 2) the family's attitude toward hospitalization; 3) the relevance of the patient's illness to the family.

Since these questions were not precategorized but answered narratively, all of the categories being reported were derived from the data itself. Although family involvement on behalf of the patient ranged from minimal or none to intense, most frequently some member of the family, usually the mother and/or spouse, cooperated with the social worker on behalf of the patient.

Table 1
Family Cooperation on Behalf of the Patient

	Total 47	Per Cent 100.0
1. Minimal or no family involvement	15	31.9
2. Family cooperated on behalf of patient	20	42.6
3. Family member cooperated on behalf of self	2	4.2
4. Family involved	10	21.3

The attitude of the family toward the patient's hospitalization was rarely indifferent. The family responded in one of five ways (see Table 2). There is a qualitative difference between categories 4 and 5—category 4 implies acceptance of the fact of illness and hospitalization without much understanding of the illness and the need for hospital care.

Table 2
Attitudes of the Family toward the Patient's Hospitalization

	Total 47	Per Cent 100.0
1. Family indifferent	2	4.2
2. Denial of illness and need for care	12	25.5
3. Discomfort or anger	9	19.1
4. Acceptance of the fact without understanding of the need	7	14.9
5. Perceived patient behavior and need	17	36.3

Half the families tended not to connect the patient's illness to any factor. Some attributed the illness to a variety of people or forces other than themselves; a few attributed the illness to their behavior; usually this kind of attribution was made by mothers who blamed their own past behaviors or child-rearing practices.

Table 3
Family Theory of Etiology

	Total 47	Per Cent 100.0
1. No connection made between illness or any factor	23	49.0
2. Attribution to people other than self or external forces	15	31.9
3. Some connection between patient's illness and self	9	19.1

The question of how the family functioned in relation to the patient's illness and hospitalization can be described only for the group as a whole, since none of the three measurements of the family's functioning in relation to the patient's hospitalization were associated with the patient groups. All of the categories were found scattered among all the patient groups.

On the whole, these families displayed a range of functioning in relation to the patient's illness. It would be unwise to infer levels of family pathology from these descriptive categories since there is no single desirable standard of family functioning in relation to the mental illness of the family member, except that some family involvement and access to family are generally considered desirable.

Family Types

The original check list of 69 traits minus a list of 29 was used to cluster the data for 47 families of origin. Traits were deleted for reason of infrequency of occurrence (five or fewer) in the group as a whole. On this basis all traits dealing with the question of how the family functions in relation to other social systems were discarded.

The 40 remaining traits were analyzed by a clustering program designed to handle dichotomous data developed at the New York Scientific Center of IBM by Jerrold Rubin (1965, Chapter 5). The criterion function which is used to measure the structure of a grouping of the data is based on a similarity coefficient, which is a measure of the number of matches between two subjects on the traits under study. The presence of a trait for both of a given pair of subjects is a match, and the absence of a trait for the same two subjects is also a match. Hence both the presence and absence of traits enter into the measure of structure.

The 40 traits resulted in six family clusters (families of origin) present among the four patient groups as shown in Table 4.

Table 4
Family Type and Patient Group

Family Type			Patient Group				
			I	II	III	IV	Total
		Total	17	10	13	7	47
I			4	6	9	—	19
II			3	—	3	—	6
III			6	—	—	3	9
IV	Residue		3	2	—	2	7
V	Residue		—	1	1	2	4
VI	Residue		1	1	—	—	2

Type I families were found more frequently among Group II and III patients than among Group I and IV patients. There is no one kind of family associated with one kind of patient group. Family types I, II and III are different from each other and from the 47 families as a whole.

Clusters IV, V and VI should be considered residues. The small clusters V and VI separated out as misfits with any of the others. Cluster IV was unique in that it was primarily formed by the nonoccurrence of the traits under study. This cluster of families matched each other, with one exception, on the absence of the traits studied. The one exception was the presence of overdevotion on the part of the father. This result is of interest since the patients whose families were in this cluster were females (5 of 7).

Family Type I—19 Members

This group of families clustered on the presence of a set of traits which describe the pathological way the family maintained its integration. The occurrence of the traits shown in Table 5 was more frequent among this group of 19 families than among the remainder of the sample.

Here and for the remainder of the discussion of family types the chi-square is presented to give the reader an index to the difference in the proportion of the trait present in the specific family type compared with the proportion of the trait present in the remainder of the sample. For example, the proportion of trait 9, "Family is not a mutually protective unit," present for type I was 19/19 compared

Table 5
Family Type I

Trait		Type I N = 19	Frequencies Total N = 47	Chi-square*
1	Marriage is highly discordant	18	30	11.04
7	Family relationships marked by chronic overt conflict or competition	17	28	9.85
9	Family is not a mutually protective unit	19	25	24.24
15	Outright rejection of parenthood or excessive conflict over parenthood	16	27	7.60
25	Mother-child relationships are problematic	15	28	3.71
37	Quality of mother's affect was predominantly negative	7	7	9.39
47	In general, communication may be characterized as confused	12	19	5.35

* Adjusted by Yates' correction.

with 6/28 for the remainder of the sample. The *P* values usually associated with the chi-square test of significance are not shown, since to show them would be misleading. The *P* values usually associated with the chi-square assumes under the null hypothesis that the groups were random samples from the same population. The groups produced by the clustering procedure were not selected at random but according to a criterion that maximized the difference between them (Chapter 5).

As trait 9, "Family is not a mutually protective unit," was present for all 19 families of this type, it serves as an anchor point of description of type I families in contrast with the other family types. The other traits on which family type I clustered are consistent with trait 9 as the anchor point: discord, conflict, role rejection and confusion. The nonoccurrence of traits also contributes to clustering; type I families also matched on the absence of traits that describe any resistance to the process of family disintegration which, we will now see, characterized type II families.

Family Type II—6 Members

This group of families clustered on the presence of a set of traits that describe how the families resist the natural process of disintegration, a polar opposite kind of pathology from type I families. Trait 10, "Family is excessively protective," was present for all six members of family type II, in contrast to the anchor trait for family type I. The remainder of the traits for family type II consistently describe the smothering, suffocating static family. The occurrence of the traits shown in Table 6 was more frequent among this group of six families than among the remainder of the sample, and they were not found at all in type I.

Table 6
Family Type II

Trait		Type II N = 6	Frequencies Total N = 47	Chi-square*
5	Parents and/or spouses are deficient in achieving reciprocal role relationships	5	16	5.14
10	Family is excessively protective	6	17	9.18
39	The quality of the mother's affect was overdevotion	6	14	12.59
45	Contact among family members is excessive and intrusive, very involved	6	24	4.54
50	The family has not set eventual separation of parent and child as a goal	6	13	14.08
52	Static state of the family is due to self-interest of one of the parents	6	16	10.17
54	Static state of the family is due to overinvolvement with children	6	17	9.18
57	Self-identity of children has been submerged by the family	6	14	12.59

* Adjusted by Yates' correction.

All six of the patients whose families are described by family type II were unattached males. We found in follow-up that none of the six were ever married, a testimonial to the resistance of the families to disintegration.

Type III—9 Members

Type III families are described by a few traits that occur more frequently for them as a group than for any others. The anchor point of contrast with types I and II is trait 8, "Family life marked by denial

Table 7
Family Type III

Trait		Type III N = 9	Frequencies Total N = 47	Chi-square*
8	Family life marked by denial of problems	6	9	12.66
35	The quality of the mother's affect was mixed	7	18	5.42
36	The quality of the father's affect was mixed	7	20	4.01
57	Self-identity of children has been submerged by the family	6	14	5.22

* Adjusted by Yates' correction.

of problems." These families are also characterized by the absence of discordant marriages and the dominance of extremes of parental affect; there were no checks for either parent of overdevotion or predominantly negative affect. The absence of these traits is consistent with the denial of problems and the presence of mixed affect, defined as the existence of both positive and negative affect with neither one nor the other being dominant.

In conclusion, it is possible to say that our sample of borderline patients came from three varying types of pathological families, differentiated from each other but unassociated significantly with the four patient groups.

Nuclear Families

Data were available for 20 nuclear families, 16 of whom had children. Traits are presented in Table 8 for the 16 families that had children of their own. Over one-half of the patients from the 16 nuclear families came from type I families of origin. None came from type II families of origin, since none of the patients from type II families of origin were ever a party to a nuclear family. It thus comes as no surprise that the traits in Table 8 more closely resemble the profile of type I families, marked by the trait, "Family is not a mutually protective unit." The nuclear families were predominantly marked by discord and conflict, the hallmarks of type I families.

It can be seen clearly that, in addition to the fact that more than half of our patients on admission had never married, 16 of the remaining patients who had married and had had children experi-

Table 8
Sixteen Nuclear Families with Children

Trait		Number
1	Marriage is highly discordant	14
7	Family relationships marked by chronic overt conflict or competition	13
15	Outright rejection of parenthood or excessive conflict over parenthood; family does not provide adequate nurturant care for children	12
37	The quality of the wife's and/or mother's affect and emotionality in this family may be characterized as predominantly negative	12
3	Partners unable to achieve a mutuality of purpose in major areas of living; conflicting demands remain unresolved	10
9	Family is not a mutually protective unit	10
38	The quality of the husband's and/or father's affect and emotionality in this family may be characterized as predominantly negative	10
2	Partners engage in mutual devaluation and criticism	8
5	Partners and/or spouses are deficient in achieving reciprocal role relationships	5

enced great difficulty in achieving a satisfactory union. Even more important than the discordant marriage and the overt conflict between spouses was the negative attitude toward children when they existed. In other words, the borderline marries infrequently and when he does he is an inadequate spouse and a poor parent.

Discussion

It is apparent that the family's functioning in relation to the patient's hospitalization (question 1) was not specific for the borderline or, for that matter, any mental or physical illness. The family was sometimes involved and sometimes not. The highest per cent cooperated on behalf of the patient. Some denied the patient's illness and need for care; others perceived the patient's needs. Few families connected the patient's illness with the behavior of a member of the family; most made no connection between the illness and any internal factor and attributed the fault to others or external forces.

Forty of the available traits were utilized to discriminate family types which were then arranged in frequency of appearance in the four patient groups described in Chapter 6. Family type I occurred most frequently in patient Groups II and III. The traits of family type I indicate that the family is not an integrated protective unit; overt conflict and discord were present, the mother's affect was negative and there was outright rejection of the children. The patient Groups II and III were respectively the "core borderline" and the "adaptive, defensive" patients. The two groups stemming from this family type are sufficiently differentiated from each other so that the family type cannot predict the type of borderline patient, just as the family's functioning is not specific for the borderline altogether.

Nevertheless the family types I, II and III are clearly differentiated. Type II is static (resistive to healthy abandonment of control), dominant and generally intrusive. Although patients stemming from this type did not belong to a specific patient group, all were males and never married. Clearly they preferred to remain attached to their family of origin probably held by the family's domination and intrusiveness.

Family type III was characterized by denial and mixed parental affects. The patients from this type were in greatest number among Group I, the sickest and closest to psychotic.

It must be emphasized that the study of the family was an afterthought, not included in our original design. We neither interviewed the family directly nor observed the family interaction with the patient. Therefore we were dependent on data derived from routine psychiatric social workers' observations. The data available were adequately rated and statistically analyzed. Significant differences isolated three family groups, but none was specific for a patient group nor were the family functions and attitudes specific for the syndrome. We cannot, therefore, utilize family data from which to draw etiological conclusions except to state that all the families were "sick," which is no surprise in view of the sickness in at least one of its progeny. Furthermore, as spouses and parents in their own nuclear families, the patients carried on the deviant behavior.

As Fleck (1966) has stated, we would wish to relate specific family constellations to specific psychiatric entities—in this case the borderline—but this is not possible with our present concepts and methods applicable to family functions. If as Birdwhistell (1966) states, culture communicates information and devices for coding messages around a central theme, direction and order, then we as yet do not know the code.

Differential Diagnosis
and Treatment

Otto F. Kernberg, M.D.
(1975)

A Critical Review of Recent Literature

Diagnosis

A review of the literature on the diagnosis and treatment of borderline conditions is to be found elsewhere (Chapters 1 and 3). I will limit myself here to reviewing more recent contributions to these issues.

Regarding the diagnosis of borderline conditions, Grinker et al.'s book, *The Borderline Syndrome* (1968), constitutes a major contribution to the delimitation of this clinical entity. Grinker et al. define the overall characteristics of the borderline syndrome as including "anger as the main or only affect, defect in affectional relationships, absence of indication of self-identity, and depressive loneliness" (p. 176). They define four subgroups within this clinical constellation: Group I—"The psychotic border," characterized by inappropriate and negativistic behavior and affects toward other patients and hospital staff; Group II—"The core borderline syndrome," characterized by negativistic and chaotic feelings and behavior, contradictory behavior and a strong acting out potential; Group III—"The adaptive, affectless defended, 'as if' person," characterized by bland adaptiveness with an "as if" quality, with superficially adaptive but affectively deficient interactions; and Group IV—"The border with the neuroses," which presents childlike clinging depression.

Grinker et al. conclude that, in general, and in contrast to schizophrenia, the borderline syndrome does not present disturbances in intellectual associational processes, nor autistic or regressive thinking, nor a characteristic family structure with "pseudo-mutuality" or "skewing," nor delusions or hallucinations, nor any deficit in the connotative aspects of language (p. 93). In comparing the borderline syndrome to the neuroses, Grinker et al. state that "although depression as an affect is found in several of the borderline categories, it does not correspond with that seen in the depressive syndrome. The borderline depression is a feeling of loneliness and isolation" (p. 95).

Grinker et al.'s efforts to differentiate the borderline syndrome from other personality or character disorders seems less satisfactory. They point (accurately, it seems to me) to the tendency on the part of some authors to use various characterological labels for what are essentially borderline patients, and imply that a better definition of the borderline syndrome will help clarify the vague field of diagnosis of character pathology. It may well be that because the research design of Grinker and his co-workers focused particularly on overt behavior and interaction of borderline patients within a hospital setting, the underlying structural characteristics of these patients which differentiate borderline personality organization from less severe types of character pathology were not fully explored in this study. In spite of this limitation, I think that Grinker et al.'s study is a most important research contribution to the delimitation of the borderline syndrome. Werble (1970) reported a follow-up study of the patients of Grinker et al.'s experimental population. He concluded that over a five-year period after the completion of the original study, there had been little individual change in the social functioning of these patients; they were able to adapt themselves within narrowly constricted limits, with very few human object relations in their lives, and (very importantly) these former patients did not present evidence of schizophrenia at the follow-up time.

Several authors have contributed to the clinical analysis of borderline conditions. Collum (1972), combining the viewpoints of Grinker et al. and those suggested in my papers on this subject, focuses upon the central nature of identity diffusion as characteristic of borderline patients. Cary (1972) develops further the structural-dynamic analysis of borderline conditions, stressing the following characteristics: "Depression" within the borderline syndrome is characterized by a sense of futility and pervasive feeling of loneliness and isolation—a feeling of isolation and angry demandingness rather than neurotic and psychotic depression which would be characterized by feelings of guilt and self-derogation. He also stresses schizoid detachment as a major defense of borderline patients. I think that both Grinker et al. and Cary's analysis point to the predominantly early ego organization of borderline patients within which self and object images have not become integrated (and, therefore, where a state of "total" object relationships has not been reached). This primitive ego organization explains the primitive nature of depressive reactions of borderline patients, their lack of capacity for fully experiencing concern and their pervasive experience of emptiness (Chapter 7).

Bergeret (1970, 1972) has examined the structural and dynamic characteristics of borderline states from a psychoanalytic viewpoint. After reviewing both the Anglo-Saxon and recent French psychoanalytic literature, and examining clinical case material, he concludes that borderline conditions are characterized by a predominance of pregenital conflicts and a predominance of primitive structural and defensive characteristics of the ego and superego. He stresses that borderline conditions are characterized by the ego's immaturity of object relations and constitute a psychopathological category different from both neurotic structures and psychotic structures. Duvocelle (1971) integrates Bergeret's and my viewpoints into an overall clinical and theoretical overview of borderline personality organization.

Mahler (1971) has recently proposed that, during the rapprochement subphase of the separation-individuation process, children whose normal resolution of the rapprochement crisis fails may develop a "bad" introject, which becomes infiltrated with the derivatives of aggressive drive and may evolve into a more or less permanent split of the object world into "good" and "bad" objects. She states (p. 413), "These mechanisms, coercion and splitting of the object world, are characteristic in most cases of borderline transference." This pathological development is in contrast to the normal consequences of the resolution of the rapprochement subphase in the form of normal identity formation in the third year of life.

While all of the authors mentioned for the most part agree on the overall descriptive and perhaps even dynamic-structural characteristics of borderline conditions, the differential diagnosis of borderline conditions from other types of character pathology on the one hand, and from psychotic, particularly schizophrenic reactions on the other, has not been explored extensively in the recent literature. One paper (Weisfogel et al., 1969) reviews the literature on the differential diagnosis of borderline conditions and concludes that "those authors who classified these patients as psychotic presented the most cogent conceptualizations and data, and it appears that these patients should best be considered as psychotic" (p. 34). This paper represents a thoughtful review of the literature, but, on the basis of the evidence reviewed, I cannot agree with the conclusion.

Kohut (1971) has commented on the differentiation of borderline structures from narcissistic personalities, and I deal with the complex interrelationships between borderline condition and narcissistic personalities in Chapter 9. In more general terms, I attempted an overall classification of character pathology which includes borderline conditions as the most severely regressed level of character disorders (1970).

Bellak and Hurvich (1969) and Hurvich (1970) have recently explored the assessment of ego functions as a major dimension in the differential diagnosis of schizophrenic from nonschizophrenic conditions. The function of reality testing—a crucial variable in the differential diagnosis of borderline from psychotic conditions (Frosch, 1964; Chapter 1)—has been comprehensively reviewed by Hurvich (1970). Later in this chapter I will explore the utilization of reality testing in the differential diagnosis of borderline from psychotic conditions.

In addition to the English and French reviews of the borderline constellation, some Spanish reviews have also been published (Meza, 1970; Paz, 1969). A good overall review of the literature on borderline conditions can be found in Arlene R. Wolberg's recent book (1973).

Treatment

There has been an increase of papers in the psychiatric and particularly psychoanalytic literature of recent years dealing with treatment of borderline conditions. As before, opinions are divided on whether borderline patients should be treated supportively, or with an expressive, psychoanalytic approach, or with nonmodified psychoanalysis. There has been a gradual shift away from the recommendation that these patients should be treated with supportive psychotherapy, and only Zetzel (1971) has recommended "regular but limited contact (very seldom more than once a week)" in order to decrease the intensity of transference and countertransference manifestations, and a stress on reality issues and structuralization of the treatment hours, all of which constitute jointly an essentially supportive approach. Zetzel acknowledged that (with her approach) "for many borderline patients, however, it may be necessary for the therapist to remain at least potentially available over an indefinitely extended period." The implication is that this supportive approach, while effective in permitting the patient to adjust better to reality, may contribute to an interminable psychotherapeutic relationship.

Various authors have recommended a modified psychoanalytic procedure or expressive psychotherapeutic approach commensurate with what I proposed in Chapter 3. Frosch (1970) has spelled out the clinical approach to borderline patients within a modified psychoanalytic procedure, and, more recently (1971), summarized his overall strategy of treatment with these patients. Greenson (1970) proposes a similar approach, illustrating his modified psychoanalytic technique with clinical cases. Both Frosch and Greenson stress the importance of clarifying the patient's perceptions in the hours, and his attitude toward the therapist's interventions. Their approach (with which I basically agree) implies a basically neutral technical position of the the therapist, and only a minimum deviation from such a position of neutrality as might be necessary. In contrast, other psychoanalytically derived psychotherapeutic approaches to borderline conditions involve more modifications of technique.

Thus, Masterson (1972) suggests that "the borderline syndrome is a result of the feelings of abandonment which are in turn created by the mother's withdrawal of supplies when the patient attempts to separate and individuate. The patient's need to defend himself against his feelings of abandonment produces the developmental arrest and the clinical picture" (p. 35). On this basis, he designs a special psychotherapy as specifically geared to "the resolution of the acute symptomatic crisis (the abandonment depression) and the correction and repair of the ego defects that accompany the narcissistic oral fixation by encouraging growth through the stages of separation-individuation to autonomy." It seems to me that his approach does not consider sufficiently the differences between conflicts around and defenses against symbiotic fusion (related to pathological refusion of self and object images) and conflicts related to structural conditions centering around splitting (related to the incapacity to integrate aggressively determined and libidinally determined self and object images). His approach also neglects the importance of conflicts around pregenital aggression in the etiology of borderline personality organization. In addition, one finds various characterological structures at the level of borderline personality organization, and the individual treatment technique should take into account these and other more individually determined genetic-dynamic characteristics.

Arlene R. Wolberg (1973) suggests that early interpretation of the hostile transference may gratify the masochism of borderline patients rather than be helpful in the working through of the transference. She proposes that conflicts around hostility be interpreted indirectly "by projective therapeutic techniques" which focus on the expression of these conflicts onto other objects. She states that "a projective therapeutic technique allows the relation with the here and now to be handled through the use of the 'other person' emphasizing the defensive aspects of the transference behavior of the 'other' and letting the patient avoid the personal confrontation with the analyst until he is able to tolerate the anxiety he feels in the interpersonal relationship, without resorting to massive defense. The aim of treatment is to help the patient let up on the creation of defenses rather than to force him by premature confrontation to increase his defenses." I disagree with this approach, and would stress instead that the direct but noncritical focus upon both positive and negative transference aspects is most effective in helping the patient reduce his own fears over his aggression. However, many other aspects of Wolberg's technical approach to the treatment of borderline conditions are related to the approach taken by other authors who apply a modified psychoanalytic procedure. The same is true, it seems to me, with the psychotherapeutic approach for borderline conditions recommended by Chessick (1971).

Masterson (1972) has pointed out the need for hospitalization of some borderline adolescent patients, and suggests specific designs of the milieu to deal with their defenses and conflicts (pp. 105–109). Adler (1973) has succinctly described the basic structure required for borderline patients hospitalized in short-term treatment units. He stresses the danger of permitting unchallenged regression to occur to such an extent that the acting out of conflicts within the hospital setting perpetuates the patient's gratification of pathological needs, and the danger of excessive limit setting that obscures the patient's psychopathology. The area of long-term inpatient treatment for some borderline patients who cannot be treated on an outpatient or short inpatient basis seems to me still largely unexplored in the literature.

Boyer and Giovacchini (1967) recommend a nonmodified psychoanalytic approach to schizophrenic and characterological disorders. They state that the broadening of technical understanding and technique in recent years has made it possible to deal analytically with those severely regressed patients who are able to enter a regular, purely outpatient treatment setting. Although Giovacchini, in chapters dedicated to character disorders, does not refer specifically to borderline conditions (in contrast to severe character pathology in general), his observations focus upon the technical problems posed by what I would consider patients with borderline personality organization. He acknowledges that some patients "may act out with such violence that the analytic decorum is disrupted and analysis cannot proceed" (p. 258). In practice, Giovacchini would set limits to the patient's acting out in the hours, and utilize parameters of technique which he would attempt to resolve through interpretation later. He recommends, for some cases, temporary discontinuation of treatment (p. 261). He acknowledges "that there are some patients who need someone to manage some facet of their chaotic situation to effect sufficient stabilization so therapy can proceed. Whether this can be done by the analyst while preserving the necessary conditions for therapy . . . is still an unsettled question" (p. 286).

Boyer (1971) stresses the importance of interpreting early in the analytic treatment of patients with severe characterological and schizophrenic illness the aggressive drive derivatives, and reiterates his earlier thinking that an essentially nonmodified psychoanalytic technique can be maintained with these patients. Paz (1969) also stresses the possibility of maintaining an essentially unmodified psychoanalytic approach with borderline conditions, and a similar approach is implied in Khan's (1964, 1969) papers on specific defensive operations in borderline schizoid patients.

On the basis of the final outcome study of the quantitative data of the Psychotherapy Research Project of The Menninger Foundation (Kernberg et al., 1972), I feel strengthened in my conviction that the majority of borderline patients require a modified analytic approach while a minority may be suitable for a standard psychoanalytic procedure. In what follows, I will first briefly summarize my earlier work on the psychopathology, diagnosis, and treatment of borderline personality organization, and then present some further clinical contributions regarding the vicissitudes of the transference in these cases, the long-range treatment strategy, and the differential diagnosis with schizophrenia.

Summary of Previous Work

The two terms most frequently used to designate structural alterations of a patient's ego which raise the question of limits of effectiveness of psychoanalysis are "ego distortion" and "ego weakness." For all practical purposes, these two terms are applied to the same type of patients; ego distortion focuses on the highly pathological, rigid character patterns these patients present, while the term ego weakness focuses upon these patients' inadequacy or lack of certain normal ego functions. From a research viewpoint, the term ego weakness is preferable because of its quantitative implications; indeed, this term was utilized in the Psychotherapy Research Project of The Menninger Foundation to evaluate the relationship between structural alterations and inadequacy of ego functions on the one hand, and the effectiveness of psychoanalysis and psychoanalytic psychotherapy on the other (Kernberg et al., 1972). My work on diagnosis, prognosis and treatment of borderline conditions stems from that project.

In this chapter, I use the term ego weakness to refer to structural alterations of the ego derived from early ego disturbances, and will examine briefly, 1) the clinical manifestations of ego weakness which is typical for borderline personality organization, 2) some hypotheses regarding the origin of ego weakness, 3) complications arising from efforts to analyze patients with ego weakness and some technical implications for the treatment of these patients, and 4) some conditions improving or worsening analyzability in these cases. I will introduce at several points new material to the respective analyses developed in earlier chapters, emphasizing the diagnostic and therapeutic features of borderline personality organization. Finally, I will summarize some clinical and theoretical implications of transference psychosis and clarify further the differential diagnosis with schizophrenia.

The Clinical Manifestations of Borderline Personality Organization

Clinically, when we speak of patients with borderline personality organization, we refer to patients who present serious difficulties in their interpersonal relationships and some alteration of their experience of reality but with essential preservation of reality testing (Chapter 1). Such patients also present contradictory character traits, chaotic coexistence of defenses against and direct expression of primitive "id contents" in consciousness, a kind of pseudo-insight into their personality without real concern for nor awareness of the conflictual nature of this material, and a lack of clear identity and lack of understanding in depth of other people. These patients present primitive defensive operations rather than repression and related defenses, and above all, mutual dissociation of contradictory ego states reflecting what might be called a "nonmetabolized" persistence of early, pathological internalized object relationships. They also show "nonspecific" manifestations of ego weakness. The term "nonspecific" refers to lack of impulse control, lack of anxiety tolerance, lack of sublimatory capacity, and presence of primary process thinking, and indicates that these manifestations of ego weakness represent a general inadequacy of normal ego functions. In contrast, the primitive defensive constellation of these patients and their contradictory, pathological character traits are "specific" manifestations of ego weakness. In short, they represent highly individualized, active compromise formations of impulse and defense.

Hypotheses Regarding the Origin of Ego Weakness

Two essential tasks that the early ego has to accomplish in rapid succession are: 1) the differentiation of self-images from object-images, and 2) integrating libidinally determined and aggressively determined self- and object-images.

The first task is accomplished in part under the influence of the development of the apparatuses of primary autonomy: perception and memory traces help to sort out the origin of stimuli and gradually differentiate self- from object-images. This first task fails to a major extent in the psychoses, in which a pathological fusion between self- and object-images determines a failure in the differentiation of ego boundaries and, therefore, in the differentiation of self from nonself. In contrast, in the case of borderline personality organization, differentiation of self- from object-images has occurred to a sufficient degree to permit the establishment of integrated ego boundaries and a concomitant differentiation between self and others.

The second task, however, of integrating self- and object-images built up under the influence of libidinal drive derivatives and their related affects with their corresponding self- and object-images built up under the influence of aggressive drive derivatives and related affects, fails to a great extent in borderline patients, mainly because of the pathological predominance of pregenital aggression. The resulting lack of synthesis of contradictory self- and object-images interferes with the integration of the self-concept and with the establishment of object-constancy or "total" object relationships. I will now examine these hypotheses in more detail.

Good enough mothering implies that mother evokes, stimulates and complements ego functions which are not yet available to the infant. For example, mother's intuitive handling of the baby permits the early detection of sources of pain, fear, and frustration, in addition to providing an optimum of gratifying, pleasurable experiences while satisfying the baby's basic needs. Intrapsychically, this means that a core experience of satisfaction and pleasure is set up in the baby, powerfully reinforced by the pleasurable affects thus released and gradually also by the proprioceptive and exteroceptive perceptions linked with such experiences. Out of this core will come the basic, fused self-mother image which in turn determines basic trust. Basic trust involves recognition, and, later, anticipation of a pleasurable mother-child relationship. The basic ego disturbance is the failure to build up a sufficiently strong fused "all good" self-object image or "good internal object."

The libidinally determined good self-object image permits some attentuation or neutralization of the anxiety producing and disorganizing effects of excessive frustration, with which "bad," fused self-object images are set up. The normal relationship with mother reinforces, as well as depends upon, the buildup of this good internal fused self-object image.

Severe frustrations and the consequent predominance of aggressively-determined, "all bad" fused self-object images may interfere with the next stage of development, namely the gradual sorting out of self from object components in the realm of the good self-object image. As Jacobson (1954) points out, defensive refusion of primitive, all good self- and object-images as a protection against excessive frustration and rage is the prototype of what constitutes, if prolonged beyond the early infantile stages of development, a psychotic identification.

If and when self-images have been differentiated from object-images in the area of libidinally determined ego nuclei and, later, in the area of aggressively-determined ego nuclei, a crucial step has been taken which differentiates future psychotic from nonpsychotic ego structures. The next step is the gradual integration of contradictory (that is, libidinally determined and aggressively determined) self-images, with the crystallization of a central self surrounded, we might say, by object-images which in turn become integrated (in the sense that good and bad object representations related to the same external objects are integrated). This is also the point where tolerance of ambivalence begins to develop. When such integration is achieved, an integrated self-image or self-concept relates to integrated object-images and there is also a continuous reshaping and reconfirmation of both self-concept and object-images by means of mechanisms of projection and introjection linked with actual interpersonal relationships with mother and other human beings surrounding the child.

The integrated self-concept and the related integrated representation of objects constitutes ego identity in its broadest sense. A stable ego identity, in turn, becomes a crucial determinant of stability, integration, and flexibility of the ego, and also influences the full development of higher level superego functions (abstraction, depersonification, and individualization of the superego).

Failure to integrate the libidinally determined and the aggressively determined self- and object-images is the major cause for nonpsychotic ego disturbances which, in turn, determine limits in analyzability. Such lack of integration derives from pathological predominance of aggressively determined self- and object-images and a related lack of establishment of a sufficiently strong ego core around the originally fused good self-object image. However, in contrast to conditions in which self-images have not been differentiated from object-images (the psychoses), there has been at least sufficient differentiation between self- and object-images for the establishment of firm ego boundaries in cases of ego distortion which are generally designated as borderline conditions. The problem at this point is that the intensity of aggressively determined self- and object-images, and of defensively idealized all good self- and object-images, makes integration impossible. Bringing together extremely opposite loving and hateful images of the self and of significant others would trigger unbearable anxiety and guilt because of the implicit danger to the good internal and external object relations; therefore, there is an active defensive separation of such contradictory self- and object-images; in other words, primitive dissociation or splitting becomes a major defensive operation.

Lack of integration of self- and object-representations is at first a normal characteristic of early development; but, later, such lack of integration is used actively to separate contradictory ego states. Splitting refers to the active, defensive separation of contradictory ego states. Primitive defensive operations linked to splitting (denial, primitive idealization, omnipotence, projection and projective identification) powerfully reinforce splitting, and protect the ego from unbearable conflicts between love and hatred by sacrificing its growing integration. Clinically, the child who is going to become a borderline patient lives from moment to moment, actively cutting off the emotional links between what would otherwise become chaotic, contradictory, highly frustrating and frightening emotional experiences with significant others in his immediate environment.

There are several significant structural consequences of these primitive defensive operations set up to protect the ego against unbearable conflict and the related pathology of internalized object relationships. First, an integrated self-concept cannot develop, and chronic overdependence on external objects occurs in an effort to achieve some continuity in action, thought, and feeling in relating to them. Lack of integration of the self-concept determines the syndrome of identity-diffusion. Second, contradictory character traits develop, representing the contradictory self- and object-images, further creating chaos in the interpersonal relationship of the future borderline patient. Third, superego integration suffers because the guiding function of an integrated ego identity is missing; contradictions between exaggerated, all good ideal object-images and extremely sadistic, all bad superego forerunners interfere with superego integration. Therefore, the superego functions which would further facilitate ego integration also are missing and this reinforces the pathological consequences of excessive reprojection of superego nuclei in the form of paranoid trends. Fourth, a lack of integrated object-representations interferes with deepening of empathy with others as individuals in their own right; lack of integration of the self-concept further interferes with full emotional understanding of other human beings; the end result is defective object-constancy or incapacity to establish total object relationships. Fifth, nonspecific aspects of ego strength (anxiety tolerance, impulse control, sublimatory potential) suffer because of the weakness of ego and superego integration. Ego strength depends on the neutralization of instinctual energy; such neutralization takes place essentially in the integration of libidinally and aggressively derived self- and object-images.

Complications in Analyzing Patients with Borderline Personality Organization, and Technical Implications for Their Treatment

In patients with ego weakness, primitive, early conflicts are not repressed; conscious mutual dissociation among contradictory primitive contents replaces repression and the normal "resistance versus content" organization of defenses and impulses. Consciousness of primitive material does not reflect insight but the predominance of splitting mechanisms—a different set of defensive constellations from those centering around repression seen in neurotic patients.

Also, deficit in nonspecific manifestations of ego strength interferes with the necessary tolerance of increased conflict awareness during treatment, and provokes excessive acting-out tendencies.

In addition, lack of differentiation of the self-concept and the lack of differentiation and individualization of objects interfere with the differentiation of present from past object relationships. Transference and reality are confused; also, the analyst is not differentiated from the transference object because of the prevalence of primitive projection. Furthermore, the lack of capacity for seeing the analyst as an integrated object in his own right, and the pathologically increased, alternating projection of self- and object-images (so that reciprocal roles are easily interchanged in the transference), weakens ego boundaries in the transference and promotes transference psychosis.

Finally, the therapeutic relationship easily replaces ordinary life, because its gratifying and sheltered nature further intensifies the temptation to gratify primitive pathological needs in the transference and acting out.

This summary reflects the typical structure of borderline personality organization and the typical treatment difficulties these patients present. Although some authors believe that a standard psychoanalysis can and should be carried out under these conditions, others, including myself, question this. However, the treatment I suggest as ideally suited for these patients is a psychoanalytically derived procedure which strongly emphasizes the interpretation of resistances and of the transference and the adherence to an essentially neutral position of the analyst.

I have suggested the following technical requirements for the psychoanalytic psychotherapy of borderline patients (Chapter 3): 1) systematic elaboration of the negative transference in the "here and now" only, without attempting to achieve full genetic reconstructions; 2) interpretation of the defensive constellations of these patients as they enter the negative transference; 3) limit-setting in order to block acting out of the transference, with as much structuring of the patient's life outside the hours as necessary to protect the neutrality of the analyst; 4) noninterpretation of the less primitively determined, modulated aspects of the positive transference to foster the gradual development of the therapeutic alliance.

Some Conditions Under Which Analyzability Improves or Worsens

Improvement or worsening of the prognosis for psychoanalysis within the context of serious ego distortions of borderline personality organization depends on structural developments which complicate borderline personality organization and which, in turn, largely depend upon further vicissitudes of internalized object relationships (Chapters 4, 8, 9).

If the borderline patient has achieved some higher level of superego integration, abstraction, and depersonification, the superego may still be sufficiently strong to carry out functions fostering ego integration at large, thus compensating for the lack of integration of the self-concept (identity diffusion). Some infantile personalities have developed surprisingly good internalized value systems; the capacity to identify with ethical, professional, and/or artistic values beyond satisfaction of their own needs; and a personal integrity in dealing with these values, professions, or arts. Although a high intelligence and particular talents may be helpful elements, most important for such a development to occur seems to be the availability of object relations at the height of the development of advanced superego structures (around ages 4 to 6 and/or throughout adolescence) which were not completely controlled by their primitive conflicts and which permitted more harmonious integration of some realistic superego demands and prohibitions. Honesty and integrity in the ordinary sense of these words are also valuable prognostic factors which may permit some infantile personalities and other borderline personality structures to undergo a nonmodified psychoanalytic procedure.

A prognostically negative development complicating borderline personality organization is a pathological fusion of "all good" self-images with early ideal self-images and early ideal object-images. Such a pathological fusion of all the "good" aspects of internalized object relationships crystalizes into an idealized, highly unrealistic self-concept which, if fostered by some realistic circumstances (such as an unusual talent, physical beauty, or intelligence), may be reinforced by reality and, paradoxically, foster better reality adaptation to "specialness." This development characterizes the narcissistic personality (Chapter 8, 9). Social functioning may improve greatly under these circumstances, but at the cost of the loss of the normal differentiation between self on the one hand, and ego ideal on the other (at the cost, therefore, of a most important superego structure). Serious superego defects are typical of narcissistic personalities and compromise their analyzability.

It hardly needs to be stressed that the idealized self-concept requires even stronger activation of primitive defensive operations to deny and project the devaluated, bad aspects of the self; therefore, these defenses perpetuate a lack of realistic integration of the self-concept. However, the very improvement in surface functioning may obscure the severity of the underlying psychopathology, and narcissistic personalities may undergo years of psychoanalysis without change. Elsewhere, I refer to the fact that these patients should, however, be treated with psychoanalysis, and I also stress the special technical requirements of their analysis (Chapter 8).

A particularly ominous development worsening the prognosis for both psychoanalysis and psychoanalytic psychotherapy is the development, within the character structure of borderline patients, of identification with primitive superego forerunners of a highly sadistic kind. Under these circumstances, primitive destructiveness and self-destructiveness are built into the ego structure, are sanctioned by the superego, and permit direct expression of aggressive impulses under conditions which can seriously threaten the physical as well as the psychic life of these patients. Self-destruction, originally expressing primitive, pregenital aggression, may become an ego ideal and gratify the patient's sense of omnipotence in that he no longer needs to fear frustration and suffering (suffering is now an enjoyment in itself). Such aggression is expressed not only by random destructiveness, but by selective destructiveness toward those on whom the patient depends for his gratification (and his improvement). Therefore, he particularly envies those on whom he depends because these objects have an internal sense of love and they even want to provide goodness for others, including the patient. These patients represent prognostically the most ominous type of identification with the aggressor (Chapter 4).

Further Considerations about Treatment

Transference Interpretation, Regression and Reconstruction

I would now like to stress the following aspects of the treatment of these patients: first, one has to keep in mind that ego weakness does not reflect absence of a solid defensive organization of the ego, but represents the very active presence of a rigid constellation of primitive defenses; these defenses by their effects contribute to producing and maintaining such ego weakness. Second, rather than attempting to reinforce higher level defenses or to support the patient's adaptation directly, it is helpful to consistently interpret these primitive defensive operations, especially as they enter the transference, because the interpretation of these defenses permits ego growth to resume and higher level defensive operations to take over. Third, interpretations have to be formulated so that the patient's distortions of the analyst's intervention can be simultaneously and systematically examined, and the patient's distortion of present reality and especially of his perceptions in the hour can be systematically clarified. This clarification does not mean suggestion, advice giving, or revelation regarding personal matters of the analyst to the patient, but a clear explanation of how the analyst sees the "here and now" interaction with the patient in contrast to how the analyst assumes the patient is interpretating this "here and now" interaction. Clarification of perceptions and of the patient's relationship to the interpretation is, therefore, an important component of an essentially interpretive approach which attempts to systematically analyze the primitive defensive constellation as it enters the transference.

Often, in advanced stages of treatment of borderline patients, it turns out that while the traumatic circumstances patients reported earlier were unreal, there were other, very real, chronically traumatizing parent-child interactions which they had never been consciously aware of before. It turns out that the most damaging influences were those which the patient had taken as a matter of course, and the absence of these influences is often experienced by the patient as an astonishing opening of new perspectives on life. The following case illustrates the relationship between distortion of present reality and distortion of the past in the transference of a borderline patient, and the need to clarify the patient's perceptions in the hours.

A patient reminisced about having intimate physical contact with both parents which in her mind amounted to a family shared orgy. Gradually she became aware of the fantastic nature of these memories but later she recalled experiences she had not reported because they seemed such a matter of course. The patient reacted angrily whenever the analyst stated he did not understand some verbal or nonverbal communication of hers. She did not believe him; she thought he really could read her mind and that he only pretended he could not because he wanted to make her angry. After she consistently explored her assumption that the analyst could read her mind, she remembered that her mother had told her that she could indeed read the patient's mind. The patient's rejection of interpretations that seemed false to her was experienced by her as rebelliousness against mother. The implicit omnipotence of mother, her sadistic intrusion, the patient's passive acceptance of such a style of communication during childhood and adolescence, and her secondary omnipotent utilization of this pattern, turned out to reflect the real, highly traumatic aspects of her childhood. After working through in the transference the fantastic experiences with the parents—and the defenses against them—the patient was able to perceive the more realistic aspects of the therapeutic relationship. She became aware of the real, pathological interactions with her parents, which previously had seemed natural to her.

The implications of this observation that I wish to stress are that the disturbance in reality testing of this patient was related to a double layer of transference phenomena: a) the highly distorted transference (at times of an almost psychotic nature) reflecting fantastic internal object-relationships related to early ego disturbances, and b) the more "realistic" transference related to real experiences—the highly inappropriate parent-child interactions.

Interpretation of primitive defensive operations as they are activated in the therapeutic relationship may bring about immediate, impressive improvement in the patient's psychological functioning to such an extent that such a method in itself may be used in the diagnostic process when trying to differentiate borderline from psychotic patients. Systematic probing of primitive defensive operations, such as interpretation of splitting mechanisms in the hour, will tend to improve immediately the functioning of the borderline patient, but will bring about further regression into manifest psychotic symptomatology in the psychotic patient. The following cases illustrate such improvement or regression in the diagnostic process:

In the hospital, I examined a college student, a single girl in her early twenties, with awkward and almost bizarre behavior, childlike theatrical gestures, emotional outbursts, suicidal ideation, and breakdown in her social relations and scholastic achievements. Her initial diagnosis was hysterical personality. She was very concerned about social and political matters, cried over the fact that she needed to be in the hospital, but simultaneously acted completely indifferent while talking about her suicidal fantasies, acted as if she were drowsy or drugged, gave clear indication of boredom with the interviews, and complained about her inability to make up her mind about herself. I pointed out to her the displacement of her concern over herself to the social and political situation, the expression of depreciation of the interviewer, the effective avoidance of taking responsibility for herself by dissociating her concern for herself from the chaotic, easy-go-lucky behavior geared to force others to take over for her.

In technical terms, I interpreted primitive defensive operations (splitting, denial, omnipotence and devaluation) as they were apparent in the "here and now" interaction with me. In the course of the interviews, the patient changed from an almost psychotic appearance to that of a rather thoughtful, perceptive although highly anxious neurotic patient. The final diagnosis was: infantile personality, with borderline features.

In contrast to this case, I examined another college student in her early twenties, also single, whose initial diagnosis was that of an obsessive-compulsive neurosis, probably functioning on a borderline level. The entire interaction was filled with highly theoretical, philosophical considerations, and efforts to examine more personal, emotional material only intensified the abstract nature of the comments that followed. I attempted to interpret to the patient the avoidance function of her theorizing, and explored some of the emotional experiences which she expressed in theoretical, philosophical terms. I also wondered with her whether the direct, personal impact of those experiences was too much for her, her theorizing providing her with some safety by distance. For example, when exploring the unhappy nature of a relationship with a boyfriend, she discussed the theological theories about guilt; and I wondered whether it was hard for her to explore guilt feelings she might have had in connection with that relationship. As I confronted the patient with her defensive maneuvers, she became more disturbed, openly distrustful, and even more abstract. Toward the end of the interviews, there was direct evidence of formal thought disorder and the diagnosis of schizophrenic reaction was eventually confirmed.

The implications of these observations that I wish to stress are: 1) interpretation of the predominant defensive operations in borderline patients may strengthen ego functioning, while the same approach to psychotic patients may bring about further regression; 2) the intimate relationship between reality testing, the effectiveness of defensive operations, and the immediate interpersonal interaction.

The fact that interpretation of these defensive operations may increase regression in psychotic patients does not imply that interpretive approaches should not be attempted with them; but such approaches do require particular modifications of the analytic technique which contraindicate both psychoanalysis as such, and the modified approach recommended for borderline patients. The psychotic patient, with his blurring of limits between self- and object-images and the subsequent loss of ego boundaries, also utilizes splitting and other related primitive defensive operations; but he uses them to keep a surface adaptation in the face of threatening primitive dangers of complete engulfment or ego-dissolution. His problem is not only to separate hatred and love completely from each other but to avoid any intensification of awareness of affects, because the very intensity of any emotional relationship in itself may trigger off the refusion of self- and object-images. Therefore, interpretation of the psychotic patient's primitive defensive operations may bring about further loss of reality testing and psychotic regression.

Primitive defensive operations, and especially pathological forms of splitting and projection which bring about total dispersal of emotional awareness, protect the tenuous social adaptation of the psychotic patient: the underlying lack of self-object differentiation is thus obscured. Intensive psychotherapy with psychotic patients highlights this self-object fusion and requires a therapeutic approach which is different from that required with borderline conditions.

The intensive, psychoanalytic psychotherapy of psychotic, particularly schizophrenic, patients requires a tolerance, on the therapist's part, of the powerful countertransference reactions triggered off by the patient's fusion experiences in the transference. The therapist has to make maximal use of his countertransference experiences to understand the patient's experience, to convey to the patient his understanding in verbal communications, and to map out gradually in these communications the implicit differences existing between the patient's experiences and the therapist's reality, and between the patient's past and the present in the transference. In contrast, the therapist working with borderline patients needs to interpret the primitive projective mechanisms, particularly projective identification, which contribute powerfully to the alternating projection of self- and object-images, and therefore, to blurring the boundary between what is "inside" and "outside" in the patient's experience of his interactions with the therapist. Acting out of the transference and excessive gratification of primitive emotional needs in the transference of borderline conditions need to be controlled while preserving an essentially neutral attitude of the therapist.

The following, concluding comments refer specifically to border-line patients. Working through of the primitive level of internalized object relationships activated in the transference gradually permits a shift in the transference into a predominance of the higher level, more realistic type of internalized object relations related to real childhood experiences. In order to achieve improvement in distorted ego functions, the patient must come to terms at some point with very real, serious limitations of what life has given him in his early years. Here the issues of coming to terms with physical and psychological defects converge. It is probably as difficult for borderline patients eventually to come to terms with the fact of failure in their early life as it is for patients with inborn or early determined physical defects to acknowledge, mourn, and come to terms with their defects. Borderline patients gradually have to become aware of how their parents failed them—not in the distorted, monstrous ways which existed in their fantasies when beginning treatment, but failed them in simple human ways of giving and receiving love, and providing consolation and understanding, and intuitively lending a helping hand when the baby, or the child, was in trouble. Borderline patients also have to learn to give up the highly idealized, unrealistically protective fantasies about perfect past relationships with their parents; for them to really separate from their parents is a much more difficult and frightening prospect than for the neurotic patient. These patients also have to work through the corresponding idealizations and magical expectations in the transference, and learn to accept the analyst realistically as a limited human being. This painful learning process is achieved by means of eventual analysis of parameters of technique, or by means of realistically examining in the treatment situation modifications of technique and why the analyst used them. Coming to terms with severe defects in one's past requires the capacity to mourn and to work through such mourning; to accept aloneness; and to realisti-cally accept that others may have what the patient himself may never be able to fully compensate for. Hopefully, such capacity will develop throughout the treatment, but it is hard to foretell to what extent this development will take place.

Transference Psychosis

I mentioned earlier that the lack of differentiation of the self-concept and the lack of differentiation and individualization of objects interfere with the differentiation of present from past object-relationships, and contribute to the development of transference psychosis. Transference psychosis is a characteristic complication in the treatment of patients with borderline personality organization. There are similarities and differences between the transference psychosis that borderline patients develop and the psychotic transference characteristic of psychotic patients in intensive treatment.

The similarities of transference psychosis in borderline and psychotic patients are: 1) In both, there is a loss of reality testing in the transference situation, and the development of delusional thoughts involving the therapist; hallucinatory or pseudohallucinatory experiences may develop in the hours. 2) In both, primitive object relationships of a fantastic nature predominate in the transference; these relationships are characterized by multiple self-images and multiple object-images, that is, fantasy structures reflecting the earliest layers of internalized object relationships which represent a deeper layer of the mind than the dyadic and oedipal-triangular relationships characteristic of transference neurosis. This is in contrast to the predominance in the transference neurosis of less severely ill patients, of later, more realistic, internalized self- and object-representations in the context of an integrated ego and superego, reflecting more realistic, past interactions with the parents. 3) In borderline and psychotic patients, there develops an activation of primitive, overwhelming affective reactions in the transference, and a loss of sense of having a separate identity from the therapist.

The differences between the transference psychosis of borderline patients and the psychotic transference of psychotic, particularly schizophrenic, patients who undergo intensive psychotherapy are:

1) In borderline patients, the loss of reality testing does not strikingly affect the patient's functioning outside the treatment setting; these patients may develop delusional ideas and psychotic behavior within the treatment hours over a period of days and months without showing these manifestations outside the hours. Also, the transference psychosis of patients with borderline personality organization responds dramatically to the treatment previously outlined. In contrast, the psychotic transference of schizophrenic patients reflects their general loss of reality testing, and the psychotic thinking, behavior, and affect expression of their life outside the treatment hours. The initial detachment of the schizophrenic patient is usually reflected in psychotic behavior in the

hours which is not markedly different from his psychotic behavior outside the treatment hours. It may take a long time for psychotic patients to develop a particular, intensive emotional relationship to the therapist, differentiated from all other interactions: when this finally does happen, the psychotic transference becomes particularly different from that of borderline patients, our next point.

2) Psychotic patients, particularly at more advanced states of development of their psychotic transference, have fusion experiences with the therapist by which they feel a common identity with him. In contrast to borderline patients, this identity confusion in the transference is not due to rapid oscillation of projection of self- and object-images (so that object relationships are activated with rapidly alternating, reciprocal role enactment on the part of patient and therapist), but is a consequence of refusion of self- and object-images, so that separateness between self and nonself no longer obtains: this reflects their regression to a more primitive stage of symbiotic self-object fusion. Borderline patients, even in the course of a transference psychosis, do experience a boundary of a sort between themselves and the therapist: it is as if the patient maintains a sense of being different from the therapist at all times, but concurrently he and the therapist are interchanging aspects of their personalities. In contrast, psychotic patients experience themselves as one with the therapist at all times; however, the nature of this oneness changes from a frightening, dangerous experience of raw aggression and confused engulfment (without differentiating who engulfs and who is the engulfed) to that of an exalted, mystical experience of oneness, goodness, and love. In short, the underlying mechanisms determining loss of ego boundaries, loss of reality testing, and delusion formation are different in the psychotic transferences of borderline and psychotic patients.

Differential Diagnosis of Schizophrenia and Borderline Conditions

We often face the task, in the early states of the evaluation of patients, of making a careful differential diagnosis between borderline conditions and schizophrenia. It is important to make such a differential diagnosis because of the differences in the prognosis and treatment of the two conditions: I have become optimistic about the prognosis of borderline patients in a specially designed treatment program that combines intensive, psychoanalytically oriented psychotherapy with a highly structure hospital milieu program—during the initial phase of treatment for many cases, and during more extended periods of time for some. In contrast, the prognosis for chronic schizophrenic patients is, of course, always serious.

The two major considerations in differentiating schizophrenia from borderline conditions are the issues of reality testing and transference psychosis. Having already considered transference psychosis, I will limit myself to the discussion of reality testing.

When a patient comes into the hospital with a typical history of chronic manifestations of formal thought disorder, hallucinations and delusions, bizarre behavior and affect, and disintegration of the connection between thought content, affect, and behavior, the diagnosis is usually that of a schizophrenic reaction. However, many borderline patients who present severe, chronic disturbances in their interpersonal relationships and a chaotic social life, and who have undergone psychoanalysis or intensive psychoanalytic psychotherapy on an outpatient basis, may have developed transitory psychotic reactions which raise the question of schizophrenia. Also, both borderline and schizophrenic patients who have received intensive drug treatment over a long period of time, or have socially stabilized in the form of chronic withdrawal from interpersonal interactions (while still functioning relatively appropriately in some isolated, mechanical work situation), require this differential diagnosis.

I have pointed out earlier that, while both borderline and psychotic patients present a predominance of pathological, internalized object relations and primitive defensive operations (which distinguish these two categories of patients from less disturbed neurotic and characterological conditions), the functions of these primitive defensive operations in borderline conditions are different from those in schizophrenia. In patients with borderline personality organization, such primitive operations (particularly splitting, projective identification, primitive idealization, omnipotence, denial, and devaluation) protect the patients from intensive ambivalence and a feared contamination and deterioration of all love relationships by hatred. In contrast, in schizophrenic patients, these defensive operations, and particularly the pathological development of splitting mechanisms (leading to generalized fragmentation of their intrapsychic experiences and interpersonal relations), protect the patients from total loss of ego boundaries and dreaded fusion experiences with others which reflect their lack of differentiation of self and object images.

Clinically, the implications of these formulations are that while interpretation of the predominant primitive defensive operations in borderline patients tends to strengthen ego functioning and increase reality testing, the same approach may bring about further regression (uncovering the underlying lack of differentiation between self and nonself) in psychotic patients. As I have stated earlier, while interpretation of these primitive defensive operations may increase the psychotic regression in schizophrenic patients, this does not imply that a psychoanalytic or expressive approach should not be attempted. The regressive effect of interpretation of primitive defenses in the transference is only a short-term one; in the long run, intensive psychoanalytic psychotherapy with psychotic patients may develop their capacity to differentiate self from nonself, and strengthen their ego boundaries.

The temporary increase in disorganization that occurs in schizophrenic patients when primitive defensive operations are interpreted in the transference enables the clinician to differentiate these cases from borderline conditions, whose immediate functioning, particularly their reality testing, tends to improve when primitive defensive operations are interpreted in the transference. In practice, this approach means that diagnostic interviews with patients who require the differential diagnosis of borderline conditions versus a schizophrenic reaction should be structured so that this testing of defensive operations can be carried out.

It is, of course, useful to explore first whether, in the diagnostic interviews, there is any formal thought disorder, hallucinations and/ or delusions; if present, these would confirm that the patient is psychotic. If the interviews reveal no formal thought disorder, no clear-cut hallucinations or delusions, I would then focus upon the more subtle aspects of the patient's thinking, affect, and behavior which would indicate some inappropriate or bizarre quality within the context of the interpersonal situation of the interviews. Confronting the patient with such subtly inappropriate or bizarre aspects of his behavior, affect, or thought content is usually anxiety provoking for him. However, when done tactfully and respectfully, and with an effort to clarify the confusing, disruptive or distorting influence of this aspect of his behavior upon the relationship with the interviewer in the "here and now," this confrontation may provide an opportunity for meaningful support of the patient.

The interviewer, following such an approach, actually carries out a boundary function between the patient's intrapsychic life which the interviewer tries to reach empathically, and the external reality represented by the social relationship between the patient and the therapist. This approach is in contrast to: 1) the classical, descriptive search for isolated symptoms in order to establish the diagnosis of schizophrenia; and 2) the psychoanalytic effort to empathize with the intrapsychic experience of the patient regardless of whether the patient can maintain reality testing of this experience.

For example, if the patient presents a strange lack of affect in the face of an emotionally meaningful subject matter, this discrepancy may be pointed out to the patient and its implications explored. A borderline patient will be able to recognize this discrepancy, while identifying with the reality implications of the interviewer's question, and will become more realistic in this regard. In contrast, the schizophrenic patient confronted with the same discrepancy may be unable to grasp the therapist's point, or may interpret it as an attack, or may react by further increasing the discrepancy between affect and thought content. In other words, reality testing increases in borderline patients with such an approach, and decreases in schizophrenic patients.

This same approach may be applied in focusing upon an inappropriate gesturing (a behavior manifestation which may reflect a psychogenic tic or a stereotype), or upon any specific content which appears to be in serious contrast with other related thought contents, affects, or behavior. Often, multiple discrepancies among affect, thought content, and behavior are present, and the total emotional situation of the interpersonal relationship between patient and therapist will determine which of these elements represent highest priorities for investigation in terms of their urgency or their predominance in distorting the "here and now" relationship.

If this confronting approach indicates that reality testing is, indeed, maintained in all areas, a second line of exploration would be to focus directly upon primitive defensive operations and their interpretation in the transference. For example, if the patient seems highly concerned about philosophical or political matters on the one hand, and completely unconcerned about a serious immediate problem in his daily life on the other, the denial (the dissociation of concern from his immediate life situation) may be interpreted; or, if the patient indicates massive projection of aggression plus tendencies to exert sadistic control of the interviewer, a tentative interpretation of projective identification in the transference may be formulated. Again, borderline patients usually react to such interpretations with an improvement in reality testing and in their general ego functioning in the hour; schizophrenic patients tend to regress, and to experience such interpretation as frightening intrusions which threaten or blur their self-boundaries.

Often the interviewer intuitively senses that such regression may occur as a response to his interpretive efforts; thus it needs to be stressed that this approach is indicated only for diagnostic purposes. If excessive anxiety is aroused in the patient with such an approach, the psychotherapist, after reaching his diagnostic conclusion, should decrease the patient's anxiety by clarifying the relationship between the psychotic distortions and the therapist's interventions. The psychotherapist acting as a diagnostician has to balance the need to remain objective enough to arrive at a diagnosis, with the need to remain sufficiently empathic with the patient to protect him from excessive anxiety.

In summary, using the total interpersonal relationship in order to explore discrepancies among thought content, affect, and behavior leads to clarifying the presence or absence of reality testing. Also, the interpretation of primitive defensive operations, particularly as they enter the transference situation, further intensifies the exploration of the presence or absence of reality testing.

Loss of reality testing in any one area indicates psychotic functioning. It should be stressed that this conceptualization of reality testing is a restricted, delimited one, referring exclusively to the presence or absence of the patient's capacity to identify himself fully with the external reality represented by the patient-therapist relationship. This formulation implies that there is no continuum, no gradual shift from presence to absence of reality testing, and that there are qualitative as well as quantitative differences between the structural organization of borderline and psychotic conditions. As mentioned before, this essential qualitative difference derives from the particular vicissitudes of self- and object-images in borderline and psychotic conditions, and the related capacity to differentiate self from nonself, which, in turn, determines the capacity to differentiate perception from fantasies and intrapsychic perceptions from those of external origin and the capacity to empathize with social criteria of reality.

Discriminating Features of Borderline Patients

John G. Gunderson, M.D., and Jonathan E. Kolb, M.D.
(1978)

Borderline patients were compared with schizophrenic patients, neurotic depressed patients, and a group of patients with differing diagnoses. The purpose of this comparison was to find out whether borderline patients could be discriminated from other psychopathological groups and whether a discrete list of recognizable characteristics discriminating borderline patients could be isolated. According to the results of the comparison, borderline patients can be discriminated with high accuracy from matched comparison groups with whom diagnostic confusion is common. Seven criteria provided a clinically sensible and practical means of approaching the diagnosis of borderline disorder.

The first step in defining a clinical syndrome is to demonstrate that it is a recognizable entity that can be discriminated from other disorders. This is particularly relevant to borderline disorder because of its presumed position between psychosis and neurosis and the arguments that persist as to whether it is really a subtype of

Presented at the 130th annual meeting of the American Psychiatric Association, Toronto, Ont., Canada, May 2–6, 1977. The authors wish to acknowledge the statistical assistance of Murray Dalziel. Reprinted with permission from *The American Journal of Psychiatry, 135,* 792–796. Copyright © 1978 American Psychiatric Association.

schizophrenia or a variant of affective disorder. In a previous report (Gunderson & Singer, 1975) the descriptive literature on borderline patients was reviewed and those characteristics of borderline patients about which there is consensus were summarized. We have also demonstrated which of those consensus characteristics were actually found and which were not found in a systematic study (Kolb & Gunderson, 1968). In this report we ask two new questions. First, can borderline patients be discriminated from other psychopathological groups with whom diagnostic confusion often exists? The failure to do so would cast doubt on the rationale for continuing use of borderline disorder as a separate diagnostic entity in our clinical parlance. A positive result could lend support to the inclusion of borderline disorder in our standard nomenclature. The second question addressed in this study is, Can a discrete list of readily recognizable characteristics that are highly discriminating be isolated? Such a list could be useful in selecting a sample of borderline patients in a replicable way.

Method

All of the patients included in this study were given clinical diagnoses by the admitting physician at McLean Hospital. All of the patients were hospitalized, were between the ages of 16 and 35, and had no evidence of organicity. Only patients given an initial diagnosis that was considered certain for schizophrenia, neurotic depression, or borderline personality were included. Patients given a primary diagnosis of alcoholism or drug habituation, even if they were considered to have a borderline personality organization, were not included. Each sample was further screened using independent research criteria and/or clinical diagnoses to prevent overlapping diagnoses (Gunderson, 1977). The samples were matched for age, sex, race, and marital status (Kolb & Gunderson, 1968) (see Table 1). The patients were generally young, white, middle-class people from the Boston area; approximately two-thirds of them were women.

After giving informed consent, the 64 patients were interviewed within one week of admission using the Diagnostic Interview for Borderlines (DIBs). The DIBs consists of 123 inquiries ("items"), from which 29 of the characteristics of borderline patients found in the literature (each presented as a "statement") are scored. These statements are distributed in the 5 areas ("sections") of the interview as follows: 4 for social adaptation, 5 for impulse/action patterns, 5 for

Table 1
Demographic Variables and Diagnoses of 64 Inpatients*

| | Diagnosis | | |
| | Borderline Disorder | Schizophrenia | Neurosis |
Variable	(N=31)	(N=22)	(N=11)
Mean age	23.7	23.7	25.5
Sex			
Men	9	8	4
Women	22	14	7
Marital status			
Ever married	11	4	2
Never married	20	18	9

*All of the patients were white except 1 black patient, who was in the borderline group.

affects, 8 for psychosis, and 7 for interpersonal relations. The statements are added and converted into a scaled score for each of these 5 sections. Reliability and scoring characteristics of this instrument have been reported elsewhere (Gunderson & Kolb, 1976).

A stepwise discriminant function analysis was used to compare the borderline sample (N=31) with three different comparison groups.[1] The first comparison group was composed of 22 schizophrenic patients. The second comparison group was composed of 11 patients with neurotic depression. The third comparison group, called "all others," consisted of a combination of the schizophrenic and neurotic depressed patients plus a mixed group of nine patients with other diagnoses. For each of these three comparisons discriminant functions were done on two sets of variables. The first discriminant function was done on the 29 summarizing statements. The second analysis was a discriminant function using the scores from each of the 5 sections of the interview. One further discriminant function analysis was done on the comparison between the borderline patients and all others. This function was done on 10 items selected because we have found them especially helpful in our clinical experience. Other reasons for selecting these items were that they reflected independent areas of function and were among the most significantly discriminating according to t tests. The best overall discriminators were then synthesized on the basis of clinical and conceptual overlap into a discrete list of clinically sensible discriminating characteristics.

Results

The borderline patients were first compared with the schizo-phrenic patients, then with the neurotic depressed patients, and then with the group of patients with differing diagnoses.

Borderline versus Schizophrenic Patients

Together, the eight statement variables listed in Table 2 were able to discriminate the borderline sample from the sample of schizophrenic patients with 100% accuracy. The most useful dis-criminator was flat affect. It was unusual to find flatness in our borderline sample, but it was common in the schizophrenic patients. This difference was more obvious in terms of affect within the interview than as it was reported in the patients' recent histories. As found previously (Gunderson et al., 1975; Grinker & Holzman, 1973), although schizophrenic patients actually evidenced considerable depression and reported recent histories of other affects, unlike borderline patients they were often flat at the time of the interview.

The variable of devaluation/manipulation reflects qualities of the close interpersonal relationships of borderline patients that are less evident in schizophrenic patients. In fact, as the "loner" variable indicates, the schizophrenic patients were more likely to be socially isolated and to lack the intense relationships of the borderline patients. The fact that derealization was more frequent in the schizophrenic patients than in the borderline patients was also found in a previous study using other samples (Gunderson et al., 1975). Both the extensiveness of drug abuse and the fact that some of the borderline patients had psychotic experiences only while on drugs were also useful discriminators. The final two statement variables reflect the greater degree of social aggressiveness and more active social life involving groups of people found in the borderline patients than existed for the schizophrenic patients.

Although all five areas of assessment were represented in locating the most discriminating groups of variables, the psychosis section did not provide useful additional information when the section total scores were analyzed (see Table 2). These four variables were able to discriminate the two groups of patients with 85.45% accuracy. The most useful section totals were for interper-sonal relations and impulse/action patterns, both of which reflect more enduring behavioral patterns. This analysis suggests that the

Table 2

Standardized Coefficients in Comparison of Borderline versus
Schizophrenic Patients and DIBs Statement and Section Scores*

Variable	Standardized Coefficient
Statement description	
Flat/elated**	.482
Devaluation/manipulation	.397
"Loner"**	.273
Derealization***	−.184
Drug abuse	.130
Psychotic experiences on drugs	.188
Aggressiveness	.154
Active social life	.136
Section description	
Interpersonal relations	.512
Impulse/action patterns	.271
Social adaptation	.325
Affects	.228

* For the DIBs statements, Wilks' Lambda was .200, the group centroid for
the borderline patients was .776, and the group centroid for the schizophrenic patients was −1.012. For the DIBs sections, Wilks' Lambda was
.418, the group centroid for the borderline patients was .662, and the
group centroid for the schizophrenic patients was −.863.
** A low score on this variable was expected to characterize borderline
patients.
***This variable was higher in the comparison group (i.e., not in the
expected direction).

least useful information in discriminating borderline from schizophrenic patients can be expected to come from the sign and
symptom information.

Borderline versus Neurotic Depressed Patients

The 14 scored statements listed in Table 3 were able to discriminate the borderline from the neurotic depressed sample with
95.45% accuracy. As in the comparison with the schizophrenic
patients, both drug abuse and the occurrence of psychotic experiences while using drugs were helpful discriminators. The only
discriminator from the affect evaluation was that borderline patients
reported more frequent and sustained dysphoria and anhedonia.
Borderline patients were more frequently found to have a sexually
deviant pattern (usually promiscuity) or antisocial pattern, and they

Table 3
Standardized Coefficients in Comparison of
Borderline versus Neurotic Depressed Patients and
DIBs Statement and Section Scores*

Variable	Standardized Coefficient
Statement description	
Drug abuse	.411
Dysphoria/anhedonia	.307
School/work achievement**	−.541
Devaluation/manipulation	.353
Paranoia	.233
Past therapy regressions	.443
Antisocial	.297
Psychotic experiences on drugs	.281
Difficulty being alone	.222
Instability	.357
Hallucinations/delusions***	.281
Mania, delusional***	.195
Past therapy relationships	.211
Sexual deviance	.228
Section description	
Impulse/action patterns	.590
Interpersonal relations	.621
Psychosis	.236

* For the DIBs statements, Wilks' Lambda was .167, the group centroid for the borderline patients was .546, and the group centroid for the neurotic depressed patients was −1.489. For the DIBs sections, Wilks' Lambda was .530, the group centroid for the borderline patients was .410, and the group centroid for the neurotic depressed patients was −1.119.

** This variable was higher in the comparison group (i.e., not in the expected direction).

***A low score on this variable was expected to characterize borderline patients.

had lower school or work achievement records. Borderline patients were more intolerant of being alone, but their interpersonal relations were more unstable and marked by more devaluations and manipulation. Such problems were often evident in their previous treatment experiences, which indicated countertransference problems, staff splitting, and frequent reports of "getting worse." A final major area of difference is that the borderline patients were more likely to report brief paranoid experiences and occasionally had experiences that resembled hallucinations but proved difficult to evaluate. The neurotic depressed patients were more likely to have had possible manic episodes.

With respect to the section scores (see Table 3), once again more enduring patterns (impulse/action patterns and interpersonal relations) proved more valuable than signs and symptoms. The section scores discriminated the two groups of patients with 84.09% accuracy. Neither social adaptation nor affects added much when the other three sections were taken into consideration.

Borderline Patients versus All Others

The comparison between borderline patients and all of the other patients sharpened the focus on those characteristics of borderline patients which are the best overall discriminators for use in a variety of differential diagnostic problems. The 14 DIBs statements shown in Table 4 were able to discriminate the borderline patients from all other patient groups with 86.84% accuracy.[2] Because of clinical and conceptual overlaps within the 14 variables they can be condensed into the following seven criteria:

1. Low achievement. The typical level of the school and work achievement in the two years before hospitalization was quite low in borderline patients. This was so despite apparent talent or ability to do better and was quite similar to the achievement levels attained by schizophrenic patients.

2. Impulsivity. The principal form this took was a pattern of serious alcohol or drug abuse. Sexual deviance was highly related to impulsivity because it consisted largely of the promiscuous behavior of borderline patients under the influence of alcohol or other drugs.

3. Manipulative suicide. This refers to those suicide efforts or gestures which seemed designed to exact a "saving" response from a significant other. This commonly occurred as wrist slashing or overdosing and was the most frequent precipitant for hospitalization.

4. Heightened affectivity. Borderline patients displayed multiple intense affects. Anger may be the most discriminating of these. Even more important in discriminating borderline patients from others was the absence of flat affect and the relative absence of satisfied feelings.

5. Mild psychotic experiences. These most commonly took the form of drug-free paranoid ideation, derealization experiences, and a history of regressions or getting worse in previous treatment. Occurrence of any of these in the absence of severe widespread psychotic symptoms of any type in the patient's past life was a strong indicator for the borderline diagnosis.

Table 4
Standardized Coefficients in Comparison of Borderline Patients
versus All Others and DIBs Statement and Section Scores*

Variable	Standardized Coefficient
Statement Description	
Devaluation/manipulation	.163
Drug abuse	.460
Flat/elated**	.176
"Loner"**	.214
Paranoid	.283
Manic, delusional**	.380
School/work achievement	.185
Hallucinations/delusions**	.253
Derealization***	−.257
Sexual deviance	.324
Dependency/masochism	.219
Past therapy regressions	.222
Manipulative suicide	.222
Angry, hot-tempered	.155
Section description	
Impulse/action patterns	.485
Interpersonal relations	.468
Psychosis	.194
Affects	.175
Social adaptation	.154

* For the DIBs statements, Wilks' Lambda was .309, the group centroid for
the borderline patients was .965, and the group centroid for all of the
other patients was −.706. For the DIBs sections, Wilks" Lambda was .537,
the group centroid for the borderline patients was .790, and the group
centroid for all of the other patients was −.578.
** A low score on this variable was expected to characterize borderline
patients.
*** This variable was higher in the comparison group (i.e., not in the
expected direction).

6. High socialization. Borderline patients were definitely not
socially isolated ("loners") and were, in fact, intolerant of being
alone, i.e., compulsively social.

7. Disturbed close relationships. Devaluation, manipulation,
dependency, and masochism characterized and caused instability in
the intense attachments of borderline patients. Devaluation refers to
the tendency to discredit or undermine the strengths and personal
significance of important others. Manipulation is used here to
describe those efforts by which covert means were used to control
or gain support from significant others. Some typical ways included

Table 5

Standardized Coefficients in Comparison of Borderline Patients
versus All Others and DIBs Items*

Item Description	Standardized Coefficient
Do your significant others complain that you are mean (e.g., teasing, beating, withholding)?	.329
Have you ever hurt yourself deliberately—other than suicide?	.232
(After making inquiries for delusions) How do you explain (the delusion) to yourself? How do you experience the belief that (the delusion)? (Judge whether ego dystonic)	.571
Do you suffer chronic feeling of emptiness or loneliness?	.343
(After inquiries for delusions) How does your belief in (the delusion) affect you? (Judge whether delusions are widespread)	.219
Have you ever been dependent on any drug?	.201
Have you developed special relationships with any of the staff or psychotherapists you have been involved with?	.248

*Wilks' Lambda=.382; the group centroid for the borderline patients was .823; the group centroid for all the other patients was −.738.

somatic complaints, provocative actions, or misleading messages. Masochism refers to the pattern in which borderline patients repeatedly, knowingly, and avoidably found themselves hurt in their close relationships (i.e., they saw themselves as victimized). The dependency issues of borderline patients were frequently manifest in receiving actual caregiving or directions from their important other.

A discriminant function by section scores showed that for this comparison all five areas provided valuable discriminatory information (see Table 4). The section scores discriminated the patient groups with 81.58% accuracy. As in the previous comparisons, sign and symptom areas (psychosis and affects) were less helpful than the impulse/action patterns and interpersonal relations.

The third function on this comparison was derived from 10 highly specific items that had shown differences on t tests. The seven items included in the function are shown in Table 5 in the form in which they are asked on the DIBs. This function discriminated the borderline patients from all others with 85.35% accuracy. This is very similar to the function that was derived from statements. Sadism reflected a habitual pattern of being hurtful in relationships despite conscious knowledge of the effect. Two other items had to do with the fact that the delusions reported by borderline patients were circumscribed and ego alien (patients felt disturbed about them, i.e., they were experienced as symptoms). Loneliness and emptiness were very frequent complaints and quite specific to the borderline patients. Another useful discriminator was the frequency with which borderline patients reported having formed special relationships with previous therapists or others in caregiving positions. Other items that resembled aspects of the previous function include the history of self-mutilation and drug dependence.

Discussion

This study has shown that borderline patients can be discriminated with high accuracy from matched comparison groups with whom diagnostic confusion is common. The fact that there were fewer variables but with slightly higher power for discriminating borderline patients from schizophrenic patients than from neurotic depressed patients may reflect the fact that the diagnosis of neurotic depression is likely to be a more difficult differential diagnosis. If so, this would apply only to hospitalized neurotic depressed patients, who are a much more disturbed group than non-hospitalized neurotic patients.

The advantage of a list of the best overall discriminators developed from items over one developed from statements is that the items are more discrete and simpler to evaluate or quantify. The list of 14 variables derived from the statements was condensed into seven criteria that provided a clinically sensible and practical means of approaching the diagnosis of borderline disorder. These have the advantage of being more broadly applicable and conceptually enlightening.

Two unresolved questions about this study are the degree to which the discriminating variables found in this study are generalizable to other settings in which diagnostic habits may differ and to what extent they would hold up if other comparison groups were employed. A potentially more difficult control group would be one made up of patients with personality disorders not considered borderline. Even more demanding would be to examine a sample from consecutive admissions or a cross-section of the general population.

There are several ways in which we foresee these results can be used. The acceptance of a reasonable and replicable approach to the use of the term "borderline" can help clinicians anticipate certain clinical problems and subtypes. Among these are the probable contraindications for unmodified psychoanalytic treatment (Kernberg, 1976; Zetzel, 1971), the questionable advisability of antipsychotic medications (Klein, 1975), the risks of staff splits (Adler, 1973), and the temptation to underestimate or overestimate the patient's potential level of functioning. A major implication of several of the recent reports (Carpenter & Gunderson, 1977; Gunderson & Carpenter, 1975) on the social functioning of borderline patients also targets the low level of work and school achievement as a major problem for such patients and points to the role that social learning programs (groups, rehabilitation, milieu) can have in comprehensive treatment planning.

A second advantage of a practical and replicable guide for diagnosing borderline patients is that it would allow research to proceed into questions whose answers are controversial or unknown. Among these questions are the following: 1) Are borderline patients a heterogeneous group containing subgroups that could more appropriately be placed in other standard diagnostic categories? 2) do borderline patients have common genetic linkages with chronic schizophrenic patients, as suggested by the adoptive studies (Kety et al., 1968)? 3) do formulations employing splitting and projective identification as the predominant defenses (Kernberg, 1967) or abandonment depression (Masterson, 1976) reflect our understanding of these patients; or, as others have suggested, are different formulations required (Robbins, 1976)? 4) do these patients have specific psychopharmacological sensitivity to antidepressants or lithium (Klein, 1975)? 5) Is an expressive supportive psychotherapeutic approach (Kernberg et al., 1972) preferable to a more limited ego-directed approach (Friedman, 1975; Zetzel, 1971)? 6) Are there characteristic interactional patterns or parental psychopathology in the families from which these patients originate? 7) Does the course of these patients parallel that of schizophrenic patients (Carpenter & Gunderson, 1977; Gunderson & Carpenter, 1975)? 8) do the children of patients designated borderline by these criteria have a high risk for growing up to be chronic schizophrenics (Mosher & Gunderson, 1973, p. 25; Nameche & Ricks, 1966)?

These results provide evidence supporting those clinicians who have argued that borderline patients have a recognizable personality disorder. As Grinker and associates (1968, 1977) have shown, these results also indicate that a definite syndrome exists. The results clarify what the most discriminating aspects of that syndrome are and provide a replicable means for identifying borderline patients. Further studies that use these criteria are under way to search for external validators in terms of treatment responsivity, course, and etiology; such studies could further establish this syndrome as a coherent psychiatric disorder.

Notes

1. This method uses Rao's V to indicate the separation between groups. The first variable entered is one that maximizes V. This proceeds sequentially unless the variable correlates highly with all other variables in the function. In that case the V will decline and that variable is excluded.

2. Application of this function to an additional independent sample of 29 clinically diagnosed borderline patients accurately identified 76%. In another analysis, 81% of 27 patients who were classified by this function as having borderline disorder had been given this clinical diagnosis.

Theoretical Perspectives

W. W. Meissner, M.D.
(1984)

An even more complex and perplexing thicket of problems in our attempts to understand the borderline phenomenon may be found in the bewildering array of theoretical approaches and perspectives. Although thoughtful clinicians can readily come to terms with the idea that borderline pathology may involve multiple defects, it is not always clear how various formulations are related, to what extent they are mutually coherent, and even that they are, in fact, addressing the same data.

The current state of thinking about the borderline personality disorders has been relatively complacent following as it has upon a period of much chaos and confusion. Kernberg (1966, 1967, 1968, 1970, 1971), in a series of important contributions, finally culminating in a more or less definitive volume (1975), has offered formulations that have a comprehensiveness and a sweep that makes them seem both formidable and definitive. Uncertainties and ambiguities necessarily remain, and a sense of uneasy dissatisfaction has been expressed—having to do not only with diagnostic uncertainties, but also with conceptual difficulties in the understanding of the borderline syndrome (Dickes, 1974; Klein, 1975; Gunderson & Singer, 1975; Guze, 1975), as seen in Chapter 1.

In review, these include terminological ambiguities over whether the borderline entities represent forms of shifting patterns of symptom and defense or more or less stable personality configurations; inconsistent descriptions of borderline syndromes, with dramatic shifts in symptoms and behaviors and general fluidity at all levels of borderline psychopathology; and the need to distinguish between borderline conditions and the more established neuroses and psychoses. Were they *formes frustes* of psychosis, essentially psychoses with a covering neurotic facade, as seen in descriptions of latent schizophrenias, pseudoneurotic schizophrenia (Hoch & Cattell, 1959; Hoch et al., 1962; Hoch & Polatin, 1949), ambulatory schizophrenia (Zilboorg, 1941, 1956, 1957), or even the psychotic character (Frosch, 1964, 1970)? Over against this, other analysts were increasingly forced to confront the question of whether such patients were essentially neurotics and, therefore, in some degree, analyzable (Knight, 1953). Given the dominant dichotomy between neurosis and psychosis, what was not clearly definable as neurosis tended to be regarded as essentially psychosis.

Only gradually did the view emerge that borderline psychopathology was neither neurotic nor psychotic. Since the attempts to describe borderline conditions as both psychotic and neurotic were unsatisfactory, they gave way to a view of such conditions as constituting persistent forms of personality organization or character structure that had to be conceptualized and dealt with in their own terms. Kernberg's work has served to consolidate this perspective.

Other realignments in thinking followed, with the appreciation that transient regressive episodes in such personalities did not necessarily reflect an underlying psychotic process. Zetzel (Rangell, 1955; Zetzel, 1971) delineated borderline states from borderline personality organization, emphasizing that in the borderline states the overt clinical picture, whether acute or chronic, represents a group of conditions in which the patient is initially in a state of regression, which challenges the therapist from the outset. The borderline personality, however, initially presents with few or no disabling symptoms, but rather shows a variety of disturbances during the course of analysis. In a later elaboration, Zetzel (1971) commented that in the borderline states, both neurotic and psychotic phenomena are manifested, but neither fit unequivocally in either of those diagnostic categories. The patient cannot be described as overtly psychotic or as presenting any of the generally accepted personality disorders; no specific organic disease may be manifested, and symptoms and character structure are not consistent simply with a diagnosis of neurosis or neurotic character structure. Consequently, one is left with a borderline diagnosis.

Clinically, the distinction between borderline states and a borderline personality is important. The subsequent history of a patient presenting in a borderline state, including response to appropriate treatment, may lead to a revised diagnosis, since the patient may have been seen in an acute regressive crisis. Borderline patients, however, may not always present initial symptoms that suggest a borderline diagnosis and may, in fact, only reveal such a personality configuration during psychoanalysis or psychotherapy. To establish the diagnosis of borderline personality and to differentiate it from borderline states or other regressive manifestations may require an extended evaluation of the patient's response to therapy, and the evaluation of the nature of the doctor-patient relationship may play an essential role. In contrast to the potentially healthy or the neurotic patient in an acute crisis, the borderline patient has great difficulty establishing a secure and confident therapeutic relationship. Magical expectations, failure to distinguish adequately between fantasy and reality, episodes of anger and suspicion, and fears of rejection characterize a borderline therapeutic relationship, and they may persist over an extended period of time. In a favorable treatment situation, however, the borderline gradually will be able to acknowledge and partially relinquish such unrealistic and magical expectations, fears, and suspicions.

A parallel shift in diagnostic emphasis occurred—from a phenomenological or symptomatic evaluation to an evaluation of the organization and integration of structural aspects of the personality. Kernberg's (1967) perspective, as we have already noted (see Chapter 1), emphasized the specific stable form of pathological ego structure found in borderline patients. The pathology was specifically different from the neuroses and less pathological character structures on one side and from psychoses on the other. He opted for the structural determination of a borderline personality over the symptomatic or phenomenological borderline state. The organization of the personality was itself stable, rather than a form of transitional state, fluctuating between neurosis and psychosis.

The important point here is that these issues and ambiguities still affect our attempts to describe and formulate our understanding of borderline conditions. They also reflect and contribute to diagnostic ambiguities, which raises the possibility that variant theoretical accounts have focused on one or another of the diagnostically heterogeneous entities that form a spectrum of borderline conditions. This diagnostic spectrum has not been well articulated or differentiated. We shall take up the diagnostic issues more extensively in Part II. Although these considerations reflect a certain uneasiness with the current approaches to the borderline pathology, only a minority are dissatisfied; the question remains as to the extent to which the different theoretical formulations can be successfully integrated into a clearer, more encompassing description of this pathological spectrum.

Consequently, in thinking about borderline formulations, the question of the extent to which specific theoretical formulations tend to mask an underlying diagnostic heterogeneity must be addressed. A multitude of theories, each covering only a fragment or subsection of the borderline pathology, cannot explain the whole, although they may have a potential for further integration, casting light on the relationship between such theoretical formulations and the heterogeneous nature of borderline syndromes.

Thus, a first step must be to clarify the theoretical assumptions that serve as the frame of reference for particular theoretical formulations regarding the borderline personality. Psychoanalytic theory is not so much a theory as a collection of models of the mental apparatus, which, taken together, manage to span the range of modalities in which the mental apparatus can function (Gedo & Goldberg, 1973). These various models are not altogether congruent, nor are they reducible to a least common denominator. Rather, they reflect different segments and perspectives of analytic experience and are effectively differentiated by their relative success in explaining one realm of analytic date and by their comparative lack of success in generating understanding of other dimensions of analytic experience. The models can be said to have a limited base and a limited explanatory power, which constrains their usefulness in providing an understanding of the forms of psychopathology. To this perspective can be added the fact that no theory of borderline personality organization gives a satisfactory account of all aspects of the condition, but rather, that each approach tends to formulate, optimally, one or another aspect of the syndrome, while it provides a less than satisfactory account of other aspects.

Our objective in this study is a limited one. An attempt to assess the various theories as contributions to a broader psychoanalytic theory would be a monumental undertaking, quite beyond the scope of this essay and not germane to its intent. These accounts are presented only in reference to their application to borderline conditions, and even then only in a limited perspective. Even within these limitations, it is not possible to convey adequately the rich complexity of content and concept they embody. A basic familiarity and appreciation of these theoretical resources is thus assumed here, so as to avoid oversimplification in applying these formulations to gain an understanding of borderline patients.

Theories of the Borderline Personality

Before specific theories are discussed, some initial cautions and clarifications may be useful. First, our primary interest in this discussion is not to criticize or evaluate specific theories, although some points of criticism and comparison will inevitably arise in the course of the discussion. No theory can explain all aspects of a specific syndrome; in some sense, all theories are only partial truths. The emphasis here is rather on the inherent limited explanatory potential of the theoretical orientations under consideration and on the clarification of these in the interest of introducing a note of caution into our use of the available explanatory modalities and clearing away some of the theoretical obfuscations, so that our way to what needs to be understood might be seen more clearly. Not only does the strength or value of any given approach rest on its explanatory power, that is, the range of the borderline personality organization and pathology it explains, it also rests on the strength and validity of its theoretical substructure. Clarification of such theoretical substructures may lead to further specification and integration of the theoretical formulations.

It should also be noted that attempts to formulate the borderline pathology frequently draw on multiple theoretical perspectives, in order to integrate these perspectives into a coherent account (Frosch, 1964, 1970; Kernberg, 1967). Blum (1972, 1974) enlists multiple perspectives, particularly in his reconstruction of the Wolf-Man's childhood. Attempts to integrate preoedipal and oedipal factors touch on complex interactions involving ego structures and defenses, object relations, narcissistic components, etc. This diversity applies particularly in the developmental approach, in which there is a convergence of hypotheses from a number of approaches.

The plan to be followed will not focus on specific theories, but rather on areas of conceptualization of specific deficits on which the understanding of borderline pathology has been based in various theories. Consequently, authors or approaches to borderline pathology may touch on one or more of these areas of defect in their overall accounts. These areas of defective functioning may be considered in a variety of ways in different approaches, and no one approach has incorporated them all. Nonetheless, in varying degrees, specific approaches tend to see one or another of these areas of defect as central to the borderline pathology. The specific areas to be considered tend to relate the central pathology of borderline conditions to 1) instinctual defects, 2) defensive impairments, 3) impairments or defects in other areas of ego functioning and integrations, 4) developmental defects, 5) narcissistic defects, 6) defects and impairments in object relations, 7) the organization and pathology of the false self, and finally, 8) forms of identity diffusion.

None of the available accounts of borderline pathology precludes any one of the above aspects; but at the same time, it must be acknowledged that no two theories grant the same place or priority to these aspects. For example, borderline pathology is generally felt to involve significant developmental impediments. Two separate accounts may formulate the developmental deficit in somewhat similar terms, so that their descriptions of the developmental course seem to differ little. However, if one account sees the process as driven by inherent and biologically given determinants whose impact on the developing organism is programmed by a preset timetable of organically determined events, whereas the other account sees the same process as the result of the progressively modulating quality of the infant's object relationships with significant caretaking persons, entirely different theoretical accounts and understanding result. The theories render their accounts of the same developmental progression from opposite sides of the radical, nature-nurture dichotomy. Here the attempt is to delineate the basic theoretical assumptions embedded in accounts of the borderline pathology and to place in some perspective what may be called the "primary defect" and the degree of centrality ascribed to it in various approaches.

Instinctual Defects

Formulations that place the root of borderline pathology in some form of instinctual defect inevitably are caught in the dilemma as to whether the pathology can be basically attributed to an unusual titer of instinctual power or to a relative weakening or impairment of the resources of the ego to regulate, control, and modulate instinctual derivatives. Frequently, the borderline ego is pictured as helpless before the intensity of the onslaught of inner instinctual forces, so that to protect itself, the ego is forced into a position of helpless dependency or of omnipotent control (Geleerd, 1958). Such formulations frequently come out of an instinctual theory background and emphasize the continuity between border-line conditions and psychotic states. The underlying instinctual dynamics, with all their primitive force and primary process integration, seem to be postulated as given, and the ego is helplessly buffeted by these powerful internal forces.[1]

Along the same line, other authors have noted the chaotic and somewhat undifferentiated state of instinctualized energies giving rise to a sense of inner chaos. Particularly noteworthy in the evaluation of borderline patients is the manifestation of material from all phases of libidinal development, which presents a rather confused, mixed picture. This lack of instinctual phase dominance seems to reflect an interference with a normal processing of ego and id influences that allow the emergence of phallic trends in the oedipal situation. The bulk of the libido remains fixed in the oral and anal level, with little evidence of phallic maturation. Rosenfeld and Sprince (1963) have commented on this aspect of the borderline pathology in children:

> There seems to be a faulty relationship between the drives and the ego. At no stage does the ego give direction to the drives; neither does the ego supply the component drives with the special ego characteristics and coloring. It is as if the drives and ego develop independently and as if they belong to two different people. (p. 615)

Thus, the instinctual components remain fixed at a primitive level and seem unable to emerge from the domination of the pleasure principle.

An important question raised by such formulations has to do with the basic reasons for such instinctual impediments. One of the most consistently elaborated attempts to answer that difficult question has taken shape in Kernberg's formulations. A prominent element in his analysis of borderline pathology is the predominance of pregenital and specifically oral conflicts, and primarily, the intensity of pregenital aggressive impulses (Kernberg, 1967). The predominance of primitive pregenital aggression strongly influences the nature of the oedipal conflict. There is a pathological condensation of pregenital and genital aims under the influence of these aggressive needs and, in consequence, a premature development of oedipal striving (Kernberg, 1967, 1968).

The condensation of pregenital and genital aims under the influence of aggressive impulses sets the stage for primarily oral-aggressive projection, particularly onto the mother, resulting in a paranoid distortion of early parental images. The projection of both oral and anal sadistic impulses turns the mother into a potentially dangerous, persecutory object. The father is also gradually contaminated by this aggressive projection, with a resulting amalgamated image of the father and mother as somehow dangerous and destructive. This leads to a concept of sexual relationships as dangerous, and colored with aggressive and destructive themes. In an attempt to deny oral-dependency needs and to avoid the rage and fear related to them, there is a flight into premature genital strivings, which often miscarries because of the intensity of the aggression that contaminates the entire experience (Kernberg, 1967, 1968). Kernberg comments that these primitive dynamics may serve to discolor transference paradigms as well.

It is frequently difficult to see where or how Kernberg places the primary defect, whether on the level of instinctual organization or in terms of the predominance of splitting defenses or on a defect of ego capacity for synthesis or integration. Nonetheless, some unequivocal statements can be found. He comments, for example, that the ego in its early development has two essential tasks to accomplish: the differentiation of self-images from object-images, and the integration of both self- and object-images, under the influence of libidinal drive derivatives and related affects and under the influence of aggressive drive derivatives and related affects, respectively. The first task is not accomplished in the psychoses, but in the lower level of character organization, for example, the borderline personality organization, self- and object-images are sufficiently differentiated to permit an adequate integration of ego boundaries and a differentiation between self and others. With regard to the second task, however, Kernberg (1970) comments:

> . . . integration of libidinally-determined and aggressively-determined self- and object-images fails to a great extent in borderline patients, mainly because of the pathological predominance of pregenital aggression. The resulting lack of synthesis of contradictory self- and object-images interferes with the integration of the self-concept and with the establishing of "total" object relationships and object constancy. (p. 811)

The need to keep good self- and object-images from being contaminated by primitive aggressive influences leads to a basic defensive division of the ego, which serves as the basis for the defensive splitting, a concept that plays such an important role in Kernberg's thinking about borderline pathology (Wilson, 1971).

The degree to which the balance of constitutional as opposed to environmental factors is unclear in Kernberg's theory. It is clearly not exclusively a theory of nature as opposed to nurture, but one has the impression that constitutional factors play a clear-cut and decisive role. In this sense, Kernberg's developmental theory strikes a somewhat different pose from that of Mahler and her co-workers. The weighting in the direction of constitutional factors, specifically the increased titer of primitive oral-aggressive impulses in Kernberg's theory, has been detailed by Masterson and Rinsley (1975). The presence of such an unneutralized primitive aggression produces a situation in which there is a quantitative predominance of negative introjections, which have further implications for the persistence of splitting and the diminished capacity for constructive ego growth and the integration of self-concepts. Although Kernberg leaves room for the influence of early environmental frustration, the emphasis and the central role seem to be given over to a constitutionally determined heightened aggressive drive, which reflects his predominantly heredo-congenital view. Consequently, in his theory he pays little attention to the importance of maternal or interactional factors within the early mother-child exchange—an emphasis that sets his approach decisively off against the more specifically developmental approach of Mahler. Mahler's approach, by way of contrast, emphasizes the mother's libidinal availability and its role in eliciting the development of the child's intrapsychic structure (Mahler, 1968, 1971; Masterson & Rinsley, 1975).

If this more or less postulated and constitutionally given play of intensified aggression raises a suggestion of a Kleinian motif in Kernberg's thinking, the suspicion is not without substance. Kernberg (1967) has commented:

> Pregenital aggression, especially oral aggression, plays a crucial role as part of this psychopathological constellation. The dynamic aspects of the borderline personality organization have been clarified by Melanie Klein and her co-workers. Her description of the intimate relationship between pregenital and especially oral conflicts, on the one hand, and oedipal conflicts, on the other, such as occur under the influence of excessive pregenital aggression, is relevant to the borderline personality organization. (p. 678)

But the Kleinian influence extends beyond the constitutional given of a primary destructiveness, whether related to the postulation of a death instinct or not. Kernberg further postulates that the primitive instincts, libidinal and aggressive, function as the specific organizing principles in the organization of the earliest psychic structures at a point before self-object differentiation has taken place. It is not clear whether these basic instincts or their affective expression serve the organizing function at this level, since Kernberg also suggests that it is the primitive experience of pleasure and unpleasure that serves this basic function. His formulation seems to suppose an early differentiation of aggressive as opposed to libidinal instincts and their primary defusion. It is the combination of this instinctual situation with the emerging experience of part-objects that provides the basis for Klein's paranoid-schizoid position. Thus, the central formulation of Kernberg's theory, the internalized object relation, seems to occur under the influence of these instinctual organizing principles prior to any differentiation between self and object—a formulation that seems to provide its own inherent difficulties.

There is general clinical agreement that aggression plays a primary role in the borderline syndrome, particularly expressed in the ready mobilization of anger and the degree of primitive rage so often seen in such patients (Meza, 1970; Friedman, 1970; Gunderson & Singer, 1975). The clinical facts argue unquestionably to the importance of the role of aggression in understanding the borderline pathology, but they do not argue to the necessity of postulating a primary aggressive instinct or drive, nor do they force on us the theoretical conclusion that aggression is a constitutional given. Such has been the attitude expressed in early Freudian and Kleinian instinctual theory, but it may be that instinctual drives themselves can be conceptualized in terms of developmental process in which certain constitutional givens are shaped and modified by the quality of interaction with significant objects (Loewald, 1971). Nor are we compelled to think of primary aggression as essentially defused and only subsequently modified in a benign direction by fusion with libidinal inputs. It may be, for example, that the destructive and relatively "unneutralized" or "defused" quality of borderline aggression is related to the underlying vicissitudes of injured narcissism, which is threatened on a variety of fronts and for the restitution of which aggression is mobilized (Rochlin, 1973).

The appeal to instinctual factors as basic to the understanding of borderline conditions focuses on essentially economic-energic factors. The key issue then becomes the distribution, channeling, or transformation of basic energies, specifically, aggression. The psycho-economic concern is reflected in a preoccupation with disruptive states of hyperstimulation, modification of aggressive drive stimuli by fusion, and the need to protect nascent structure from overwhelming traumatic forces. This focus may have a useful application during the very early stages of development or in severe psychotic regression, but it is less useful in more evolved contexts of psychic functioning. Its explanatory range is, thus, quite limited (Gedo & Goldberg, 1973).

Defensive Impairment

In the formulation of borderline pathology, the deficits in the defensive structure of the ego are emphasized. Thus, our understanding shifts to the resources of the ego as a system of functions, but the defect in defensive functions, as opposed to other capacities of the ego, are specifically emphasized. The most dramatic failure of the defenses is seen in periods of transient psychotic regression, in which the patient decompensates and presents an apparently psychotic picture complete with helplessness, emotional collapse, and panic. At such points, the patient's vulnerability is most apparent and may provide the basis for difficult psychotic transference distortions (Giovacchini, 1973).

But even on more characterological and less regressed levels of functioning, the borderline tends to manifest relatively primitive defenses, including splitting, projection, projective identification, primitive idealization, and denial (Adler, 1974). Perhaps the strongest emphasis on defensive modalities and their role in borderline pathology is that of Kernberg. He makes adequate room in his description of borderline functioning for other modalities of primitive defensive operations, but splitting is the essential defensive activity that underlies the others, and it is essential to his understanding of borderline pathology. It is the distinction between splitting, as the crucial aspect of defensive organization of the ego at a lower level of character pathology, and repression, as a central mechanism at more advanced levels of defensive organization, that provides the basis for a diagnostic discrimination between borderline conditions and neurotic conditions. Speaking of the splitting process, Kernberg (1967) observes,

> This is an essential defensive operation of the borderline personality organization which underlies all the others which follow. It has to be stressed that I am using the term "splitting" in a restricted and limited sense, referring only to the active process of keeping apart introjections and identifications of opposite quality. . . . Splitting, then, is a fundamental cause of ego weakness, and as splitting also

> requires less countercathexis than repressions, a weak
> ego falls back easily on splitting, and a vicious circle is
> created by which ego weakness and splitting reinforce
> each other. (p. 667)

Thus the notion of ego weakness, often left unspecified in other approaches, is assigned a specific reference and cause in Kernberg's formulation, namely the underlying prevalence of the splitting mechanism that is seen as basic to other forms of ego dysfunction (Kernberg, 1967, 1971). The splitting process arises in the primary context of organizing discrete affect states around the libidinal and aggressive drives. This primitive organization is inseparably linked with the internalization of pathological object relationships, which persist in a relatively nonmetabolized condition as a result of the continuing effects of splitting. Kernberg (1966) explicitly relates this conceptualization to the concept of splitting in Fairbairn's account of the schizoid personality.

Kernberg's position has been questioned. Atkin (1974), for example, discusses the apparent splitting in a borderline patient:

> The "cleavage" in the cognitive, thought and linguistic
> functions that will be demonstrated in my patient can best
> be understood, in my opinion, as developmental arrest.
> No anxiety was produced in the analysis of the dysjunc-
> tion, a proof that it is not a defense (where no knitting into
> a whole has taken place there can be no "split" in
> Kernberg's sense). I found that only after some maturity of
> the ego occurred as a result of the psychoanalysis did
> anxiety appear when the discrepancies were analyzed.
> Only then was the dysjunction used as a defense, with
> resistance against giving it up. (pp. 13–14)

The objection posed here is fundamental in that it focuses on the issue of developmental arrest as opposed to defense. Kernberg appears to assume the differentiation and organization of specific drive states and the internalization of pathogenic internalized object relationships at a developmental stage prior to any differentiation between the infant self and the non-self.

There are inherent difficulties in the term "splitting" even beyond Kernberg's usage. Certainly, Kernberg's effort to narrow the focus of the term so that splitting becomes the fundamental defensive operation in borderline pathology and, thus its clinical touchstone, leaves something to be desired. Splitting is found throughout the broad spectrum of psychopathology. In its most dramatic and intense form, it is identifiable in the psychoses, but it can also be described in relatively healthy neurotics. The effort to focus the differentiation between borderline and neurotic pathology on the presence of splitting in the one and the reliance on repression in the other founders on clinical fact.

In an extensive review of the subject, Pruyser (1975) has pointed out the broad range of pathological expression of so-called splitting. He also criticizes the ambiguity and confusing connotations associated with use of the term. Kernberg's use of the term has a certain phenomenological or descriptive validity, but it merely describes the disjointed, mutually contradictory, and sudden shifting of patient behaviors, attitudes and emotions, transferences, and relations with important objects that seem to reflect a lack of integration. Pruyser (1975) concludes that

> The word *splitting* is both too slippery and too hard. It does not fit what we know about the mental life and is incommensurate with the temper of modern science, which has moved far and fast in the direction of process conceptions. Whatever psychic structure is, it is not hard and substantial and spatial. Splitting is too spatial, too surgical, and at the same time extremely indefinite. With all these peculiarities, its users, especially when they attempt to reconstruct the child's mind, run the risk of adultomorphic impositions. Elevated to a psychological concept, the words *splitting* and *split* create more problems than they solve. (p. 44)

If Kernberg's use of "splitting" has some descriptive value, he also relies heavily on the notion of splitting as a defense. "Splitting" thus becomes an active transitive verb denoting a defensive process by which the ego separates psychic contents, particular affects and representations. Dorpat (1979) has pointed out the lack of empirical evidence to support the notion of splitting as a defense. Kernberg's (1976) argument that the precipitating of anxiety when a patient is confronted with the unreal quality of his view of the analyst as both idealized and devalued (split representations) suggests that the defensive nature of the splitting is questionable. Dorpat (1979) points out that anxiety does not necessarily indicate that the behavior is defensive, nor does it follow that, even if it could be shown to be defensive, the defense in question would be splitting rather than, let us say, denial. This point of view is reinforced by Robbins (1976). The linkages with the Kleinian underpinnings of

Kernberg's early thinking (later revised by a more developed concept of ego formation) require the postulation of a capacity for psychic differentiation prior to the differentiation of object representations and also assume that splitting serves as a central organizing principle in mental life, a position at variance with current developmental views that the organization of mental life is effected by processes of synthesis and differentiation. All these authors agree that "splitting" can legitimately connote only descriptive divisions in the mental apparatus, and not a specific mechanism of defense.

It can be questioned whether Kernberg's formulations regarding this early developmental stage do not represent a translation of Kleinian motifs into ego psychological terms. The description of this early context has multiple resonances with Klein's description of the paranoid-schizoid position, and the healthy normal or neurotic resolution of this primitive splitting in terms of the fusion of aggressive with libidinal components seems to come very close to Klein's description of the depressive position. Kernberg is quite aware of this derivation, and he takes care to distinguish his position from that of Klein and the Kleinians (Kernberg, 1967).

Other aspects of the defensive configuration in borderlines have received attention. Modell (1961) has discussed the role of denial in borderlines, particularly in relation to separation anxiety. The denial of separation creates the illusion that the object is somehow part of the self and, therefore, cannot be lost. This creates a condition in which individuation cannot be acknowledged, since separation becomes equivalent to loss. Thus, growth to mature autonomy and individuality becomes translated into terms of separation from primary objects. Inherent in this separation is the threat of destruction or annihilation. The borderline differs from the psychotic in that psychotic denial is more severe and leads to the development of restitutional delusions or hallucinations. The psychotic then uses derivatives of internalized objects as the substitute for lost objects, and hallucinations serve as substitutes for painful reality. The borderline, however, does not take this additional step. Modell notes that quantitative factors determine the extent of the denial, particularly in relation to the degree of regression in object relationships. However, Modell's (1961) formulation does not place denial at the root of the borderline pathology, but rather sees it as another manifestation of a defect or a failure in the development of a capacity for object relationship.

The shift to an emphasis on defenses refocuses the borderline pathology in terms of the ego, but it is specifically a defensive ego that is called into play. The description of primitive defenses tends to link the borderline pathology more closely to psychotic levels of functioning. The general tendency is to think in terms of clusters of primitive defensive operations, which can then be explained in terms of some other defect, whether this is seen specifically in developmental terms or not. Thus, the role of primitive defenses in the theory of borderline pathology is generally secondary. This applies also to Kernberg's (1967, 1975) formulations regarding splitting, even though splitting seems to loom large in his general scheme. We cannot forget that it is itself a secondary phenomenon arising out of the primitive organization of internalized object relationships and in response to the predominance of pregenital oral aggression.

A perplexing aspect of borderline pathology has been the curious mixture of postoedipal defensive functions with more primitive pregenital ones, a point noted by Gitelson some years ago (cited in Rangell, 1955). Thus, it can be argued that an emphasis on splitting as a primitive defensive function does not allow for the development of higher defensive capabilities. It can even be questioned whether Kernberg's formulation tends to push out of appropriate perspective the function of higher defenses in borderline personality organization. In general, the tendency to see borderline pathology as closer to the psychotic border than to the neurotic border tends to reinforce this general inclination.

An additional point that demands consideration is the extent to which defensive defects can be read back from a more differentiated and evolved state of intrapsychic organization to early primitive developmental levels. It is by no means clear, for example, how splitting as a defensive activity arises within Kernberg's theory. Its point of departure is from the initial integration of internalized objects and their associated affects, but it is difficult to see how this then moves to the level of defensive functioning. It may be that, in order to make the model of the origin of borderline personality operative, one must postulate initial ego capacities and functions that require a greater degree of developmental maturation and intrapsychic differentiation. This is a fundamental point of divergence between theorists who base their analysis on ego functions, both defensive and otherwise, and developmental theorists.

It is worth reminding ourselves that the theoretical account of the defensive ego represents a more evolved level of ego functioning that has its reference in the topographic model. The topographic model, and later the structural model, which was meant to replace it (Gill, 1963), were derived from clinical data having to do with intrapsychic conflict and were not intended to explain earlier prestructural phenomena.

Ego Defects

Although the focus on defenses as the central aspect of the borderline pathology stems from the point of view that specifically conceptualized the ego in terms of its defensive functions, the emphasis on other nondefensive functions stems from a later and more evolved view of the ego, in which the concept of the ego centers upon notions of autonomy and adaptation. This view was specifically advanced and systematized by Hartmann (1939, 1964) and Rapaport (1958, 1967). In this context, the borderline pathology is viewed as a relatively stable form of ego pathology (Kernberg, 1967). The common denominator is viewed as the ego defect (Blum, 1972), which distinguishes the borderline from the neurotic, and in which the problems of adaptation take precedence over conflicts concerning unacceptable impulses (Giovacchini, 1973). The borderline ego is envisioned as weak, ineffectual, and vulnerable (Ekstein & Wallerstein, 1956; Frosch, 1970).

Kernberg's (1967, 1971) systematic treatment of aspects of ego weakness provides us with a framework for discussing these aspects of defective ego functioning. He lists, besides the predominance of relatively primitive defensive operations related to splitting, a lack of impulse control, a lack of anxiety tolerance, a lack of developed sublimatory channels, a tendency to primary process thinking, and finally, the weakening of the capacity for reality-testing.

The lack of the capacity to delay impulse discharge, normally regarded as a function of the ego, had been previously noted (Rangell, 1955) and related to the general fluidity of borderline cathexes and the inability to establish libidinal object constancy (Frank, cited in Robbins, 1956). But, as Kernberg (1966) points out, the borderline pathology represents a form of selective impulsivity and an acting-out character disorder. The patient may manifest relatively good impulse control in all but one area in which impulse control may be defective. He suggests, however, that rather than diminished impulse control we may be seeing an alternating activation of contradictory aspects of the patient's psychic life, as for example in the switching back and forth between intense sexual fears and impulsive sexual acting-out, both apparently ego-syntonic. Borderlines will alternately express complementary sides of a conflict, on the one hand, acting-out a libidinal impulse, and on the other, acting in terms of a specific defensive character formation erected against the impulse. They tend to be conscious of the contradiction, but blandly deny the implications of this contradiction, with a lack of concern over the apparent compartmentalization. Kernberg relates this phenomenon to the underlying defense of splitting, which he sees as lying at the root of ego weakness. Thus, the impulsive behavior may represent the emergence into consciousness of a dissociated identification system, in which the impulses are expressed in impulsive behavior, but have lost contact with the rest of the patient's experience and undergo subsequent denial. He also points out that this pattern of specific loss of impulse control is different from the more nonspecific and erratic dispersion of intrapsychic tension seen in infantile personalities (Kernberg, 1967).

The inability to tolerate frustration, tension, or anxiety to any significant degree has also been frequently noted as a characteristic of borderline patients (Brody, 1960; Kernberg, 1967, 1971; Rangell, 1955; Robbins, 1956; Worden, 1955). As Kernberg notes, the important variable here is not the degree of anxiety in itself, but rather the extent to which any additional anxiety added to the patient's habitual level of anxiety experience tends to induce an increase of symptoms or a pathological regression or other forms of pathological behavior. He regards this as a highly unfavorable prognostic indicator (1971).

Ego weakness is also reflected in a lack of sublimatory channels, specifically expressed in a capacity for work and an enjoyment of living, the capacity for creative achievement, and the ability to invest oneself in activities or in a profession that reach beyond mere narcissistic satisfactions. Although sublimatory capacities are frequently expressed in creative activities and achievement, it should be noted that borderline personalities often are attracted to, and find narcissistically gratifying, enjoyment in creative activities, whereas they find it difficult to deal with and master the day-to-day routine of more humdrum work situations (Fast, 1975).

Similarly, the tendency to primary process thinking, or to regress to levels at which primary process contaminates the secondary process thought processes, is an important index of ego weakness. This particular manifestation of ego weakness plays a particularly telling role, since it is one of the more frequently relied on indices, clinically, for identifying borderline personalities (Kernberg, 1967). Patients rarely manifest a formal thought disorder on clinical examination, but quite regularly, primary process manifestations in the form of primitive fantasies or peculiar verbalizations or other idiosyncratic responses may show up on projective testing. The importance of this indicator as the most important single structural index of borderline organization highlights the importance of the use of projective tests in the diagnosis of such patients. It is not at all clear, however, what a regression in such thought processes may mean, since the evaluation of it as an indicator must be considered in the context of the discrimination from an underlying psychosis.

The most critical index of ego dysfunction is the weakening of reality-testing or the loss of a sense of reality. This is particularly important, since the capacity to maintain reality-testing is one of the most useful discriminatory indices separating borderlines from psychotics (Frijling-Schreuder, 1969). Modell (1963) has noted the loss of a sense of reality in borderlines, but also noted that it was more subtle and less advanced than in schizophrenics. Other authors have noted the weakening in the capacity for reality-testing and in reality sense, noting that the impairment in these capacities may be transient, although in some patients it may be a permanent aspect of their functioning (Adler, 1970; Buie & Adler, 1972; Klein, 1975).

Frosch (1964, 1970) differentiates the quality of the patient's involvement with reality in terms of the relation to reality, the feeling of reality, and finally, the capacity to test reality. All of these aspects of the reality function of the ego are impaired, but the best preserved tends to be reality-testing. It is this relative preservation of the capacity to test reality that distinguishes the borderline syndromes from psychotic states (Frosch, 1964; Giovacchini, 1965). Disturbances in the patient's reality function are usually relatively easily reversible and are facilitated in this by the relative intactness of the capacity to reality test. Even patients who experience hallucinations or depersonalization may still be able to recognize these phenomena as derived from their internal experience, so that their reality-testing remains functional (Frosch, 1970).

Kernberg (1971) reinforces this view by noting that reality-testing involves the capacity to differentiate intrapsychic and external perceptual events. Such reality-testing in borderline patients undergoes transient impairment, particularly under the influence of emotional stress, alcohol, drugs, or when the patient is caught up in a transference psychosis. It is the preservation of reality-testing under ordinary circumstances and in most contexts of ordinary living that differentiates the borderline from the psychotic. A persistent impairment in this capacity in any area of psychological functioning and/or the production of psychotic manifestations must be taken as a manifestation of psychosis. Thus, Kernberg (1971) notes, if these are not present, the patient is not psychotic. He also notes that the frequency or intensity of the loss of reality-testing is not an important prognostic indicator, since the borderline in a regressive transference psychosis usually will respond favorably to treatment and to the increase of structure, either in therapy or in the life situation. This does not hold true for the psychotic loss of reality-testing. Attention has also been called to the capacity of the ego to control or to regulate inner psychic states as defective in borderline patients. Ekstein and Wallerstein (1954) have compared this function of the ego to that of a thermostat—neurotic patients undergo minimal fluctuations under the control of the secondary process, but in borderline and psychotic patients, the fluctuations are wide-ranging and unpredictable. Thus, the ego is battered back and forth by fantasies and unconscious instinctual derivatives so that the state of the ego fluctuates rapidly and radically from one state to another through the course of the day (Blum, 1972; Dickes, 1974; Ekstein & Wallerstein, 1954; Klein, 1975).

Various authors have focused on the lack of integrative or synthetic function as central to borderline pathology. The defect in this essential function has been related to the incapacity to integrate sensory stimuli (Rosenfeld & Sprince, 1965), the susceptibility to dedifferentiation under stress (Frosch, 1967), the uneven binding of instinctual energies and the failure of neutralization (Rosenfeld & Sprince, 1963), and the failure to coordinate perceptual stimuli, both inner and outer, with executive responses (Giovacchini, 1973). Atkin (1974) has further pointed out that the capacity for integration and synthesis, which normally creates an integrated inner world, is defective in borderline patients and is responsible for lapses and discontinuities in the cognitive sphere, so that primary process influences on language and thinking, as well as predominant pregenital sexual and aggressive responses, may result. The failure to integrate leads to a bland toleration for contradictory states of thought and action in which there is no need to unify or reconcile them. It should be noted that theorists who focus on the lack of capacity for integration and synthesis seem to write out of a background that is more or less developmental.

A latent issue in the discussion of defective ego functions and their relevance to borderline pathology has to do with the question of the degree to which they are considered as discrete, that is to say, the extent to which they are regarded as present or absent or as functional or impaired, as against the extent to which they are seen to function on a continuum, that is, subject to various degrees of operation or levels of functioning. The synthetic function, for example, tends to be conceptualized in terms of gradations of function, whereas reality-resting is often used as a discriminator of the presence of or absence of psychosis.

But reality-testing itself may be conceived in terms of degrees of alteration or impairment (Modell, 1963). Thus, the function of reality-testing may itself be a complex function, which may be subject to contextual variations in the sense that it may be relatively impaired in specific contexts of the patient's experience, but relatively unimpaired in others. The tendency to see these functions operating discretely in the borderline tends to dichotomize thinking and to push the concept of borderline pathology in the direction of linking it with the psychoses. Conceptualizing these functions in terms of gradients offers the opportunity of a more refined conceptualization of the borderline pathology as neither psychotic nor neurotic, while it forces us to a more specific and refined sense of intermediate gradations of functioning within which the borderline pathology occurs. The question is discussed in greater detail in Chapter 6.

In general, the approach to an understanding of the borderline pathology in terms of specific ego defects has only limited explanatory power. The approach, in general, is generated from Hartmann's (1939, 1964) perspective on the relative independence of ego functions, in which he implied that impairment or relative dysfunction could appear in one or another ego function, while other capacities of the ego would be relatively unimpaired. It somehow seems too simplistic, or "neat," that the multiple impairments found in the borderline pathology can be attributed to a single ego defect. Rather, we may be forced to a position that recognizes that ego deviations and defects are a vital and integral part of the understanding of the syndrome, but that we cannot think solely in terms of specific defects. We need to think of multiple deviations in many areas of ego functioning, possibly operating on a different level of disturbance in each area. Such ego functions, which may involve a series of gradations of impairments or levels of functioning, may also be subject to a partial reversibility in their level or integration of functioning, which is particularly labile in the borderline (Rosenfeld & Sprince, 1963).

The conceptualization of impaired, non-defensive ego functions derives from the more evolved concept of the autonomous ego. The defects considered to be central to the borderline pathology take their toll in the diminished autonomy of the patient's ego and its function and a diminished capacity to relate and adapt to reality. The focus on the ego defects has a certain descriptive validity, although even here the attempt to reduce the multifaceted borderline syndromes to a single defect seems weak. Not only do the specific ego defects not explain all manifestations of the borderline pathology, but they also stand in need of explanation themselves. These defects must be constitutionally given, or they must be explained. Thus, ego defects tend to serve as an intermediate explanatory concept that must give way usually either to a developmental or to a more specifically object relation conceptualization.

Moreover, the frame of reference, the Hartmann-Rapaport ego model, tends to place all capacities for adaptive or autonomous functioning in the ego and sets the ego over against the undisciplined and unmodified id impulses. The function of the ego, therefore, becomes one of regulation and control in the interest of adaptive functioning. The model postulates a radical dichotomy between the undifferentiated energetic and chaotic impulses of the id and the regulating, controlling, modulating, and directing capacities of the ego. The model dictates, then, that the developmental achievement enlarges the capacities of the ego and establishes their jurisdiction over the id. Any defect in this regimen causes the ego to yield to the power of instinctual impulses. It should be noted that this is not the only developmental model that can be envisioned, nor is it the only frame of reference within which the interrelation and integration of id impulses and ego controls can be envisioned (Apfelbaum, 1966). Consequently, just as all healthy and adaptive functioning need not be exclusively a function of ego capacities, so the borderline pathology may not necessarily be a function simply of ego defects as such.

Developmental Defects

Within the developmental perspective, there is a decisive shift away from a reliance on specific defects, whether of an instinctual or a structural nature, to explain the borderline pathology. The basis for understanding rests rather on multiple defects affecting a variety of psychic subsystems and related to the developmental failures involved in a relatively specific phase or level of the child's growing experience. Although the developmental approach rests uneasily on the assumption of constitutional factors, it primarily emphasizes the vicissitudes of the child's object relationships, so that it is, in essence, emphasizing experiential factors over constitutional factors. Further, the explanation depends on the quality of the infant's object relations experience, so that there is a significant degree of overlap between developmental perspectives and specific object relations theories.

To this extent, the developmental approach provides a frame within which multiple perspectives can be organized. It adds a specific and important dimension to other theoretical accounts, namely, progression through time, which allows for the emergence of certain deficits in phase-specific sequence that may undergo a variety of developmental vicissitudes in subsequent phases. As applied to borderline pathology, however, as in any other pathology, the issues of specific and primary defects remain operative. To this extent, current developmental formulations remain usefully eclectic as theoretical commitments. In this degree, then, the developmental orientation shares in and reflects the general theoretical tensions and uncertainties regarding borderline pathologies.

In proposing a developmental approach to borderline pathology a few years ago, Zetzel (1971) envisioned the borderline defect in terms of the developmental failure to achieve adequate one-to-one relationships with the respective parental objects, so that the borderline was prevented from entering into and successfully resolving a triadic oedipal involvement that simultaneously included both parental objects. The borderline may thus show a relative, but not necessarily equal, failure in specific developmental tasks. The affected tasks may include the establishment of a definitive self-object differentiation; a capacity to recognize, tolerate, and master separation, loss, and narcissistic injury; the internalization of ego identifications and self-esteem, which permits genuine autonomous functioning; and the capacity to maintain relatively stable object relationships. The borderline's vulnerability in the differentiation of self and object is illustrated by his difficulty in maintaining the distinction between fantasy and reality, particularly under emotional stress or during a regressive transference reaction. Thus, the borderline's capacity to internalize a stable ego identification and to achieve a genuine autonomy is severely limited and quite vulnerable.

The failure to achieve satisfactory one-to-one relationships points to a relatively early developmental failure. Margaret Mahler (1968, 1971, 1975) has made the most consistent attempt to specify this defect, relating developmental failure to the separation-individuation process. The failure of that process tends to produce a relatively unassimilated bad introject around which the child's inner experience is organized. Specifically, it is the upsurge of aggression in the rapprochement phase of the separation-individuation process that provides the conditions for the organization of the borderline intrapsychic economy (Mahler, 1971).

The rapprochement phase is characterized by increased separation. Development is favorable when the separation reaction is characterized by modulated and ego-regulated affects and where the titer of libido predominates over that of aggression. The child's need to separate is accompanied by a wish for a symbiotic reunion with the mother, but this wish is also attended by a fear of re-engulfment.[2] The child's attempts to ward off maternal impingement on his recently acquired and fragile autonomy tend to mobilize the aggressive response. The two-year-old toddler's autonomy is defended by the vigorous use of the word "No" and the increased aggressiveness and negativity of the anal phase. The rapprochement conflict is brought to an end by the developmental spurt of the relatively conflict-free autonomous ego, which sets the stage for the attainment of libidinal object constancy in the third year (Mahler, 1971).

The upsurge of aggression thus tends to undermine the good self and object representations and to increase ambivalence. The result is a rapid alternation of clinging and negative behavior, reflecting a split in the object world and an attempt to preserve the good object. Mahler emphasizes the child's interaction with the mother, particularly the mother's libidinal availability and responsiveness as the determinants of the development of the child's intrapsychic structure. Formation of self and object representations is based on the internalization of the interaction with the mother. Generally, the child's early developmental experience in the symbiotic phase may have been relatively untroubled, but initiation of the attempts to separate and individuate is met by maternal withdrawal of supports. It is this abandonment on the part of the mother that becomes powerfully introjected.

As Masterson and Rinsley (1975) have extended this theory, it is the maternal withdrawal of libidinal availability in the face of the child's efforts to separate, individuate, and achieve some degree of relative autonomy that forms the leitmotif of the borderline child's development. The postulate that the mother herself manifests borderline qualities in that she is excessively gratified by her symbiotic involvement with the child. Thus, the child's separation, especially during the rapprochement phase, creates a crisis in which the mother is unable to tolerate the toddler's ambivalence, assertiveness, and independence. The mother is available to the child only if the child continues to cling and behave in a regressive manner. The borderline child's dilemma is that he needs maternal support in order to continue the process of separating, individuating, and growing, but this very process leads to the withdrawal of that support. Consequently, the child tries to sustain the image of the good, supportive and nurturing mother by splitting it from the image of the bad, rejecting, withdrawing, and abandoning mother of separation.

It should be noted that the "splitting" in this developmental perspective should be distinguished from the notion of splitting advanced by Kernberg as a specific and active defensive function. Splitting here has much more to do with the sense of a failure of developmental integration. The contrast with Kernberg's more defensively oriented view can again be seen in terms of the relative emphasis on the constitutionally determined role of aggression in one approach, as opposed to the emphasis on an environmentally determined reaction to the withdrawal of maternal libidinal availability in the other. The child's intense oral dependence and absolute need for affection and support from the mother result in rage and frustration because of the mother's depriving response. The resulting fear that these intense feelings will destroy both the needed object and the self requires that the image of the mother be split into good and bad portions. Thus, the child constructs the fantasy or illusion of being cared for and loved by a good mother and projects the bad, frustrating, and depriving aspects onto other objects. Since these images remain unintegrated, objects are either good and gratifying or bad and frustrating, without ever being amalgamated into a single object experience. Thus, the child, in Kleinian terms, remains mired in the paranoid-schizoid position and is unable to achieve a more integrated depressive position in which the ambivalence to the object can be tolerated. In these terms, the borderline fails to achieve genuine object constancy (Masterson, 1972). Here again, there is tension between the tendency to view object constancy as a discrete developmental accomplishment and a view of such constancy as relative, involving different degrees or gradients.

It should be noted that although Mahler tends to place the impediments in the separation-individuation process somewhere in the second and third years of life, other authors have placed the developmental defect even further back in the symbiotic phase of development, somewhere in the first year of life (Chessick, 1966; Giovacchini, 1973). As Horner (1975) has noted, the splitting becomes apparent in the separation-individuation phase, but its genetic roots can be traced to earlier levels of the symbiotic merger with an ambivalent object. Moreover, there are some suggestions in Mahler's own formulations that the beginnings of splitting and the forming of good and bad centers of frustration-deprivation or satiation-gratification are taking place even before separation plays its part. Thus, the earliest failures of maternal symbiosis in the hatching phase of separation or before may set the stage for pathological introjections that underlie borderline pathology (Mahler, 1968, 1971).

The developmental approach tends to focus on a particular level of developmental impairment as the specific locus of pathological defect in the borderline syndrome. It must be remembered, however, that the developmental course is subject to a variety of vicissitudes and a sequential elaboration of both progressive and regressive potentialities, which tend to diversify significantly the effects of developmental impediments at any level. Thus, for example, the dilemmas of separation and individuation are critically reworked on the adolescent level, so that the borderline adolescent is again trapped in the conflict between his striving for autonomy, on the one hand, and his fear of parental abandonment, on the other (Zinner & Shapiro, 1975). Consequently, it must be remembered that whatever deficits can be traced to specific developmental phases, these need to be thought out more carefully in terms of the sequential progression of the developmental achievements and failures as the child moves from, let us say, the conflicts embedded in the rapprochement phase of separation-individuation through subsequent phases of reworking similar issues on into adolescence and young adulthood. It cannot thus be said that a developmental failure at a specific phase, such as the rapprochement phase, can be related, with any consistency or clarity, to a specific configuration or pathological characteristics in the borderline personality on an adolescent or adult level. Mahler (1971) herself has introduced a cautionary note:

> My intention, at first, was to establish in this paper a linking-up, in neat detail, of the described substantive issues with specific aspects of borderline phenomena shown by child and adult patients in the psychoanalytic situation. But I have come to be more and more convinced that there is no "direct line" from the deductive use of borderline phenomena to one or another substantive findings of observational research. (p. 415)

Thus, the simplistic conceptualization of a link between a phasic developmental failure and a specific form of psychopathology cannot be consistently maintained. Rather, a more careful study of sequential development may suggest meaningful patterns in which sequences of developmental variability can be related more meaningfully to patterns of psychopathology. This demands not only a more intensive and more refined exercise in careful diagnosis, but also more extensive and observational longitudinal data.

It should also be noted that there is a tendency in the developmental literature, particularly in Mahler's work, to relate developmental impediments to a failure of the integrative capacity or synthetic function of the ego. Again, this approach seems to reflect a tendency to organize the complexities of developmental data in terms of a specific ego defect. This reflects a more or less implicit adherence to a Hartmannian frame of reference, in which significant developmental attainments and functional capacities are located in the ego, to the exclusion of other aspects of psychic functioning.

Narcissistic Defects

The emphasis on the role of narcissism in borderline pathology shifts the locus of the pathology to the self. The metapsychological status of the self is still open to considerable question and debate, but the attempt to define borderline pathology in terms of the defects of self-structure leads to a completely new emphasis on pathological impairments and brings the function of narcissism to the center.

Issues of pathological narcissism have often been viewed in terms of narcissistic entitlement (Murray, 1964). Narcissistic entitlement dictates that the patient has a right to life on his own terms. A developmental fixation at narcissistic levels can reflect either excessive gratification or deprivation; either the patient's wishes were always granted, so that he assumes they should be, or they were never satisfied, and he feels the world should make it up to him. Such narcissistic entitlement plays a central role in borderline pathology, since the borderline sees himself as a special person with special rights and entitlements, such that any frustration of these entitled desires tends to undermine and often shatter the patient's self-esteem.

But it must be remembered that there is more that one level of entitlement (Buie & Adler, 1972). The patient's emotional deprivation because of the emotional unresponsiveness and withdrawal of the mother threatens the borderline patient's survival. Such survival entitlement is related to maternal abandonment and its inherent threats of destruction or annihilation and is the basis of the patient's terror and rage. The persistence of such archaic ego states, and their early narcissistic vicissitudes, is often expressed in a sense of fragmentation, confusion between self and object, coexisting or alternating grandiosity and terror, and alternating or tangled states of dread and rage, humiliation and triumph, megalomania and devastation (Moore, 1975).

Much of this approach owes its impetus to the work of Kohut (1971), but the amalgamation of primitive, pregenital object libido and narcissism was appreciated previously. For example, Reich (1953) noted that it is characteristic of early phases of object relations that objects tend to be used primarily for the gratification of the self, and that objects exist only to the degree that they provide such gratification and are destroyed in frustrated rage when such gratification is withheld. The narcissistic omnipotent need to control such objects is often not outgrown and may be regressively revived, so that when the narcissistically invested object fails to provide the needed gratification, problems in self-esteem arise.

The central concept on which Kohut's approach focuses is that of the "cohesive self." The narcissistic personality disorders, as he describes them, have attained a relatively stable and cohesive self, which remains more or less stable, although precariously balanced; but it shows a tendency for transient temporary fragmentation in response to narcissistic injury or loss (Kohut, 1971; Ornstein, 1974). The discrimination between narcissistic personalities and borderline or psychotic patients is cast in terms of the failure of the latter group to attain a cohesive self, so that such patients are unable to mobilize cohesive narcissistic structures to form consistent and analyzable transferences. The borderline patient has a less cohesive self that is subject to fragmentation so that he is unable to maintain the boundaries between self and object. Thus, the central vulnerability of the narcissistic personality is the danger of fragmentation or disintegration when a narcissistic relationship is disrupted, but these individuals possess a resilience that is missing in borderlines, which allows them to repair the shattered narcissism. The threat of disintegration is more central and critical in borderlines, whereas disruption of the narcissistic relationship plays the more prominent role in narcissistic personalities.

It should be remembered that narcissistic vulnerability occurs in the context of the important object relation with the mother. The infant is caught between the threat of symbiotic engulfment, on the one hand, and loss or abandonment, on the other. The usual picture is that of the narcissistic mother who withdraws her love when the child attempts to define himself as somehow separate from her. She becomes emotionally unavailable when he tries to individuate and to establish his own narcissistic equilibrium independently of her. The threat of object loss and abandonment depression leads to a narcissistic oral fixation, which impedes the establishment of a cohesive self (Horner, 1975). It should also be remembered that narcissistic impediments that impinge on the organization and stabilization of the self take place within a more complex family context, in which the child's dependence, and failure to achieve narcissistic differentiation, can be an important function in maintaining the delicate balance of narcissistic equilibrium within the family system (Zinner & Shapiro, 1975).

It should be noted that formulations in terms of the cohesiveness of the self are not very helpful in distinguishing between borderline pathology and psychotic levels of organization. In fact, Kohut's (1971) description of the temporary regressive fragmentation of the self in narcissistic personalities is strikingly similar to the borderline regression as described in other orientations. It is also noteworthy that formulations in terms of the self put the basis of the pathology on an entirely different footing than in other approaches. The potential of this approach is considerable, since it leaves open the possibility of reasonably well integrated functioning in the structural components of the tripartite theory, while the pathology develops and is rooted in the organization and functioning of the self. In most borderline cases, however, such a discrimination cannot be cleanly made, and there is evidence of defects in all the psychic systems.

It should be emphasized that the shift to a narcissistic basis introduces a quite distinct theoretical paradigm. Understanding of the pathology is shifted from a concern with structural integrity or the autonomy of ego/superego function to the organization and stabilization of the self as the significant principle of intrapsychic integration. The shift in emphasis to the centrality of the self follows the lead of the notion of "identity theme," as proposed by Lichtenstein (1964, 1965). Some of the implications in this alteration of basic reference point have been suggested by Gedo (cited in Meissner, 1976).

However, the shift in perspective raises the question of what defects may be primary, and what defects secondary, as well as the interesting diagnostic question of whether certain borderline categories may involve a pathology of the self, with minimal disruption of ego and superego functions. In addition, the approach through the pathology of the self may link the pathology more specifically to the object relations context, insofar as defects of the self may involve only one side of the self-object differentiation. Within that frame of reference, then, defects in the organization of the self and impairments in object relations may be envisioned as two sides of the same coin. Here again, the emphasis on narcissism seems to focus on an internal frame of reference, which gives rise to a series of economic preoccupations regarding the distribution and stabilization of narcissistic cathexes, rather than an emphasis on the context of interaction, within which narcissistic vicissitudes are worked out vis-à-vis the interaction with objects.

Defective Object Relations

The contextual framework within which such primitive narcissistic issues are elaborated and worked out is provided by a consideration of object relations. Thus, the object relations theory considerably overlaps and interdigits with the approach to the vicissitudes of early archaic narcissism and the developmental approach. These various approaches tend to be mutually reinforcing and complementary within the confines of their respective emphases. The disturbance and fragility of object relations have frequently been noted (Reich, 1953; Rangell, 1955; Frosch, 1964, 1967, 1970; Knight, 1953), and perhaps earliest of all by Helene Deutsch (1942), in her description of the "as-if" characteristics. The need-satisfying quality of such relationships, and the intense dependence on objects for the satisfaction of narcissistic oral needs, is characteristic (Adler, 1975; Blum, 1972; Frijling-Schreuder, 1969; Keiser, 1958; Klein, 1975). Thus, borderline patients characteristically feel empty and hungry, demanding to be nurtured by new objects with an overwhelming immediacy and insistence, so that, if these demands are not met, there is an experience of intense rage, which threatens to destroy the needed good object relationship (Adler, 1970). Thus, the libidinal object constancy is fragile and vulnerable, so that object cathexis is maintained poorly and with relative instability (Frijling-Schreuder, 1969; Rosenfeld & Sprince, 1963, 1965). Following a suggestion of Anna Freud, Rosenfeld and Sprince describe borderline children as "constantly on the border between object cathexis and identification" (p. 619). Thus, these children easily revert to identification with the object, which may lead to a sense of merging with the object. The child's incapacity to maintain an object cathexis thus threatens the integrity of the ego, and personality characteristics become merged with those of the object.

It should be noted that Kernberg's theory is explicitly and specifically a theory of pathological internal object relationships. Yet Kernberg's argument concerns itself very little with object relations as such, but rather with the internalized derivatives of object relations, while he designates these internalized derivatives as "internalized object relationships." They seem to come much closer to what has been described, in other contexts, as "introjects" (Meissner, 1971, 1978; Schafer, 1968). Rather than a theory of object relations as such, it propounds a theory of object representations. Thus, Kernberg's theory addresses itself to the vicissitudes and instability of such internalized objects, with little or no attention to the relationships with objects as such.

One of the most important contributions to the object relations approach to borderline states was based on Winnicott's (1953) formulation of the transitional object. The notion was further elaborated by Modell (1963, 1968) into the concept of transitional object relationships, and then applied to borderline pathology. Although there are remnants of such object relationships in everyone, to some degree, the borderline personality is character- ized by an arrest of development at the stage of the transitional object; the healthier neurotic has been able to pass beyond that stage to the experience of the loved object as somehow separate from the self. As Winnicott had already suggested, the remnants of earlier transitional phases can be found in a variety of normal experiences, including creative and imaginative processes, cultural manifestations, and religious experiences. The arrest of object relationship development at this transitional phase is not due to an actual loss of the significant object, but rather to a more subtle failure of mothering in which the mother is unable to make emotional contact with the child and becomes libidinally unavailable. Conse- quently, there is an absence or a diminished amount of the usual holding and cuddling, so that the mother's attitude toward the child is distorted and she is unable to experience and respond to the child as a separate individual. Modell's formulation does not distinguish adequately between borderline and psychotic forms of transitional relatedness. More recent formulations, however, have enlarged on the potential and utility of the transitional form of object relationship for a more mature capacity for object relations (Coppolillo, 1967). Nonetheless, the dominant concept is Modell's, namely, borderlines suffer from a pathology of object relations based on a developmental fixation in the stage of transitional object relatedness (Fast & Chethik, 1972; Fintzy, 1971; Modell, 1968).

The object relations approach fills an important gap in psycho- analytic theory in focusing on and articulating the early developmen- tal experiences that lie at the root of the child's emerging psychic structure. Consequently, its risk lies in its reductionistic tendency to read the development of later and more differentiated pathology in terms of the primitive vicissitudes of object relatedness. The theory borrows from the developmental perspective in terms of concepts of fixation and developmental deviation or arrest. Although these concepts have their appropriate application and a wide explanatory significance, their application in the more developed and structuralized context of evolved character structure and character pathology involve a radical presumption that demands validation and explanation. Thus, a critical area in this frame of reference that is passed over with only a nod is that of internalization. The theory must explain how object relations become internalized and provide the structural components out of which adult character and its associated pathology is formed and expressed.

The False Self

A brief comment about the false self concept is necessary here. It is another genial contribution of Winnicott (1960), but neither its theoretical underpinnings nor its relationship to the borderline concept have been established. Winnicott's description seems to lie closer to the range of schizoid character pathologies, and forms a schizoid subvariant in which the real or true self is dissociated from the false self that is caught up in compliant submission to the demands of external reality. The false self serves, in part, to protect the true self from affective interactions with other people. The threat to the autonomy of the true self arises from the proximity to objects, which carries with it the risk of engulfment.

The description of the false self is phenomenologically apt and often clinically accurate. The false self configuration is identifiable in some borderlines, or at least in those schizoid characters who fall within the borderline spectrum. Borderline compliance is closely related to the intense clinging dependence and seeking of narcissistic gratification from objects, but the relationship between these conditions needs to be further explored. The "as-if" compliance so often seen in borderlines is another manifestation of this phenomenon.

However, Modell (1975) has recently linked Winnicott's false self organization with Kohut's narcissistic personality. There are striking similarities, and the dynamic issues may be closely juxtaposed, particularly the underlying narcissistic dynamics. Unfortunately, the false self concept covers a wide range of psychopathology, all the way from the frankly schizophrenic to the relatively healthy and normal. Modell particularly addresses the illusion of self-sufficiency, by which he characterizes narcissistic personalities, and which also seems to be at issue in the guardianship of the false self over the true self. The compliance of the false self insulates the true self from commerce with objects and allows the true self to maintain its relatively grandiose illusion of self-sufficiency. However, similar features are often seen in borderline disorders, and we are left with a need to better define the role of false self characteristics in the borderline personality. Winnicott's formulation has certainly gone further in the direction of offering a basis for understanding borderline compliance than any other.

Identity Diffusion

Loss of identity has frequently been attributed to borderline pathology (Rosenfeld & Sprince, 1963; Frosch, 1970). The loss of ego identity, or its vulnerability, is also an aspect of Kernberg's theory, in that ego identity represents the highest level of integration of internalized object relations. However, the organization of identification systems at a level of ego functioning in which splitting is the crucial and central defensive mechanism makes whatever sense of identity has been attained precarious (Kernberg, 1966). Similarly, the loss of identity in borderline patients can precipitate urgent emergency states as reparative maneuvers. The borderline may then feel a sense of inner emptiness, having nothing inside, no individuality or originality. The acute anxiety in this state of identity diffusion can give rise to feelings of depersonalization and derealization. The patient may resort to various forms of acting-out or self-inflicted pain or create other emergencies in order to help restore the sense of reality and the sense of self (Collum, 1972).

The original description of acute identity diffusion was given by Erikson (1956) and specifically related to problems in adolescent turmoil and borderline psychopathology. Acute identity diffusion occurs in a context in which experience demands a commitment to adult contexts of physical intimacy, occupational choice, competition, and psychosocial self-delineation. The individual is caught between conflicting identifications, such that every move may establish a binding precedent and a concretization of psychosocial self-definition. Thus, the subject avoids significant choices, with the result that he is left in a situation of outer isolation and inner emptiness. Fast (1974) has spoken of these in terms of the multiplicity of identities, whose identity characteristics stem from the period in development in which the infant is making the transition from narcissism to a commitment to objective reality. The narcissistic sense of unbounded possibility and marked libidinization are characteristic of such partial identities.

In the face of failing identity, there are regressive attempts to delineate identity by a mutual narcissistic mirroring, so that the ego loses its capacity for abandoning itself to a sexual or affectionate relationship with objects. The object thus becomes the guarantee of the continuity of identity and raises the threat of fusion with its inherent risk of engulfment and loss of identity. The subject then often retreats to a position of distantiation, in which he is ready to repudiate, ignore, or destroy any forces that threaten the integrity of self. The need to repudiate lies at the basis of the fanatical embracing of causes or the merging with a "leader" in enthusiastic discipleship. This is an attempt to restitute identity in the face of the inability to gain genuine intimacy because of an incomplete or fragmented sense of identity. The failure of this process many lead to a paralyzing borderline state, in which there is an increasing sense of isolation and withdrawal, a sense of fragmented and diminished identity, a sense of shame and doubt, an inability to derive any sense of gratification or accomplishment from any activity, and a sense of being under the control of powerful forces and lacking the capacity to control or direct, by one's own initiative, the course of one's life. Narcissistic themes of lost opportunities and unfulfilled potentials of greatness are common themes (Erikson, 1956).

The conceptualization in terms of identity seems to be dealing with the outer face of what is dealt with in more internalized terms in the frame of reference of narcissism and the coherence of the self. Thus, although the external frame of reference of the issues of self-cohesion can be articulated in terms of object relations and the psychosocial engagement of the individual, the inner structure of the problems of identity and identity diffusion can be quite adequately spelled out in terms of the structuralization of narcissism and the organization of a stable coherent self-system. It should be noted that the complex of theories having to do with narcissism, object relations, the vicissitudes of false self-organization, and the vicissitudes of identity, in general, tend more in the direction of emphasizing the role of experiential factors over constitutional givens. Each of those approaches seems to be emphasizing aspects or dimensions of the complex developmental experience, particularly its experiential rather than hereditary, or nurture rather than nature, aspects. Thus, the concept of identity diffusion accomplishes little more than to spell out the external implications in terms of the

quality of involvement with the environment of the inner fragmentation of the self, which is defined and delineated in narcissistic terms.

Here it would be extremely useful to clarify the quality of
organization of self-systems, vis-à-vis the psychosocial environment,
and embracing a complex of states reaching, on the one hand, from
the forms of identity diffusion described by Erikson and others,
through a variety of false self states in which a pseudo-identity
consisting of a compliant false self facade is maintained in the
interest of protecting the inner autonomy of the true self, to the more
mature forms of stable achieved identity, in which the radical split
between true and false self has been somehow overcome and
integrated. As yet, this complex of ideas involving identity and false
self organization remains on a phenomenological level and lacks the
theoretical underpinning that would facilitate further integration.

Recapitulation

The various theoretical approaches take their point of departure
from different reference points within the spectrum of psychoanalytic explanations and models. Consequently, they offer differing
theoretical accounts of borderline pathology, so that the different
approaches have varying degrees of explanatory power and range.
Specific approaches vary in their capacity to explain different
aspects of the complex symptomatology, behavior, defensive configurations, and character structure found in the borderline spectrum.

Without being exhaustive, a balance sheet of these relative
strengths and weaknesses can be attempted. The approach through
instinctual theory provides a good basis for understanding the role
of aggression, the lack of libidinal phase dominance, the predominance of primitive oral motifs, the polymorphous-perverse sexual
manifestations, the tendency to volatility, the frequently seen
hypomanic behavioral patterns, the sense of vulnerability, and the
frequently noted, overwhelming traumatic anxiety experience of the
borderline. However, instinctual components are not a good basis for
understanding the lack of synthetic capacity or regulatory control of
inner states, the sense of entitlement and specialness so frequently
found in borderlines side by side with a sense of worthlessness and
emptiness, or the frequently observed sense of fragmentation and
conflictual involvement with objects.

The approach through defenses offers a convincing explanation
of the alternation and dissociation of ego states, the tendency to
controlling behavior, the role of traumatic anxiety, and the tendency

to act-out, as well as the significant role of projection in the borderline clinical picture. This approach, however, is less successful as a basis for understanding the predominance of aggression, the failure of phase dominance, the defects in autonomy, the problems related to narcissism, the fragility of identity and self-cohesion, and, even within the consideration of defenses themselves, the peculiar mixture of pregenital and genital defensive organization.

The approach through ego defects has considerable relevance to understanding ego weakness and the lack of synthesis, the failure of control mechanisms, and the capacity to regulate inner psychic states, as well as the loss of the capacity to test reality. This approach is also useful in understanding regression and the general impediment to autonomous functioning, as well as the pervasive sense of vulnerability. There is little in this approach, however, that allows an understanding of the predominance of aggression and primitive orality, the narcissistic issues of emptiness and worthlessness, side by side with tendencies to idealization, or finally, the characteristic compliance so frequently found in borderline patients.

The emphasis on narcissism deals quite effectively with the concomitant tendencies to idealization and devaluation, the tendency to self-fragmentation and narcissistic vulnerability, the sense of emptiness and worthlessness, as well as the propensity to feelings of grandiosity, specialness, and entitlement. But the narcissistic approach offers little in the direction of understanding the perverse sexuality, typical borderline volatility, and the tendency to acting-out, as well as the impairment of reality-testing and other ego functions.

An approach based on object relations emphasizes the early developmental experience and the more primitive layers of psychic organization. It contributes to our understanding of the disturbances of object relationships and the quality of the patient's experience with objects, particularly the characteristic fear-need dilemma, which pervades the experience with objects. It also helps to articulate the difficulties in self-object discrimination and the tendency to schizoid withdrawal, with its inherent fears of annihilation and engulfment. The object relations approach, however, is less successful in explaining the peculiar dissociation and alternation of ego states, the failures in libidinal phase dominance, the lack of synthetic and regulatory capacity of the ego, and finally, the issues related to narcissism and narcissistic vulnerability.

The approach in terms of a false self organization is perhaps more successful than any in focusing and articulating the issues of submissive compliance in borderline relationships, as well as the fears of impingement and vulnerability. The extent to which these issues overlap with and can be integrated into other approaches remains to be determined, but the false self concept has a limited applicability to the understanding of aggressive and controlling behaviors, the alternation of dissociated ego states, or such commonly observed phenomena as polymorphous-perverse sexuality or hypochondriacal preoccupations.

The conceptualization of borderline states in terms of identity diffusion lends itself well to the consideration of issues of self-fragmentation and the loss of a sense of self, the peculiar borderline emptiness, and the frequent regressive confusion, as well as the tendency to act-out. But the conceptualization in terms of identity offers little for the understanding of aggressive components, the alternation of dissociated ego states, and the tendency to idealization and devaluation.

The developmental approach is less easy to classify or to evaluate in terms of these relative strengths and weaknesses. It overlaps, to a considerable degree, all the other approaches and thus tends to reflect their relative strengths and weaknesses. Its closest ties, however, seem to be to considerations of ego deviations, narcissistic vulnerabilities, and the vicissitudes of object relations. Depending on which aspect it emphasizes, it thereby gains from the explanatory strengths of that theoretical orientation, yet at the same time takes on its inherent weaknesses.

Conclusion

Our purpose here has been to cast some faint light on the variety of theoretical underpinnings to approaches to the understanding of borderline psychopathology. In spite of the divergence and variety of these approaches, the question still remains as to the potential integrability of these elements into a consistent and integrated account of greater explanatory power and range. We have noted, at a number of points, that divergent approaches overlap considerably and tend to articulate similar aspects of the borderline pathology from their divergent perspectives. This may offer an initial opportunity for further theoretical integration, but considerably more theoretical effort will be required to advance this integration to any significant degree. The task, for example, of integrating notions of structural formation and formation of ego and superego with the vicissitudes of narcissism and the developmental progression in object relations has yet to be accomplished.

Our understanding of borderline psychopathology, then, remains somewhat fragmented, limited by our current ability to achieve little more than a low-level, theoretical integration of divergent points of view. The organization of such divergent viewpoints in terms of a particular perspective, most particularly a developmental perspective, does not constitute an integrated theory, but rather a juxtaposition of incomplete points of view, each of which contributes to some fragment of the overall understanding. Even the most comprehensive contemporary attempts to articulate a general theory of borderline pathology can be similarly criticized. The underlying question of considerable significance that this reflection raises is whether, in fact, divergent theoretical approaches are not focusing on subvariants of pathological expression, which may be diagnostically differentiable. Just as we may have to think in terms of a variety of forms of schizophrenia, or a variety of forms of homosexuality, so too we may have to think in terms of a variety of forms of borderline pathology, which resist our attempts at integral theoretical formulation.

Notes

1. As an interesting example of this approach, Fisher (1965) speculated that if dreaming serves as a safety valve for the discharge of instinctual drives, one could expect that an increase of the pressure of drives toward discharge would be reflected in increased dreaming time. Thus, the increase of drive pressure and weakened ego defenses in a prepsychotic or borderline character would be manifested in increased dream time. He reports such results in a borderline patient who manifested an abnormally high percentage of dream time and later developed an acute paranoid psychosis. There are obvious diagnostic difficulties in the account, but the focus here is on the theoretical concept of increased drive intensity or pressure as lying at the root of the pathological manifestation.
2. The retention of intense symbiotic strivings, in the form of womb fantasies, associated with a dread of merging and a fear of annihilation were identifiable in the Wolf-Man (Blum, 1974) as an expression of borderline pathology.

The Interface Between Borderline Personality Disorder and Affective Disorder

John. G. Gunderson, M.D., and Glen R. Elliott, Ph.D., M.D.
(1985)

The authors review the available literature on the interface between borderline personality disorder and affective disorder. Three competing hypotheses have been offered to explain the substantial overlap between these diagnostic categories; they postulate that borderline disorder arises from affective disorder, that affective disorder arises from borderline disorder, or that the two are independent and overlap coincidentally. None of these hypotheses satisfactorily explains the existing data. The authors propose a fourth hypothesis focusing on the multiple etiologies of the signs and symptoms used to diagnose both affective and borderline disorders and suggesting that some patients in the resulting heterogeneous population have symptom clusters that fit both syndromes.

The upsurge in studies of borderline personality disorder and primary affective disorder has led to competing hypotheses about possible interrelationships between these diagnostic groups. In this review we summarize three existing hypotheses about this apparent

Reprinted with permission from *The American Journal of Psychiatry, 142,* 277–288. Copyright © 1985 American Psychiatric Association.

overlap, examine the available literature testing some of their predictive implications, and suggest a fourth hypothesis that appears to be in better accord with existing data.

Hypothesis I proposes that affective disorder, probably depression, is the primary problem in patients with both affective syndrome and borderline character pathology (Akiskal, 1981; Klein, 1975, 1977). From this viewpoint, a defect in mood regulation leads to certain pathological character traits. Thus, the impulsive drug use and sexual promiscuity frequently found in borderline patients are seen as efforts to alleviate chronic depression, and suicide attempts are viewed as indications of despair. Likewise, unstable relationships might be secondary to the poor self-esteem and morbid preoccupations arising from the primary disorder. Even the poor reality testing and thought disorder present in some borderline patients can be attributed to comparable disturbances that occur in patients who have affective disorders.

Hypothesis II posits that borderline personality disorder itself can produce diagnosable affective disorder in some individuals (Grinker, 1979; Gunderson, 1982; Kernberg, 1976; Masterson, 1972; Rinsley, 1982). In this view, the primary defect manifests itself as impulsivity, characteristic attempts to gain control of and support from important relationships, hypersensitivity to separation and loss, and a tendency when stressed to exhibit impaired reality testing. Given these difficulties, such individuals might secondarily be chronically dysphoric and develop other signs and symptoms of depression. As the hypothesis is stated, such signs and symptoms might be identical to or differ substantially from those in other types of depression.

Hypothesis III postulates that affective and borderline personality disorders are unrelated, with each having a relatively high incidence in the population (Kernberg, 1979; Pope et al., 1983). From this perspective, what appears to be a meaningful correlation is more like one that might be found in a search for tall people with blue eyes: such people exist, but not because being tall is related to having blue eyes. This hypothesis is consistent with DSM-III, which classifies the affective disorders as axis I and borderline personality disorder as axis II, with no suggestion of a particular relationship between them. However, when the two disorders occur in the same person, it would not be unreasonable to anticipate that they can interact.

To facilitate comparisons among studies, we will try throughout this review to identify whether a study used strict or broad criteria for diagnosing affective disorder and borderline personality disorder. In line with most recent research, we use the term "strictly defined affective disorder" for that diagnosed according to DSM-III criteria or Research Diagnostic Criteria (RDC) (Spitzer et al., 1975). These two diagnostic systems are quite similar, but many of the patients classified as having schizoaffective illness by RDC are diagnosed as either manic or depressed with psychotic features in DSM-III. Other definitions of affective disorders are noted in the text. "Strictly defined borderline personality disorder" refers to criteria in DSM-III or in the Diagnostic Interview for Borderlines (DIB) (Gunderson et al., 1981). Other definitions of borderline personality disorder typically include a wider range of personality disorders and are referred to as "broadly defined."

Each of the following sections addresses a different approach to the interface between major affective disorders and borderline personality disorder. In each, available evidence is described and analyzed with respect to hypotheses I–III.

Prevalence

Many clinicians have had patients with concurrent diagnoses of major depression and borderline personality disorder. The availability of reliable diagnostic criteria has enabled investigators to ask whether there are more of these patients than would be expected. They have taken two approaches—looking for personality disorders in patients with major affective disease and looking for major affective disease in borderline patients.

Table 1 summarizes four studies of the prevalence of personality disorders in patients with a major affective disorder. Using chart reviews, Charney et al. (1981) found many more patients with diagnosable personality disorders among patients with unipolar nonmelancholic depression than among those with either unipolar melancholic or bipolar affective depression. For unipolar nonmelancholic patients with a personality disorder, the most common personality traits were borderline and histrionic; in contrast, subjects with a personality disorder in the other two groups were more likely to have obsessional traits. Unfortunately, the investigators were able to assess reliably only borderline, compulsive, histrionic, and hostile traits, making it impossible to give specific axis II diagnoses. Using both chart review and patient interviews, Gaviria et al. (1982) found a similarly low prevalence of borderline

Table 1
Studies of Borderline Personality Disorder in
Patients with Affective Disorder

Study	N	Type of Affective Disorder	Percentage of Patients With Personality Disorder	
			Borderline	Other
Charney et al. (1981)[a]	30	Bipolar	0–6	17–23
	66	Melancholic unipolar	0–3	11–14
	64	Nonmelancholic unipolar	25	36
Gaviria et al. (1982)[b]	100	Bipolar	13	12
Kroll et al. (1981)[c]	39	Unspecified	8	—
Friedman et al. (1983)[a]	42	Major depressive	67	24
	7	Atypical depressive and dysthymic	43	0
	3	Bipolar[d]	100	0

[a] DSM-III criteria for affective disorder and for personality "traits," including borderline and histrionic, compulsive, and hostile ("other").
[b] RDC for affective disorder: broad criteria for personality disorders.
[c] DSM-III criteria for affective disorder, with no breakdown within that classification, and for nonborderline personality disorder; Diagnostic Interview for Borderlines (DIB) for borderline disorder.
[d] Two atypical and one mixed.

personality disorder in outpatients with bipolar affective disorder. Kroll et al. (1981), studying consecutive admissions to a general psychiatric unit, found a low prevalence of borderline personality disorder in patients with affective disorder (subtypes unspecified). In contrast, Friedman et al. (1983), assessing consecutive admissions to an adolescent depression unit, reported that most met DSM-III criteria for major depression and borderline personality disorder; however, these results probably are biased by their admission selection process. In summary, estimates of overlap range from 8% to 61%, with a suggestion that patients who have nonmelancholic unipolar depression may have an especially high prevalence of the borderline syndrome. To our knowledge, no study so far has assessed the full spectrum of axis II disorders. Also, Hirschfeld et al. (1983) indicated that diagnoses of personality disorder are artificially elevated if made when patients are clinically depressed. Efforts by Charney et al (1981) and Kroll et al. (1981) to avoid this effect may partially account for their markedly low prevalence figures.

Table 2 summarizes studies of the prevalence of affective disorder in patients with borderline personality disorder. Stone et al. (1981) reported a very high prevalence of broadly defined affective disorder in a broadly defined borderline population. Kroll et al.

Table 2
Studies of Affective Disorder in Patients with
Borderline Personality Disorder

Study	N	Type of Affective Disorder	Percentage of Borderline Patients
Stone et al. (1981)[a]	36	Unspecified	83
Kroll et al. (1981)[b]	21	Unspecified	14
Carroll et al. (1981)[c]	21	Major depressive	62
		Schizoaffective, depressed	14
		Minor depressive	5
Akiskal (1981)[d]	100	Recurrent unipolar	6
		Atypical bipolar	17
		Dysthymic	14
		Cyclothymic	7
Pope et al. (1983)[d]	33	Major depressive	39
		Bipolar	9
		Dysthymic	3

[a] Broadly defined criteria for borderline disorder and for depression.
[b] Diagnostic Interview for Borderlines (DIB) used for borderline disorder; DSM-III criteria for affective disorder, with no breakdown within that classification.
[c] DIB used for borderline disorder; RDC for affective disorder; 48% of the patients with major depressive disorder had endogenous disorder; 38% had primary disorder.
[d] DIB and DSM-III criteria for borderline disorder; DSM-III criteria for affective disorder.

(1981) found a much lower prevalence in strictly defined borderline patients. However, also using strict diagnostic criteria, Carroll et al. (1981), Akiskal (1981), and Pope et al. (1983) all found a high prevalence of affective disorder in their borderline patients. The proportion of affective disorder in the borderline populations of the above reports ranges from 14% to 83%. Pope et al. (1983) found that major depression accounted for most of the affective disorders in their subjects, as did Carroll et al. (1981). The latter study provided data on subgroups: endogenous and primary major depressions were common but not predominant; for patients with secondary depressions, alcoholism and drug abuse were common primary diagnoses. In contrast to these two studies, Akiskal (1981) suggested that atypical bipolar and dysthymic disorder were especially prevalent.

The available evidence suggests a 40%–60% overlap between major affective disorder and borderline personality disorder among hospitalized and clinic patients. The prevalence of major affective disorders in the general population is estimated to be 5%–10%

(Weissman et al., 1981). Baron has estimated the prevalence of strictly defined borderline personality disorder to be 1.6%–4% (unpublished 1983 paper); this estimate was indirectly supported by Loranger et al. (1982). According to *Medical World News* (1983), Kernberg, using a much broader concept, has suggested that the prevalence may be as high as 15%. Thus, compared with the general population, inpatients and clinic patients are at much greater risk than expected of having both diagnoses. However, patients are not reflective of the general population. For example, Kroll et al. (1981) estimated that the prevalence of borderline personality disorder for inpatients is 8.5% (DSM-III criteria) to 18% (DIB criteria). According to DSM-III criteria, the prevalence of affective disorder in psychiatric populations has been estimated to be 22% (Mezzich et al., 1982) to 40% (Spitzer et al., 1982). Important questions remain about the comparability of the patient populations of these various studies. Still, existing data indicate an unexpectedly high concurrence of affective disorder with borderline personality disorder, which argues against their being independent, overlapping syndromes (hypothesis III).

The existing evidence is inadequate to show whether any specific type of affective disorder is uniquely relevant to the borderline syndrome. To clarify this, studies are needed that assess the prevalence of borderline and other axis II diagnoses among patients with each of the axis I diagnoses, including particularly the subtypes of the affective disorders. Studies are also needed to assess the prevalence of affective disorders among patients representing the full range of axis II diagnoses. However, even these studies would not control for the likely tendency of patients who fulfill criteria for both an affective and a borderline disorder to be especially prone to be in psychiatric treatment. Measurement of the overlap of these disorders in the general population is needed, combined with accurate estimates of the prevalence of each alone, to resolve this issue conclusively.

Phenomenology

Grinker et al. (1968) first noted the importance of depressive symptoms in the presentation of many borderline patients, a finding confirmed by Gunderson et al. (1975). Typically, such patients have signs and symptoms of depression that closely resemble those of unipolar nonmelancholic depression (Akiskal, 1981; Carpenter et al.,

1977; Charney et al., 1981; Kroll et al., 1982). However, these and many other studies showed that other, nonaffective signs and symptoms—especially impulsive and interpersonal ones—readily discriminate unipolar depressed patients from borderline patients (Gunderson, 1977; Gunderson & Kolb, 1978; Kroll et al., 1981; Snyder et al., 1982; Soloff & Ulrich, 1981). Borderline patients have these latter characteristics whether or not they have prominent affective symptoms, and unipolar depressed patients with no personality disorder do not, making them unlikely to be secondary effects of depression.

Hypothesis II suggests that affective symptoms in borderline patients are a result of the character pathology but does not specify whether these symptoms are identical to those of primary depression. In fact, several investigators have identified important qualitative differences: the depressive experience of borderline patients is marked by loneliness, emptiness, and boredom rather than by guilt, remorse, and acute failures in self-esteem (Cary, 1972; Grinker et al., 1968; Hartocollis, 1977; Kernberg, 1967). Gunderson (1977) found that depressed borderline subjects often complain of chronic dysphoria, boredom, and loneliness, but, in addition, many report more typically depressive themes of major loss and sustained feeling of worthlessness and hopelessness. Such a heterogeneous result might be expected, because the sample contained a mixture of patients with and without concurrent affective disorder (Pope et al., 1983). Still, such features as the inner sense of badness, deprivation, and conscious rage from early life seem to be distinctive components of depression in borderline patients.

There have been a few comparisons of affective symptoms in nondepressed borderline patients and nonborderline depressed patients. Conte et al. (1980) administered a self-report questionnaire to inpatients diagnosed according to DSM-III as having either nonpsychotic major depression or borderline personality disorder. With respect to affectively relevant material, the two groups resembled each other in feeling hopeless, out of control, unhappy, lonesome, empty, overwhelmed, and indecisive. Borderline patients were much more likely than depressed patients to feel disappointed in and let down by others close to them and to view themselves as failures. Of special interest was the statement, "I want to hurt myself." None of the depressed patients but 40% of the borderline patients answered yes to this question. In an analogous study, Snyder et al. (1982), also using DSM-III criteria, obtained MMPI profiles of 26 borderline patients and 19 patients with dysthymic disorder. MMPI depression scales were elevated in both groups, but the former appeared to experience boredom and emptiness more intensely than did the latter. Kroll et al. (1981) obtained comparable MMPI results for their borderline populations.

Overall, existing research does not confirm hypothesis I—that major affective disorder is necessary to generate other aspects of the borderline syndrome. Insofar as the affective symptoms of affective and borderline personality disorder have both similarities and differences, no strong conclusion can be reached about whether depression arises from the borderline syndrome (hypothesis II) or the two are independent disorders (hypothesis III).

Course

The first studies of the longitudinal course of patients with borderline personality disorder were flawed with idiosyncratic methods of subject recruitment, making it difficult to generalize the findings (Table 3). In a 6–8-year follow-up study from the Michael Reese Hospital, Werble (1970) described the outcome of 28 of an original 51 broadly defined borderline patients; the rest of the sample either refused to provide information or could not be found. She concluded that the patients showed no substantial change over that time. Gunderson et al. (1975) and Carpenter et al. (1977) studied the 2–5-year course of an operationally defined sample of borderline patients and a matched sample of schizophrenic patients at the National Institute of Mental Health (NIMH). The borderline patients showed little change over time in the type or amount of dysfunction; the only reported difference between the two patient groups was that, at 5 years, the former had a better quality of social contacts. Both of these studies indicated that the borderline disorder was associated with substantial morbidity but that, contrary to expectations at the time, the patients did not go on to develop schizophrenia.

Subsequent research on natural history is more directly relevant to questions about the interface of affective disorder and borderline personality disorder (Table 3). Easily the most striking evidence for an association between the two is research cited by Akiskal (1981) in a review paper. He reported on a group of 100 strictly defined borderline patients who were followed for 6–36 months. In that time, 29 had an episode of major depression; four, of mania; 11, of brief hypomania; and eight, of mixed affective disorder. Thus, within a 3-year period, 52% of this population reportedly developed some form of affective disorder. As noted, many of these patients had a

Table 3
Follow-Up Studies of Patients with Borderline Personality Disorder

Study	N	Length of Follow-Up (years)	Diagnosis of Most Patients at Follow-Up	Outcome Relative to Comparison Group
Werble (1970)	28	6–8	Borderline personality disorder	
Gunderson et al. (1975)	24	2	Borderline personality disorder	Same as schizophrenic patients
Carpenter et al. (1977)	24	5	Borderline personality disorder	Same as schizophrenic patients
Akiskal (1981)	100	0.5–3.0	Affective disorder	
Stone (1979, 1980)	27	2–3	Borderline personality disorder (2 patients had affective disorder)	Better than psychotic patients
Pope et al. (1983)	27	4–7	Borderline personality disorder; 10 of 14 patients with concurrent affective disorder still had it	Same as schizophrenic patients; borderline patients with concurrent affective disorder significantly better on some measures
McGlashan (1983)	70 or 78	15 (2–32)	Borderline personality disorder	Same as patients with affective disorder; borderline patients and patients with affective disorder better than schizophrenic patients

diagnosis of concurrent affective and borderline disorders at the onset of the study; yet, even of the 55 patients who had no initial diagnosis of affective disorder, 11 (20%) had an episode of major depression and four (7%) committed suicide. However, detailed methods and results from this work have yet to be published.

In contrast, Stone (1980) reported that only two of 33 broadly defined borderline patients went on to develop newly diagnosed affective disease; both had frank manic episodes. He also compared 2–3-year outcomes of 27 broadly defined borderline patients with 18 psychotic patients, most of whom were thought to be schizophrenic (Stone, 1979). Global ratings showed improvement for 20 borderline and four psychotic patients and no improvement or worsening in seven and 14, respectively. Problems of idiosyncratic diagnostic use and rater bias make these findings difficult to interpret; at least some of the psychotic patients had bipolar affective disorder.

Two more recent longitudinal studies of borderline patients used better-defined selection criteria. Pope et al. (1983) prospectively studied patients at McLean Hospital diagnosed according to DSM-III as having either bipolar affective disorder or schizophrenia, as well as a group of strictly defined borderline patients. They concluded that over the 4–7-year follow-up period, borderline patients generally did about as poorly as schizophrenic patients, except for having somewhat better occupational or academic functioning. Nearly half of the borderline patients in this study had concurrent diagnoses of a major affective disorder. This group did substantially better than did borderline patients without an affective disorder; their overall prognosis was intermediate between the schizophrenic and bipolar affective groups. This study confirmed the serious, long-term morbidity associated with a diagnosis of borderline personality disorder but suggested that coexistence of an affective disorder may improve the prognosis. It also offered evidence that borderline personality diagnosis itself is relatively stable over time; however, patients with a concurrent diagnosis of affective disorder can be expected to have the fluctuations in course typical of that disorder.

In an even longer-term study, McGlashan (1983) reported a 15-year follow-up of patients treated at Chestnut Lodge in which borderline patients were compared with several other diagnostic groups according to DSM-III criteria. McGlashan also found that the borderline diagnosis was stable over time but concluded that the overall course for borderline patients closely resembled that for patients with affective disorder. The outcome measures used were hospitalization, work, social activity, symptoms, and global functioning. This study is the first, to our knowledge, to employ a comparison group of patients with severe neurotic character and other personality disorders. The outcome of patients in this group resembled those of the borderline and affective cohorts; patients in all three groups fared better on all measures than did the schizophrenic group.

The differences between the McLean and Chestnut Lodge studies probably arise from a combination of characteristics of the latter treatment setting: 1) the schizophrenic patients may have been especially unresponsive to treatment, 2) the borderline patients may have responded to the unusually extensive treatment provided, which included more than 3 years of hospitalization and intensive psychotherapy, and 3) the patients with affective disorder, most of whom were chronically depressed, may have been somewhat less responsive to treatment compared with the patients with primarily bipolar affective disorder used in the McLean study. Thus the McLean study may inadvertently have emphasized differences in the borderline and affective patients, and the Chestnut Lodge study may have minimized them. Alternatively, borderline patients may have especially bad outcomes only for the first 5 years or so, followed by some remission in their subsequent course according to usual measures of clinical outcome.

To date, Akiskal (1981) stands virtually alone in identifying the affective disorders as a common outcome for many patients with borderline personality disorder. Other investigators have found that the borderline syndrome is relatively stable over time. It seems most likely that Akiskal's result reflects the effects of concurrent affective disorder. As has been reported (Pope et al., 1983), such patients appear to be stable with respect to the personality diagnosis but may have repeated episodes of affective disease. Available evidence in this area best supports the suggestion that the two disorders are unrelated (hypothesis III). However, attention still should be given to possible developmental considerations, especially in late adolescence. In 1983, for example, Gossett et al. noted that some adolescents who present with character problems—especially those with "excited and expansive behavior alternating with periods of lethargy" (p. 143)—later develop a full-blown affective syndrome as young adults.

Most of the studies described in this section were devised to test whether the illness of patients with borderline personality disorder eventually resolves into some discrete form of affective disorder (hypothesis II), and most failed to support that idea. So far, no one has done a comparable test for hypothesis I, to see how many depressed patients, especially those with a nonmelancholic unipolar depression, subsequently manifest other features of the borderline syndrome.

Family Prevalence

Since 1977, there have been six reports on the familial prevalence of psychiatric disorders in relative of borderline patients (Akiskal, 1981; Andrulonis et al., 1981; Loranger et al., 1982; McGlashan, 1983; Pope et al., 1983; Soloff & Millward, 1983a; Stone, 1977, 1980; Stone et al., 1981) (Table 4). The aim of these studies was to highlight clusters of specific diagnostic categories within families. Most available studies looked at first-degree relatives (parents, siblings, and children) of identified patients. This approach can demonstrate an excess occurrence of specific disorders but cannot

Table 4

Psychopathology in First-Degree Relatives of Borderline Patients[a]

Study	Diagnosis of Subjects	Diagnosable First-Degree Relatives	
		Diagnosis	Percent
Stone (1977, 1979, 1980)	Borderline personality organization, including various forms of personality disorder (N=23)	Affective disorder	19.0
	Psychotic personality organization, mainly schizophrenia, including schizoaffective and psychotic affective disorders (N=23)	Affective disorder Schizophrenia	13.0 6.7
	Borderline personality, loosely corresponding to DSM-III borderline personality disorder (N=13)	Affective disorder	27.4
Stone et al. (1981)	Borderline personality, loosely corresponding to DSM-III borderline personality disorder (N=39)	Affective disorder Schizophrenia	14.1 2.2
	Psychotic personality organization, mostly schizophrenia, including schizoaffective and psychotic affective disorders (N=36)	Affective disorder Schizophrenia	11.0 14.4
Akiskal (1981)	Borderline personality, loosely corresponding to DSM-III borderline personality disorder (N=100)	Unipolar affective disorder Bipolar affective disorder Schizophrenia	17.0[b] 17.0[b] 3.0[b]
Andrulonis et al. (1981)	Borderline personality, loosely corresponding to DSM-III borderline personality disorder (N=106)	Unipolar affective disorder Schizophrenia	32.1[b] 3.8[b]
	Affective disorder (unipolar, N=32; dysthymic, N=19; bipolar, N=4) (N=55)	Unipolar affective disorder Schizophrenia	45.5[b] 5.5[b]
	Schizophrenia (N=55)	Unipolar affective disorder Schizophrenia	37.7[b] 20.0[b]
Loranger et al. (1982)[c]	Borderline personality disorder (N=83)	Unipolar affective disorder Bipolar affective disorder Borderline personality disorder	6.4 0.5 11.7
	Bipolar affective disorder (N=100)	Unipolar affective disorder Bipolar affective disorder Schizophrenia Borderline personality disorder	7.4 2.3 0.2 0.7
	Schizophrenia (N=100)	Unipolar affective disorder Bipolar affective disorder Schizophrenia Borderline personality disorder	2.0 0.4 2.9 1.4

| Study | Diagnosis of Subjects | Diagnosable First-Degree Relatives | |
		Diagnosis	Percent
Soloff & Millward (1983a)	Borderline personality disorder (N=48)	Unipolar affective disorder	8.7
		Schizophrenia	2.6
		Antisocial personality disorder	7.0
	Unipolar affective disorder (N=32)	Unipolar affective disorder	15.0
		Schizophrenia	1.9
		Antisocial personality disorder	4.4
	Schizophrenia (N=42)	Unipolar affective disorder	5.0
		Schizophrenia	4.5
		Antisocial personality disorder	3.5
Pope et al. (1983)[c]	Borderline personality disorder (N=33)	Affective disorder	7.2
		Antisocial, borderline, histrionic personality disorders	7.7
	Borderline personality disorder with affective disorder (N=17)	Affective disorder	10.1
		Antisocial, borderline, histrionic personality disorders	5.8
	Borderline personality disorder without affective disorder (N=16)	Affective disorder	1.6
		Antisocial, borderline, histrionic personality disorders	9.8
	Bipolar affective disorder (N=16)	Affective disorder	7.5
		Antisocial, borderline, histrionic personality disorders	0.6
	Schizophrenia (N=31)	Affective disorder	0.6
		Antisocial, borderline, histrionic personality disorders	2.2

[a] All diagnostic categories are consistent with DSM-III unless otherwise indicated.
[b] Percent of patients who had at least one relative with the disorder, as opposed to percent of first-degree relatives with the disorder.
[c] Relatives were assessed by raters who were blind to the diagnosis of the index subject.

distinguish between purely genetic effects and environmental factors of growing up in a particular setting.

Stone made the groundbreaking studies in research on families of borderline patients (Stone, 1977, 1979, 1980, 1981). His reports derived from three sequential sample populations—his clinical practice, the New York State Psychiatric Institute, and the Westchester Division of Cornell. These studies documented that first-degree relatives of patients with broadly defined borderline personality disorder were at greater risk of having an affective disorder than were relatives of a control group of patients with psychosis (primarily schizophrenia but also some psychotic affective disorders) and introduced the idea of a genetic affiliation between borderline personality and affective disorder. From a somewhat different viewpoint, Akiskal (1981) reported that 17% of his sample of borderline patients had at least one first-degree relative with unipolar affective disorder; another—possibly overlapping—17% had at least one relative with bipolar affective disorder.

These initial reports provided incentive for several methodologically superior studies. Andrulonis et al. (1981) initially reported that first-degree relatives of a sample of patients with strictly defined borderline disorder appeared to have a greater-than-expected prevalence of affective disorder. However, Andrulonis and Vogel (unpublished paper) subsequently concluded that the rates observed were comparable to those for relatives of a schizophrenic comparison group and much less than those for relatives of a sample of patients with affective disorders. They tried explicitly to exclude borderline patients who had a concurrent affective disorder, and their relative success in doing so may account for some of the differences between their results and those of the earlier studies.

Loranger et al. (1982) were the first to use raters blind to the diagnosis of the patient to assess relatives; for comparison, they used patients with bipolar affective disorder and patients with schizophrenia as controls (Table 4). Due to problems of obtaining information about relatives, the investigators used the same criteria but a lower threshold for diagnosing relatives than for diagnosing the index subjects. With respect to affective disorder and schizophrenia, first-degree relatives of borderline patients more closely resembled relatives of bipolar patients than they did relatives of schizophrenic patients, although their prevalence of bipolar disease was closer to that of the latter group. Most strikingly, they were at least 10 times more likely than relatives of either comparison group to have been treated at some time for a "borderline-like" disorder.

Soloff and Millward (1983a) also studied first-degree relatives of borderline patients and of control subjects with unipolar depression and schizophrenia (Table 4). They too found a higher prevalence of affective disorder in families of borderline patients compared with those of schizophrenic patients but much less than with families of unipolar depressed patients. Looking at antisocial personality disorder, they found that the families of borderline patients had almost twice the prevalence of either comparison group. Unfortunately, they did not assess patients with other types of personality disorder, including borderline personality disorder, so no comparisons can be made with the results of Loranger et al. (1982). Within the borderline sample, however, they identified an index group of patients with schizotypal personality disorder. There was no evidence of an increased prevalence of schizophrenia in first-degree relatives of these patients either; the prevalence of affective disorder was comparable to that of the entire borderline group. This argues against the idea that studies of borderline patients with schizotypal features may artificially lower the prevalence of affective disorder in relatives.

Finally, Pope et al. (1983) assessed relatives of several groups of carefully diagnosed patients, including borderline patients with or without concurrent affective disorder, patients with schizophrenia, and patients with bipolar affective disorder (Table 4). Raters blindly assessed the relatives for schizophrenia, affective disorder, and three personality disorders. Again, relatives of borderline patients had an increased prevalence of affective illness—but only if the patient also had an affective disorder. Without this distinction, the rate of affective disorder in the first-degree relatives of borderline patients resembled the results of Loranger et al. (1982) and Soloff and Millward. Comparison within the group shows that the presence of an affective disorder in the identified patient is associated with a fivefold increase in the prevalence of affective disorder in the family. This suggests that research results might be greatly affected by selection criteria changing the percentage of effective disorder in samples of borderline patients. Pope et al. (1983) also found more people with personality disorders among the relatives of patients with borderline personality, with a trend toward a greater prevalence among relatives of borderline patients without affective illness.

Taken together, these studies are informative but incomplete. Relatives of borderline patients have an increased prevalence of personality disorders compared with those of patients with affective disorder or schizophrenia, but neither the overall magnitude nor the distribution among types of personality disorders is known. Also, it is unclear how these relatives would differ from those of patients with nonborderline personality disorders. It seems likely that much of the observed increase in prevalence of affective disorders in families of borderline patients results from the concurrent presence of affective disorder in the borderline patients, but what types of affective disorder? The data suggest that bipolar disorder probably is not involved. Much of the variability among studies results from idiosyncracies in sample populations, diagnostic criteria, and methodological approaches. The studies do not support the idea that either disorder arises from the other (hypotheses I and II). The results of Pope et al. (1983) are consistent with their being mutually independent (hypothesis III).

Psychodynamic Factors

Major depression is diagnosed in DSM-III on the basis of specific signs and symptoms, without regard to their etiology. Thus, even though some borderline patients meet such criteria, they may differ from other depressed patients on the basis of such important psychodynamic factors as underlying meanings, circumstances that lead to depression, and the effect of the depression on the person's ongoing self- and world view. Data for this area of investigation derive largely from the clinical observations and theoretical inferences drawn from psychotherapy. Therefore, the conclusions here must be understood in the context of possible observer and sampling biases present in such work.

There have been two somewhat varying psychodynamic formulations of depression in borderline patients. The first and most widely known is "abandonment depression," proposed by Masterson (1972). He posited that traumatic separations during the rapprochement subphase of early development create a basic depressive nexus in borderline patients that is then defended against with rage, primitive psychological defenses, action, and withdrawal. This depression is thought to underlie many of the behaviors that typify the borderline syndrome and to endure as a chronic part of the character, breaking through only at times into symptomatic expression. The content of this depressive experience—emptiness, despair, and hopelessness—has been compared with Spitz's concept of anaclitic depression (Grinker et al., 1968; Masterson, 1976). Masterson's formulation was essentially reiterated in later accounts by Hartocollis (1977) and Rinsley (1982).

A second formulation emphasizes the pervasive sense of "inner badness" that many borderline patients experience. It too conceives of depression as a part of the borderline character structure, this time as a result of an enduring self-image as evil and destructive. This formulation gives a central role to dissociated anger: depression is both a reaction to and an introjected expression of this affective state (Buie & Adler, 1982; Gunderson, 1984). Kernberg (1967) viewed this self-accusation as the product of a primitive superego and posited that the depression of borderline patients characteristically is accompanied by ego disorganization. This formulation emphasizes the central importance of anger toward needed others: anger that is experienced as dangerous is redirected inward and finds its introjected expression in depression.

According to the first formulation, borderline patients use anger and other types of "acting out" to defend against an anaclitic-like depression, but not always successfully. According to the second, their depression is characterized by self-condemnation that is thought to represent a defensive reaction to aggressive impulses toward others. In both these formulations, the depressive affect is symptomatic only intermittently and is intimately connected to the current state of object relationships. However, the personality structure contains a lasting vulnerability such as poor self-image or the need to avoid the experience of depression.

Few investigators have attempted to categorize depressions according to differentiating psychological features (Val et al., 1982). This is true even for such large subgroups as chronic versus reactive and melancholic versus nonmelancholic depressions. One exception is that both of the above formulations differentiate the depression of borderline patients from those depressions characterized by guilt, remorse, or a sense of failure, i.e., those depressions believed to be characteristic of a healthier personality and a more integrated superego. Yet, even in this instance, the difference may be mainly one of degree, insofar as healthier depressed individuals have only partial aspects of the self under attack, but borderline patients experience attacks on the entire self.

A second inroad into this area is offered by a recent empirical study by Soloff and Millward (1983b), which indicates that a pathological sensitivity to separation experiences is twice as common among borderline depressed patients as among nonborderline depressed patients. This finding confirms the central hypothesis of the first formulation and is consistent with the predictions of the second one. This and other studies (Bradley, 1979; Walsh, 1977) also implicate early parental loss as especially prevalent in borderline patients. Such work suggests that identifiable pathogenic developmental processes may help to differentiate depression in borderline patients from primary depression.

Clearly, the above material supports the idea that borderline personality disorder can produce depression (hypothesis II), but it is not inconsistent with other hypotheses. For example, the traumatic separations emphasized in the first formulation and the warded-off rage postulated in the second might become pathological only with a preexisting biophysiological vulnerability. In this regard, Donald Klein (1975, 1977) has suggested that the usually tolerable frustrations of early life may permanently affect some people because of biological or physiological factors that mold their responses. If true, this would be consistent with the idea that the borderline syndrome arises from a primary affective disorder (hypothesis I).

Biological Factors

At present there is no independent biological hypothesis for borderline personality disorder. The clinical tests suggested as markers of depression include a nonsuppressing dexamethasone suppression test (DST) result, blunted thyrotropin (TSH) response, and altered sleep EEGs. None is sensitive or specific enough for depression to be an ideal research tool for studying a depressive component in other disorders (Baldessarini, 1983), but they do represent a theoretically attractive way of examining the overlap between borderline and affective disorders.

Carroll et al. (1981) reported that of 21 subjects with DSM-III diagnoses of borderline personality disorder, 62% had an abnormal DST. Nearly all of the nonsuppressors had a concurrent diagnosis of major depression; almost none of the suppressors had that diagnosis. Sternbach et al. (1983) studied 13 women who completely met and 11 who were one criterion short of meeting a DSM-III diagnosis of borderline personality disorder. All 24 women had unspecified "depressive features," and 17 met DSM-III criteria for major depression. A nonsuppressing DST was found in 65% of patients with major depression and 29% of the remainder, compared with 7% of 14 healthy control subjects. In contrast, Soloff et al. (1982) studied seven patients with borderline, five with schizotypal, and seven with mixed personality disorders diagnosed according to DSM-III. Fourteen of these 19 patients also met criteria for major depression. Soloff et al. found a total of three abnormal DSTs (16%) in the 19 patients, all in subjects who also had been diagnosed as depressed. These results are difficult to reconcile with each other. If, as many have suggested, the DST is a nonspecific indicator of severity of illness, they may, in part, reflect such differences among the patient populations.

Blunting of the usual TSH response to thyrotropin-releasing hormone (TRH) is even less established as a marker of depression than is the DST. However, two groups have extended its use to borderline patients. Garbutt et al. (1983) found a blunted response in seven (47%) of 15 borderline subjects diagnosed by DSM-III criteria, compared with no blunting in any of a group of matched control subjects. Five of the patients with a blunted response had concurrent diagnoses of alcoholism or depression, but two had only the borderline diagnosis. Sternbach et al. (1983) also measured TSH blunting; 41% of the depressed and 29% of the nondepressed borderline women they studied showed blunting. These results are somewhat higher than the 25%–30% typically reported in pure depression (Loosen & Prange, 1982).

Sleep EEGs in borderline patients have been more promising than either the DST or the TSH response to TRH. Akiskal (1981) first noted that REM latencies in the sample of eight borderline patients resembled those of a depressed control group. His finding was confirmed by McNamara et al. (1984), who studied 10 borderline patients who also had substantial depressive symptoms during testing. Bell et al. (1983) compared the sleep architecture of a group of eight inpatients with DSM-III diagnoses of both major depression and borderline disorder with that of 11 nonborderline depressed patients and found no differences between the groups. The cause of decreased REM latency in depression remains unknown, but, inasmuch as it is specific for depression, it suggests that the affective disorder of borderline patients resembles that of patients with other types of depression. However, all of these subject populations were selected in ways that probably assured a high prevalence of both borderline and affective disorder, so the reports do little to distinguish among the various hypotheses.

The use of biological markers may be of some utility in studying the interface between affective disorders and borderline personality, but more progress needs to be made in finding sensitive and specific markers for depression. In addition, when such tests are used in studies of borderline patients, care must be taken to distinguish between subjects with and without concurrent affective disorders and to use control groups of patients with other personality disorders. Still, given the current state of such tests, they are unlikely to be definitive in clarifying interrelationships between these two disorders in the near future.

Drug Response

Although borderline patients account for 8%–20% of hospital admissions and frequently receive medications (Cole & Sunderland, 1982; Cole et al., 1984; Soloff, 1981), controlled studies of their drug responsivity have just recently begun. Perhaps as a result of this lack of needed data, competing advice ranges from using no drugs at all to using each of the major drug classes. Antipsychotics have been used for many years in varying doses; several investigators currently advocate low doses (Brinkley et al., 1979; Leone, 1982).

Donald Klein's controversial category of "hysteroid dysphoria" (1975, 1977) is a type of recurrent, atypical depression thought to occur in some borderline patients that may be particularly responsive to monoamine oxidase inhibitors (MAOIs). Initial data suggest that MAOIs are useful primarily in decreasing the chronic feelings of emptiness or boredom and impulsive actions, including those which are self-damaging, and that they are less effective for treating other long-term borderline features (Liebowitz & Klein, 1981).

In retrospective reviews of drug responses of well-defined hospitalized borderline patients, both Soloff (1981) and Cole et al. (1984) concluded independently that drug response was heterogeneous. Some patients seemed to respond to antidepressants, others to antipsychotics. Soloff (1981) found that either class of drugs was superior to no drug therapy; 63% of medicated patients showed improvement, compared with 19% of unmedicated patients. He also found no differences in outcome of patients given antipsychotics, antidepressants, or a combination of the two.

Cole et al. (1984) found that borderline patients with a concurrent affective disorder were more responsive to antidepressants and antipsychotics than were those who had only borderline personality disorder. However, such patients did not have the response rates expected for purely depressed patients. In a study using some of the same patient population, Pope et al. (1983) found that among patients having only borderline personality disorder, only 37% were treated with drugs and none showed a clear response. However, 77% of borderline patients with an affective disorder received medications, and about half definitely responded. Responses in this latter group were equally distributed among patients receiving antipsychotics, antidepressants, or lithium. This result is in accord with the report by Charney et al. (1981) that fewer nonmelancholic depressed borderline patients responded to drug treatment than did those without a personality disorder (36% versus 76%, respectively). Similarly, Gaviria et al. (1982) found that bipolar patients with borderline personality disorder had a poorer response to lithium maintenance than did those without a personality disorder. There is no information about whether individual patients respond equally well to any of the drug classes, but that does not seem likely.

Much remains to be learned about the use of medication in borderline personality disorder. With respect to the overlap between affective disorder and borderline disorder, antidepressants appear to be useful at times, especially when an affective disorder is present. But even when they are useful, the response rate appears to be lower than expected. Such findings do not fit especially well with any of the three hypotheses about the relationship between affective and borderline personality disorders.

Discussion

Borderline and affective disorders have been under intense study during the past decade. That interest has heightened awareness of them and broadened their role in differential diagnoses. It seems clear now that both diagnostic categories include heterogeneous subgroups whose differentiating features remain to be elucidated. As a byproduct of the work in this area, the longstanding controversy about the boundaries of borderline personality disorder has shifted from schizophrenia to the affective disorders, and the longstanding interest in the relationship between personality and affective syndromes has surfaced with fresh vigor and rapidly accumulating information. The easiest summary of the data just reviewed is that more research is needed and that an assessment of the available literature can only capture the state of a field still in motion. Still, we believe that the existing research strongly suggests the inadequacy of several of the existing hypotheses about the relationship between borderline personality disorder and affective disorder. We suggest that a different viewpoint is needed.

Hypothesis I suggests that a primary depression can produce behaviors that result in a diagnosis of borderline personality disorder. This hypothesis receives little support (Table 5). The stability of the borderline diagnosis over time argues against it, as does the fact that antidepressants are not the treatment of choice for even the majority of such patients. Also, borderline patients have an increased frequency of relatives with personality disorders compared with patients with affective disorder, suggesting that the disorders can run independently in families. Furthermore, many borderline patients never display a symptom picture of major depression. Those affective disorders with which borderline syndrome seems to have the greatest overlap—unipolar nonmelancholic depressions—have the weakest evidence for biogenetic

Table 5

Evaluations of Four Hypotheses About the Interface Between
Borderline Personality Disorder and Affective Disorder[a]

	Evaluative Strategy						
Hypothesis	Incidence	Phenomenology	Course	Family Prevalence	Psychodynamic Factors	Biological Factors	Drug Response
I. Affective disorder is the primary problem; it can produce signs and symptoms of borderline personality disorder as well	+	–	– –	–	0	+	– –
II. Borderline character pathology is the primary problem; it can produce signs and symptoms of affective disorder as well	+	+	–	–	+	0	+
III. Affective disorder and borderline personality disorder are unrelated but can coexist in the same person because they are so common	– –	–	+	+ +	–	+	–
IV. Both diagnoses rely on signs and symptoms that can arise from a variety of sources; some of the resulting heterogeneous population have both syndromes	+	+ +	+	+ +	0	+	+ +

[a] Scores represent the consensus of J.G.G. and G.R.E. about whether the evidence supports or refutes each hypothesis: – – means strongly refutes, – means somewhat refutes, 0 means equivocal, + means supports, and + + means strongly supports.

determinants (Baldessarini, 1983; Gershon et al., 1976) and are relatively unresponsive to drugs (Baldessarini, 1983). Nonetheless, some borderline patients do have a concurrent major affective disorder that can respond to the expected medications.

Hypothesis II proposes that depression is secondary to the primary processes of the borderline syndrome; again, it has no compelling support (Table 5). Arguing against it is the evidence that, even for borderline patients without depression, there is some family loading for affective disorder. Also, such patients may have biological markers like those of depressed patients. However, there are differences in the depression that borderline patients experience and that of the more typical affective disorders, including qualitative aspects of symptom presentation and underlying psychodynamic etiologies. In addition, borderline patients appear to be less responsive to antidepressant medications than patients with major depressions. Perhaps, for at least some borderline patients, depression results from an interaction between the consequences of certain behavioral traits and the existence of an underlying biological or psychological vulnerability to depression.

Hypothesis III, which suggests that affective disorder and borderline personality disorder are independent but can coexist, has somewhat more support (Table 5). Both family prevalence and longitudinal studies suggest that the disorders can follow independent courses in the same person. Thus, families of borderline patients have a higher prevalence of personality disorders whether or not the identified patients have a concurrent affective disorder; but only the families of patients with an affective disorder also have a loading for affective disease. However, prevalence studies repeatedly have shown that borderline personality disorder and affective disorder coexist in patients more frequently than expected. Also, the affective symptoms of patients with both disorders ought to be more responsive to drugs than they appear to be.

We propose a fourth hypothesis that we think fits the data better than does any of the other three. Both borderline personality and affective disorder are diagnosed with signs and symptoms arising from many sources. Hypothesis IV suggests that the observed concurrence of affective and borderline symptoms results from the heterogeneity. For either disorder, individuals may start with a biophysiological vulnerability that increases their risk of being psychologically impaired in early development. Such early traumas may create vulnerability to either or both disorders, but the actual presentation varies as a function of later physiological and psychological reactions to environment and temperament. The key to the overlap and dissimilarities between these two disorders, then, may be a constellation of innate and external factors that are inconsequential individually but combine to shape depression, chronic dysphoria, or borderline behavior—alone or in any possible combination.

Hypothesis IV is supported by all of the evidence of heterogeneity within this patient population (Table 5). As noted, the actual overlap between borderline and affective disorders remains to be established, but all existing data suggest that it is higher than expected. Both the phenomenology and drug response are especially consistent with the concept of a variety of etiologies leading to a common endpoint. In the family prevalence studies, distinguishing borderline patients with a full affective syndrome from those without one simplified and clarified the data—again supporting the existence of subgroups that may have interactive effects.

Patients at the interface of affective and borderline personality disorders often present troubling and persistent problems for the clinician. These patients include not only those who fit contemporary criteria for these disorders but some who fulfill criteria for other diagnoses such as chronic dysphoria, hysteroid dysphoria, cyclothymia, and other personality disorders. Their problems tend to be chronic, with repeated exacerbations, and they often show no or only a partial response to any of the available forms of treatment. Research is needed to identify the relevant subgroups within this heterogeneous group. The evidence reviewed in this paper suggests that important factors in such analyses will include the prominence and chronicity of affective symptoms, individual variations in psychological and biological factors, longitudinal course, family prevalence, and drug responsivity. This conclusion is not critical of the existing boundary; rather, it opposes any conceptualization that call for sharply discontinuous categorical concepts of these two diagnostic groups. As such, this review points toward the broader need to accept the present divisions between axis I and II as paradigmatic, not actual.

The New Psychoanalysis and Psychoanalytic Revisionism

Book Review Essay on Borderline Conditions and Pathological Narcissism[1]

Victor Calef, M.D., and Edward M. Weinshel, M.D.
(1979)

The volume under discussion contains much that is essential in the thinking of one of the most prominent contributors to American psychoanalysis within the last decade. This essay, therefore, is intended as a critique not only of the book, *Borderline Conditions and Pathological Narcissism,* but of the continuing body of work it represents.[2]

Most of the papers which make up this book have been widely read and enthusiastically received; their subject matter enjoys a popularity and currency in the psychoanalytic marketplace (and the whole "mental health" field in general)[3] which should not be dismissed simply as transient or faddish; and the whole area of the "borderline" has become ineluctably identified with the author's name. Terms such as "splitting," "projective identification," and "internalized object relationships" which not too long ago merely evoked fuzzy associations to alien and dissident psychoanalytic

Reprinted with permission from *The Psychoanalytic Quarterly, 48,* 470–491, 1979.

schools of thought have now become an integral part of the lexicon of a large number of American psychoanalysts, candidates, residents, and other workers in allied fields. In fact, no other single colleague has been so instrumental in confronting American psychoanalysts with Kleinian concepts and theories. Similarly, while Kernberg has by no means been the only or the first analyst to concentrate his efforts in therapeutic work with the more disturbed psychologically ill patient, no other analyst has caught the imagination and aroused the interest of so many co-workers in such endeavors as has Kernberg. The impact and influence that have been exerted in the past dozen years by the theoretical and technical formulations presented in these papers constitute a social phenomenon which in many ways resembles a cult movement within the scientific community.

A particularly impressive facet of this "social phenomenon" and one not readily explicable is the relative paucity of *open* controversy which has characterized the introduction of Kernberg's ideas and formulations. While there has probably been the usual degree of "corridor criticism" in reaction to his writings, our literature has conspicuously lacked the kind of direct critical evaluations which we might have anticipated from the psychoanalytic community, the members of which are hardly known for docile acceptance of broad and significant revisions of analytic theory—be those revisions real or illusory. Only a few such evaluations come to mind. Perhaps the most comprehensive and probably still the most cogent and incisive critique of Kernberg's hypotheses of the discussion of his paper "Structural Derivatives of Object Relationships" (Kernberg, 1966) by Paula Heimann (the extended version of which can be found in Heimann, 1966) at the 1965 Amsterdam Congress of the International Psycho-Analytical Association. In this presentation[4] Heimann raised pertinent questions about Kernberg's structural models, his description of the early infantile defense mechanisms, his conceptualization of the process of internalization, the whole issue of splitting versus repression, and the problems of the "evidential value" of his strategy of interpretations. We are not aware of any other comparable critical effort in the psychoanalytic literature. Atkin (1975, p. 41, n.) appears to challenge at least the semantics of Kernberg's utilization of the concept of splitting. Both Dahl (1974) and Holzman (1976, pp. 265–267) raise brief but penetrating objections to Kernberg's methodology, his lack of clarity, and to his glossing over the place of thought processes in his theoretical formulations. The extent to which "the borderline" (alternately designated the "borderline state" or the "borderline patient" or Kernberg's "borderline personality organization") can be viewed as a reasonably discrete clinical entity (let alone a theoretical one) has never been entirely settled and some concern has been voiced that attempts to establish "the borderline" as a distinct psychopathological condition may be misleading and potentially confusing. Spruiell (1976) expresses definite doubts about the validity of Kernberg's conceptualization of idealization and the structural hypotheses which underlie such a formulation. Witenberg (1976), in referring to Kernberg's theory of narcissism, has called it a jerry-built concept that heaps metaphor upon metaphor.

While this list of critiques is incomplete, we believe that a more comprehensive one would produce a pathetically "thin soup" in comparison with the impressive enthusiasm evoked and the equally impressive number of ostensibly confirmatory scientific contributions which have been stimulated by the papers in this book. The reasons for such a relatively uncritical acceptance are neither clear nor easy to explain in a convincing fashion.

It must be evident by now that we harbor reservations and questions in regard to both Kernberg's theoretical concepts and the technical procedures which he has advocated. Both warrant, really necessitate, considerably more investigation than they have received thus far. Such an endeavor is, we submit, particularly important for psychoanalysts because Kernberg's work includes a number of significant, if not always explicit, additions to and revisions of psychoanalytic theory. Moreover, these theoretical modifications are frequently presented as if established, even though their basis and justification are not clear either from the clinical data supplied or from the theoretical discussion Kernberg offers.

The book is divided into two sections: the first is "The Borderline Personality Organization"; the second, "The Narcissistic Personality." For all practical purposes, however, this devolves into what is essentially a chronological order: the borderline papers from 1965–1971, those on narcissism from 1970–1974. We have decided, for a variety of reasons, to concentrate in our discussion on the part of the book dealing with the borderline personality organization rather than the section on narcissism. We think, however, that in a general way most of what we say about the borderline material is equally applicable to that on pathological narcissism.

One rationale justifying such a focus is the degree of repetition from chapter to chapter. There is, unfortunately, also a good deal of redundancy within chapters, and relatively little attempt has been made to describe transitions from one paper to another in terms of changes in Kernberg's thinking from one phase to another. As a result there is ambiguity and uncertainty as to whether a given position is an older or a more recent one. If a shift in thinking has occurred, what was the basis for an altered emphasis or formulation from one chapter to the next? We suggest that Kernberg would have very much enhanced both the readability and the value of his work had he made it clear from the very onset that what was being offered was the republication of these papers and, even more, had he provided the reader with a series of editorial introductions—however brief—to each of the chapters emphasizing the chief points he wished to underscore and explicating the transitions from chapter to chapter.

Kernberg has embarked on the serious venture of incorporating within his own theoretical framework object relations theory, Kleinian theory, ego psychology theory, the developmental approach, Bionian theory, and probably others as well. The very scope and complexity of such an endeavor is in itself an admirable project. Although the *idea* of such psychoanalytic ecumenism looms up as a conceptual tour de force, it is not a task which can be accomplished with ease or with simplicity. Whatever the intrinsic values and virtues of these various orientations, they are not so congenial that they blend together automatically or smoothly. As one consequence, Kernberg has to be selective. He has extracted from these various bodies of thought specific elements which have helped him to construct and then to buttress his formulations. In so doing, he has created a loose theoretical amalgam—or, to shift metaphors, a "part-object" pseudo-synthesis. In fact, has he not created theory out of theory itself? An example is his utilization of Kleinian theory, from which he has borrowed a number of basic conceptual planks while rejecting others of equal importance to the Kleinian concept. In our view, this adventitious theory-building does conceptual violence both to the old theory and the new product. For example, and without going into detail, positing a Kleinian mechanism of *active splitting* without giving equal weight to the idea of "a higher degree of ego organization than is usually postulated by Freud" (Segal, 1964, p. 13) generates potential misunderstanding and confusion. Kernberg could have attained a considerably greater degree of clarity and avoided a certain amount of that potential misunderstanding, had he more explicitly indicated the theoretical base for his various elements from other theoretical systems, together with some of the reasoning behind the particular ways in which he has attempted to weave portions of these often somewhat disparate systems into a consistent frame of reference. In short, one of our fundamental reservations is that Kernberg has not made his fundamental assumptions clear.

Another source of confusion, for us at least, lies in the clinical data which Kernberg has utilized. More often than not, it was not altogether clear to us whether those data derived from the beginning, middle, or advanced stages of treatment; from his own cases in psychoanalysis, psychotherapy (supportive or expressive), or from his modified psychoanalytic approach; from the experiences of his colleagues, or from the Menninger Research Project (cf., Kernberg et al., 1972). Although each of these approaches has its own particular rationale and value, we do not feel that the clinical data emerging from these diverse therapies necessarily have the equivalent meaning, significance, or validity for understanding the process from an analytic point of view or for the testing of psychoanalytic propositions. Further, the very brevity of the clinical material (most of which has been condensed to vignettes) makes it difficult to follow what actually takes place in the therapeutic setting. Throughout, the clinical reality of the patient remains obscure. The fact that more often than not Kernberg tends to lean on inferential data more than on descriptions of actual behavior and verbal associations actually given by the patient does not help his readers to form their own picture of what is going on in the patient and in the treatment process. It was our impression that later in the book, the clinical material became more explicit, somewhat more clear, and more useful. On the whole, though, we had considerable trouble in reconciling that material with the specific point (theoretical or technical) that Kernberg was making.[5]

In this same vein, we do not believe that it is altogether clear *what* Kernberg means by terms such as "supportive therapy," "expressive therapy," "psychoanalytic psychotherapy," "modified psychoanalysis"; what he sees as the crucial technical procedures in these therapies; how he conceptualizes the therapeutic goals and aims for each of them; and how he conceptualizes the differences between such therapies and the so-called classical or unmodified psychoanalysis. We recognize that these are, by no means, simple questions. In a sense, it may not be fair to ask them. Some of these issues are raised in the Menninger Psychotherapy Research Project Report (Kernberg et al., 1972) and, albeit rather cursorily, in this volume. Nevertheless, in view of the importance of the theoretical and technical innovations that Kernberg is advancing, a more explicit discussion of these points would have been welcome in this collection of papers.

Similarly, a somewhat more clear-cut delineation of the meaning of such items as "a micro-paranoid attitude," the "metabolism" or "non-metabolism" of internal object relationships, or of the "systematic" analysis of resistances would have been helpful. It is not always clear to us when Kernberg uses a certain term (for instance "technical neutrality") whether he is using such terms in an idiosyncratic sense.[6] Kernberg does not always make it clear whether he is deliberately or inadvertently revising such concepts as conflict, defense, transference, instinct theory, and so forth.

It is this very boldness and thrust which demands an ever sedulous determination on the part of the author to clarify precisely, and an equally assiduous but open-minded scrutiny on the part of the reader of what, in Kernberg's lavish array of ideas, is or is not in accord with one's own theoretical understanding and clinical observations. The problems to which he addresses himself and the solutions which he proffers are too important to allow us to settle for less.

In regard to the borderline personality organization, the lynchpin of Kernberg's thesis is spelled out on the first page of the first chapter when he states, "There exists an important group of psychopathological constellations which have in common a rather *specific* and remarkably *stable* form of pathological ego structure. The ego pathology differs from that found in the neuroses and the less severe characterological illnesses on one hand, and the psychoses on the other hand. These patients must be considered to occupy a borderline area between neurosis and psychosis" (p. 3, italics added). The words "specific" and "stable" denote a reasonably delineated psychological entity and presume the possibility of a reasonably accurate diagnosis granting the utilization of a "thorough diagnostic examination" (p. 4) and, at the same time, the possibility of the application of "specific therapeutic approaches" (ibid.). A very sizable portion of Part I of this book is devoted to the elaboration of these points: the specific ego pathology, its purported genesis, and the clinical manifestations which reflect that pathology; the clinical recognition, diagnosis, and differential diagnosis of the "group of psychopathological constellations" which make up the borderline personality organization; and ways in which the recognition and understanding of these phenomena can be utilized in devising a strategy which can be applied in the psychotherapy of such disorders.

There are few less enviable tasks facing the psychoanalyst than those related to psychoanalytic nosology. For that reason alone, Kernberg's effort to bring some order into at least one segment of psychopathological classification is in itself a most ambitious and prodigious agendum. Nor has Kernberg contented himself with a superficial, perfunctory lip service to the problem of diagnosis and classification. His is, indeed, a most serious and comprehensive program for the delineation of the borderline personality organization and its differentiation from related and outwardly similar conditions. His "thorough diagnostic evaluation" includes a "descriptive analysis," a "structural analysis," and a "genetic dynamic analysis." Although he does not develop this point in great detail, he calls (p. 4) for the use of psychological testing in those areas where clinical observations may be ambiguous. His discussions on differential diagnosis between borderline personality organization and the so-called classical prepsychotic personality structures (pp. 11–21) are exhaustive and pinpointed, even to atomistic distinctions. Further, in an area where he might have been, quite legitimately, vague and relatively noncommittal, he has not hesitated to be precise and concise.

Yet, after all is said and done, we cannot help but wonder if all of these efforts are successful. We must ask whether the nature and quantity of the data available to us and to Kernberg is truly amenable to the kind of precise categorization and systematization which Kernberg has undertaken. Further, we would ask whether these attempts at precision have in fact resulted in a real clarification of a "syndrome" or, rather, an obfuscation of what remains an area of obscurity. Our own reaction is that despite a number of disclaimers to the contrary, Kernberg has been too intent on isolating too many psychopathological entities and making sure that each was securely placed in its appropriate diagnostic pigeonhole. Consequently, as we studied this volume, we did not experience a comfortable feeling of conviction that these various pathologies (including, most importantly, the borderline personality organization) could be distinguished in a reasonable way on either a clinical or theoretical level utilizing the data and/or the frames of reference Kernberg suggests.

An example of the type of inevitable difficulty with which Kernberg has had to cope is evident from the beginning of his discourse in his selection of a label for the psychopathological entity he tries to describe. On page 13, for instance, one may observe the awkwardness of trying to differentiate a "personality" from a "character" from an "organization." While it is easy to go along with Kernberg's disinclination to become encumbered by the "confusion in the literature . . . caused by the fact that the term 'borderline' was used to refer both to the transitory acute manifestations of patients who were rapidly regressing from neurotic symptomatology to an overt psychotic reaction, and also to patients who function chronically in a stable way at a level which was borderline between neurosis and psychosis" (p. 5), it does not seem that he has avoided the murkiness and confusion involved in trying to separate and differentiate the personality organization from the character neurosis and character disorder. Complexity multiplies as Kernberg introduces the concepts of high, middle, and low level characters. All of these words represent the attempt to describe an apparent concatenation of groups of psychological manifestations which can be observed with a reasonable degree of predictability in certain individuals over a period of time. All of these words are, to some extent, artifacts insofar as all of these concatenations are relative and not altogether reliable. To speak of the infantile personality as a "middle range" character neurosis that actually reaches "into the typical borderline field" and to distinguish this from the narcissistic personality which is "a typical 'low level' character disorder, although it reaches up into the middle range of the continuum" (p. 13) seems to us to presume considerably greater knowledge and clinical diagnostic acumen than we really possess.

Thus Kernberg's section on descriptive analysis (pp. 8–21) repeatedly suggests the ability to make subtle differential diagnoses that we seriously question can be made in a reasonably reliable manner by even a highly experienced and skilled clinician (the same can be said of many aspects of Chapter IV on prognosis). Even though he warns that "these descriptive elements are only presumptive diagnostic signs of borderline personality organization" (p. 9), the tone of his text is not consistent with his disclaimer. Further, as one reads through the long list of overt clinical manifestations, it would appear that virtually every patient (and probably every nonpatient as well) would demonstrate two or three clinical manifestations, which Kernberg indicates "strongly points to the possibility of an underlying borderline personality organization" (p. 9).

Kernberg would appear to be on much more solid ground in his insistence that the "definite diagnosis depends on characteristic ego pathology and not on the descriptive symptoms" (ibid.). We are skeptical (and in some respects Kernberg seems to agree) that the analysis and understanding of this "characteristic ego pathology" can be carried out reliably in the initial interviews. Such determination must await the more telling and unequivocal data that can be ascertained in the ongoing therapeutic work. But here the clinician and the reader are caught in an impossible dilemma since Kernberg claims that the borderline personality organization requires, as noted earlier, "a specific therapeutic approach which can only derive from an accurate diagnostic study." How, therefore, does one apply that correct approach without a complete and accurate diagnostic study and before the therapy itself? Kernberg is not unaware of this problem. He suggests that the patient's response to certain interpretations may be used to differentiate the borderline personality organization from the psychotic (pp. 173–180). In situations which "require the differential diagnosis of borderline conditions versus a schizophrenic reaction" (p. 179), the interview should be structured "so that the testing of defensive operations can be carried out." "Interpretations of the predominant primitive defensive operations in borderline patients tend to strengthen ego functioning and increase reality testing, [while] the same approach may bring about further regression (uncovering the underlying lack of differentiation between self and non-self) in psychotic patients" (ibid.).

Superficially such a recommendation may appear quite reasonable, but we have a number of reservations about such a procedure. We assume, of course, that Kernberg is referring not just to "interpretations" but more pointedly to approximately "correct" interpretations. Granting, however, that the interpretation framed by a given therapist is sensible and seemingly appropriate, how can one accurately predict, when dealing with patients at this level of disturbance, what the impact of such an interpretation might be? We believe that trying to articulate an appropriate interpretive statement involving primitive defenses and resistances could be a particularly hazardous undertaking. All of us are aware how often in our clinical work we are quite surprised (both pleasantly and unpleasantly) at the impact a given intervention or a set of interventions may exert on even reasonably healthy patients. What may seem to the therapist a bland and innocuous remark can bring about apparently devastating reactions. Conversely, what may seem to the therapist to be a potentially disruptive and threatening statement may well have a most salutary effect. We certainly do not know nearly as much as we should about these somewhat commonplace experiences, but we do recognize that the complexity of the psychic apparatus and the fluidity of that apparatus even in more stable patients make the accuracy of our "predictions" (which is what is involved in interpretations, after all) somewhat less than foolproof. With more disturbed individuals, at the moment we embark on an interpretive effort, we are simply not really sure what the exact state of the patient's mind may be: we are not certain how the patient will "hear" and experience that particular interpretation; and we can be even less confident of what will be the reverberations of the interchange. Further, unless we study in some detail just how Kernberg would approach those primitive defenses, it becomes difficult to appreciate what he would consider to be a "correct" interpretation in such instances. Such a study would have to be based on a fairly elaborate protocol of the therapeutic process rather than the brief vignettes that are available in this volume. We submit, therefore, that to depend on the reaction to what can at best be only a subjectively determined interpretation is hardly a dependable and convincing form of diagnosis.

When Edith Jacobson (1975) states (in what is, on the whole, a very positive evaluation of the volume) that parts of Kernberg's book are not "easy reading," she echoes what we experienced in studying this material. It is true, of course, that the theory being presented is difficult and abstract. For many American analysts the concepts which derive from Kleinian and from object relations orientations are not particularly familiar, and the vocabulary is at times discomfiting. However, in addition to these factors which impose a legitimate burden on the reader, some aspects of the author's style also contribute significantly to this problem. Kernberg presents a particular point or formulation in a relatively positive, direct fashion; he then modifies or qualifies his assertion, usually, we feel, for the better; but then he reiterates his original position, ostensibly disregarding his previous modification. It was by no means an infrequent experience for us to be left either with the broad generalization or with some sense of perplexity or confusion. It is only with careful scrutiny and a number of rereadings that we could discern the more judicious reservations that Kernberg had often inserted but then overridden with a fresh assertion.

Our impression is that the core of this confusion and potential confusion resides in what we earlier called the "lynchpin" of Kernberg's thesis, namely his goal of delineating a group of psychopathological constellations with "a rather specific and re-markably stable form of pathological ego structure." However, as Kernberg proceeds to unveil the profile of that entity it is evident that there is more and more overlapping with elements from other psychopathological conditions. What appears to take place is that, unwittingly or otherwise, the overlapped area becomes incorpo-rated into the orbit of the borderline personality organization. As a consequence, the borderline personality organization becomes more and more inclusive, broader, and looser. Since it encompasses either so many elements on a behavioral-descriptive level or so many internal components which (frequently going by similar or not so similar labels) are often so widespread as to be essentially universal, it has become virtually impossible to find a case which cannot be suspected and/or considered to fall within the borderline personality organization orbit.

We have deliberately emphasized the diagnostic aspects of Kernberg's presentation because, as we stated earlier, we believe that his attempt to delineate a sharply discrete clinical and structural entity is so central to his overall theory. This is particularly important inasmuch as he argues that a rigorous therapeutic approach is necessary in dealing with such patients. Further, he emphasizes that the diagnosis can be verified on the basis of the patient's response to a particular intervention. As discussed above, we feel this to be unsatisfactory theoretically and technically, and logically to be circular reasoning. The poverty of explicit clinical data further complicates the situation for the reader.

A particularly illuminating example of the kind of mental acrobatics which Kernberg is obliged to employ in order to defend the essential discreteness of the borderline personality organization as a stable and specific psychopathological entity can be seen in his attempts to characterize the quality of reality testing in that "condition." In addition, the following material illustrates quite well the stylistic "oscillations" we described earlier.

He declares (p. 4) that "these patients usually maintain their capacity for reality *except*[7] under these special circumstances— severe stress, regression induced by alcohol or drugs, and a transfer psychosis." Allowing that the basic premise is correct, do not the exceptions undermine the point he is trying to make? Would we not at least grant the possibility of some measure of impaired reality testing under those circumstances in the widest array of personality organizations, from the more fragile psychotics to the reasonably well-put-together individuals who would fall into Kernberg's category of "high-level character neuroses"? He acknowledges the "presence of some degree of lack of differentiation of self and object images and the concomitant blurring of ego boundaries" as one aspect of "a non-specific aspect of ego weakness in the borderline field, *but* this aspect is closely linked to the pathology of internalized object relationships" (p. 22). On page 36, Kernberg states that "sufficient delimitation between self and objects (stability of ego boundaries) is maintained to permit a practical, immediate adaptation to the demands of reality, *but* deeper internalization of the demands of reality, especially social reality, is made impossible by the interference of these nonintegrated self and object images with superego integrations." On page 82, Kernberg alludes to the absence of an observing ego in the borderline personality organization; on the next page he reiterates that the differentiation between self and object images has "taken place *sufficiently*," and therefore ego boundaries are *more* stable "and reality testing is also preserved to a *major* extent." On page 129, Kernberg lists "the weakening of reality testing" as a reflection of both "a general outcome of pathological ego development and the specific results of the pathology of internalized object relationships of patients with borderline personality organization." On page 135, he asserts that "reality testing in the strict sense of the capacity to differentiate intrapsychic from externally perceived events is an ego function present in patients" with borderline personality organization; but it is a function which may be transitorily lost under the conditions mentioned earlier.

On the following page, Kernberg goes on to say that the "frequency and intensity of temporary loss of reality testing are not, in themselves, important prognostic indicators" in assessing the treatability of the borderline personality organization patient except "for deciding on the possibility of psychoanalytic treatment proper in any particular case" (p. 137). However, in the following paragraph, he points out that "there is another sense in which the term reality testing may be used, a more general, less precise, and yet more subtle reference to the extent to which the patient is aware of his interpersonal or social reality, and especially of the moral values of others. Subtle alterations in the behavior of borderline patients within their ordinary social context (such as their frequent lack of perception of subtle 'messages' from other persons, their unawareness of inappropriate appearance, of the emotional reality of others, of the influence of value judgments on the behavior of other persons, of how they themselves are perceived by others, and tactlessness), all reflect loss of the more discriminatory aspects of reality testing determined by ego and superego pathology. Reality testing in this broad sense does have some prognostic value. . . ." On page 170, in discussing the technical handling of various transference reactions (and, as far as we can determine, Kernberg is not here referring to the "transference psychosis"), he emphasizes that "interpretations have to be formulated so that the patient's *distortions* of the analyst's intervention can be simultaneously and systematically examined, and the patient's *distortions* of present reality and especially of his *perceptions* in the hour can be systematically clarified." In this instance, it would appear that Kernberg is speaking of a psychoanalytic situation.

We are in no way taking issue with Kernberg's reservations, qualifications, or modifications of his basic position that the borderline personality organization patient may possess a relatively adequate reality-testing apparatus and that this essential adequacy represents one of the principal differential diagnostic points between certain characterological disorders and the psychotic patient; on the contrary, we believe that these qualifications are judicious and important. What is less easy to accept is his statement that "loss of reality testing in *any one area* indicates psychotic functioning" (p. 182). Kernberg then pulls back a bit by stressing that "this conceptualization of reality testing is a restricted, delimited one, referring exclusively to the presence or absence of the patient's capacity to identify himself *fully* with the external reality represented by the patient-therapist relationship." His very next sentence, however, would appear to represent a reversion to a categorical position inconsistent with most of the quotations we have extracted from his papers and spelled out above (we are by no means unaware of the possible pitfalls and distortions which can occur by even carefully truncated extractions). He claims that "this formulation implies that there is *no continuum,* no gradual shift from presence to absence of reality testing. . . ."

If Kernberg accepted some sort of "continuum" between what he describes as the borderline personality organization and the psychotic, he could point to a series of quantitative and qualitative variations in the reality-testing functioning of such patients using the general formula that with increased regression and deterioration in overall ego integrity there would be a comparable decline in the efficacy of the reality-testing activities. However, since Kernberg holds fast to the idea that the borderline personality organization is a stable and specific psychopathological entity, he also wants to hold fast to the idea of more specific and more absolute distinctions in these reality-testing functions. Kernberg grants that, although these functions are more stable in the borderline personality organization than in the psychotic, the borderline personality organization patient may lose that relatively stable reality-testing capacity in certain special circumstances, particularly in the course of transference regression and the formation of a transference psychosis.[8] He would also insist that there are a number of categorical differences (as well as some similarities) between the transference psychosis that is observed in the borderline personality organization and in the psychotic. Kernberg acknowledges that in such a situation, the borderline personality organization patient will suffer a loss of reality testing, develop delusions and hallucinations, may have to be hospitalized, and that "at times it is quite difficult to separate a transference-limited psychotic reaction from a broader one" (pp. 84–85); but, in this area, he presents three crucial differences as well. First, in the transference psychotic reaction of the borderline personality organization patient, "the loss of reality testing does not *strikingly* affect the patient's functioning outside the treatment setting" (p. 176; see also p. 84). Second, the psychotic patient in the more advanced stages of the transference psychotic reaction has a "fusion experience with the therapist" (p. 177) while borderline personality organization patients "even in the course of a transference psychosis, do experience a boundary *of a sort* between themselves and the therapist" (ibid.). Third, there is the difference we noted earlier (see p. 230) in the reactions of these patients to the therapist's interpretations; notably, "while interpretation of the predominant primitive defensive operations in borderline patients *tend* to strengthen ego functioning and increase reality testing, the same approach *may* bring about further regression . . . in psychotic patients" (p. 179). We have already expressed our reservations about basing the diagnosis on the utilization of response to interpretation. But, while Kernberg recognizes that he needs to use a variety of qualifying words and phrases about these distinctions, he still concludes that there is no continuum. Further, although he does suggest somewhat different etiologies and posits different psychopathological ego structures (based essentially on differences in the "metabolism" of the internalized object relationships), it is not altogether clear that the clinical manifestations convincingly parallel those structural differences. The various qualifiers that Kernberg must introduce certainly tend to blur those distinctions. What stands out most on the clinical level in regard to the issue of reality testing is what we might call the "temporal duration of the break with reality." In the borderline personality organization, that break would appear to be related to some sort of stress, is transient and reversible, and is responsive to appropriate intervention, while there is the implication that these factors do not apply to the so-called psychotic. In the latter condition, one is led to believe that the defect in reality testing is ongoing and permanent. If this is so, then we are confronted with a somewhat "new" conceptualization of schizophrenia and the other psychoses: that these conditions are essentially the same over time, that they do not demonstrate periods of regression and/or restitution, and that they do not respond favorably to certain kinds of interventions (including those directed toward the primitive defense mechanisms). Inasmuch as our understanding of these psychoses is still confused and incomplete, it may well be that Kernberg's implications contain considerable validity; but at this time, at least, it would be difficult to draw such inferences since they would not coincide with our clinical experience and observations. Clinically, we also see breaks in reality testing in the much healthier patient, patients whom we would ordinarily place in the neurotic spectrum of the psychopathologies. Such "breaks" are anything but rare, invariably transient, and usually quite amenable to therapeutic intervention. We would submit, simply, that the relativity of reality testing (determined by a variety of dynamic, genetic, and economic factors) makes it a difficult area on which to establish hard and fast, categorical, isolated criteria for the diagnosis of a psychosis.

Finally, Kernberg's overall portrayal of the reality-testing functions of the borderline personality organization as essentially sound is complicated *logically* by his emphasis on the role of the mechanism of projective identification in these conditions. Kernberg stresses throughout this volume (see, particularly pp. 30–31, 80–84, 98–99, 170–177) the pivotal role played by "early forms of projection, and especially projective identification" in the structure of the borderline personality organization pathological ego. He indicates that this tendency to utilize "very strong projective trends" (p. 30) is important not only for "the quantitative predominance of projection but also the qualitative aspect of it. . . . The main purpose of projection here is to externalize the all-bad, aggressive self and object images. . . . While these patients do have sufficient development of ego boundaries to be able to differentiate self and object in most areas of their lives, the very intensity of the projective needs, plus the general ego weakness characterizing these patients, weakens ego boundaries *in the particular area of the projection* of aggression" (pp. 30–31). Later, he points out that these projective identification mechanisms become the main culprits during the course of therapy: they interfere with the self-observation functions and with the production of transference regression; they undermine the stability of the patient's ego boundaries; and they contribute centrally to the elaboration of a transference psychosis; in short, they act to compromise the reality-testing capacity of these patients.

To the extent that we feel comfortable about our understanding of the mechanism and the process of projective identification, these observations appear reasonable.

What becomes more difficult to reconcile with these observations is the more general position that the borderline personality organization patient usually presents a fairly stable and effect reality-testing apparatus. If what Kernberg tells us about the preponderant and predominant influence of the aggressive (particularly oral-aggressive) drive derivatives in the borderline personality organization is essentially correct, then it would appear that the utilization of such forms of projection and projective identification must, indeed, be comparably preponderant. If the operation of these mechanisms leads to a weakening of "ego boundaries in the particular area of the projection of aggression," then it would appear likely that these "areas" of ego weakness must be relatively pervasive throughout the entire personality structure. If the borderline personality organization patient can readily regress because of the prevalence of such defensive operations in the course of therapy, it becomes difficult to comprehend how such an individual can escape similar catastrophic reactions outside of therapy. It becomes even more difficult to understand how such an individual can "usually maintain" his capacity for reality testing.

Recurrent waves of proposed revisions of analytic theory and technique have characterized the history of psychoanalysis. Some of these proposed revisions have, indeed, become a portion of the psychoanalytic corpus; more often than not, however, they have enjoyed only a transient significance and popularity. It is not possible to submit a specific formula which would encompass all elements of these revisions, yet certain issues and emphases appear to be conspicuous and characteristic in each of the recurrent waves. In this same historical vein, we are, of course, aware that currently we are in the midst of a flurry of such proposals, and for us Kernberg's work provides the most conspicuous and influential representative of current revisionistic trends. The following list points to areas we believe warrant continued scrutiny in order to determine the nature and validity of his contributions.

1. The borderline personality organization concept has blurred the already unclear distinction between psychoanalysis and psychotherapy. Kernberg does not concern himself directly with these distinctions in the 1975 volume, but what emerges from these writings is a greater confusion of what constitutes the essence of analysis, the so-called psychoanalytic therapy, expressive or explo-

rative psychotherapy, and the so-called supportive psychotherapy. These are not simple differentiations, and it is difficult to fault anyone for not spelling our the clear-cut criteria on which to make such distinctions. What may be more crucial than the failure to formulate distinct differential *definitions* between psychoanalysis and psychotherapy is the failure to distinguish, and hence a blurring, between what is *psychoanalytic* and what is *psychotherapeutic*. What is psychoanalytic involves more than the *usage* of psychoanalytic language and concepts and, in terms of practice, cannot be divorced from what we call the psychoanalytic process, a topic which cannot be pursued here and one with which Kernberg barely deals in his work.[9]

2. There has been a retreat from an emphasis on the vicissitudes of sexuality, the derivatives of libido, and the centrality of the oedipal conflict. Instead, one finds a dramatic shift of emphasis to the role of aggression and pregenital factors in psychological life. Concomitantly the significance of regression tends to be overlooked. Often it is a concept to which lip service is paid without sufficient attention being given to whether the material at hand represents the product of a defensive regression (with a role played by earlier *fixations*), or whether that psychological material derives from a developmental *arrest* and/or defect.

3. More and more, "psychological" conflict is seen in terms of conflict with the external world and its representatives rather than in terms of intrapsychic conflict. Although the concession is made that the child may have "constitutional" propensities in certain directions, the greater emphasis is on the *real* activity and care of the early introjected objects *in toto,* particularly the mother. In many ways, such concepts return to the somewhat oversimplified conceptualization of "Momism" in place of the more complex implications of "the good enough mother."

4. Related to this shift in the arena of the "real"—and in "ideological" terms this may be the most conspicuous change—is a clear indication that the tripartite structural theory, with all of its derivatives and implications, is being replaced by the putative theories of object relations. Further, the attempts to reconcile the two are far from convincing, as are the related explanations for the ways in which earlier "active splitting" mechanisms give way to the higher level repressive mechanisms (and other comparable defenses). It would be presumptuous to insist that any one theory of what takes place in the first two years of life must be *the* correct one, or conversely, that an alternate theory *must* be erroneous. Thus, we cannot reject, out of hand, Kernberg's conceptualization of the early

building blocks for psychological structure. We do suggest, however, that such a conception raises many questions, does involve significant departures from previous structure-building theories, and by its very language enhances the tendency toward concretization and reification. Whatever the merit of these reservations, it is reasonable to state that when many analysts speak of "modern psychoanalysis," they are really referring to an object relations theory rather than one predicated on the centrality of instincts and their vicissitudes. We will only mention in this context that thought processes appear to play such a minor part in Kernberg's systematization. As Holzman (1976, p. 267) put it, "The person of this new theory does not think. Rather, he lives by the introjects. . . ."

5. Kernberg introduces a shift, diagnostically, from the emphasis on understanding, on the recognition of continua, and at least tacit acknowledgment that diagnostic labels are artificial and abstract. His concern is rather for the delineation of more strictly defined diagnostic entities which are not only more circumscribed hypothetically but also more concrete. We view this tendency as regressive, harking back to a sort of Kraepelinian taxonomy, and because precise diagnosis occupies such a central position in Kernberg's overall system and his technical "strategy," we return to this issue in the next point.

6. We would add, in this connection, that there is a significant tendency to depart from the very basic technical precepts of "free association," the rule of abstinence, the principle of the analyst's "freely suspended attention," and the priority given to the admonition to respect "where the patient is now." In their place, we see more and more instances in which the patient is being viewed through a prism of prefabricated ideas, and his treatment is predicated on *what* is believed contained within a given diagnostic label and preformed ideas about *how* that diagnostic label should be approached. We do not believe that the psychoanalyst is ever "passive," even when he is silent; but we do believe that the "new" analysis entails the danger of a kind of activity which is based not so much on the analyst's responsibility to maintain the analytic process but on his preconceived notion of what the patient *must* be like and by a greater tendency to permit the analyst's own value judgments to intrude on the analytic work and the analytic process.

We have not attempted to list other, often significant changes in analysis; nor have we attempted to document these assertions in any detailed way. What we do wish to underscore is that there *are* changes; and that these changes, in themselves, represent a striking "social" phenomenon, at least to the extent that psychoanalysts collectively represent a specific "social group." Whether or not these alterations are beneficial or deleterious will be determined by the test of time and, even more, by the results of careful scrutiny. It can, of course, be argued that there are not only differences between the "old" analysis and the new points of view (as exemplified by Kernberg's papers), but that there are even more similarities between the two. It would be difficult to refute such a contention, but an emphasis on the areas of similarity and commonality can often be misleading. As one of us (Weinshel, 1976, p. 451) stated in another context, "Such an emphasis, which could serve as a vehicle for a superficial reconciliation, can also become the means of blurring areas of conflict—some of which may, in isolation, appear trivial but in the aggregate loom large. These differences may not necessarily be incompatible but they do demand further careful study if we are to arrive at a scientific rather than political reconciliation."

We very much wish that we could offer convincing and comprehensive explanations for what we have referred to as the "social phenomena": the recurrent waves of efforts to introduce significant alterations in basic psychoanalytic theory and practice, the tremendous "band-wagon" popularity of Kernberg's contributions, the cult-like atmosphere that has surrounded much of his work, the reluctance (or at least, the open reluctance) to question its derivation and its validity. We do not believe, however, that we are capable of doing so. It may be necessary, perhaps, for more time and distance to intervene before a psychoanalyst can undertake such a critique; and, perhaps, only someone outside of the profession of psychoanalysis can bring both the objectivity and the necessary complex perspectives in humanistic studies to accomplish this task.

Notes

1. Kernberg, Otto: *Borderline Conditions and Pathological Narcissism.* New York: Jason Aronson, Inc., 1975.
2. Seven of its 10 chapters have been published before, a fact that is not made clear (in the publisher's dust jacket copy, the editor's introduction, or the author's preface) until the very end of the volume. As far as we can determine, the papers have been reprinted as they were at the time of their publication. If any editorial changes have been made, they have been minimal.
3. It may well be that no contribution by a psychoanalyst has been taken up so avidly and so happily by the nonpsychoanalytic segment of the mental health community, with the possible exception of Erikson's introduction of the identity concept a quarter of a century ago.

4. Most of the points Kernberg made in the Amsterdam contribution already contained the central ideas that can be found in the current collection.
5. We refer the reader to pp. 94ff., 100–101, 121–122, 197–200, 244–245 for a representative assortment of Kernberg's clinical material.
6. In his precirculated paper, "Implications of the Teaching and Practice of Psychotherapy for Psychoanalytic Training," written in advance of the Eighth Pre-Congress on Training of the International Psycho-Analytical Association Congress in New York, Kernberg does, in fact, offer an extensive discussion of what he means by the term "technical neutrality." He does this in the context of distinguishing his definition of psychoanalysis from psychoanalytic psychotherapy. This most recent paper continues the exploration of these subjects in Kernberg's presentation at the May 1978 American Psychoanalytic Association panel: *Conceptualizing the Nature of the Therapeutic Action of Psychoanalytic Psychotherapy* (cf., Nemetz, 1979, pp. 132–136) and its expanded version, "Developments in the Theory of Psychoanalytic Psychotherapy."
7. In this section, all of the italics are ours.
8. There is some inconsistency and potential confusion in Kernberg's use of the term "transference psychosis." See Weinshel (1966) for remarks by Reider, p. 546, and Frosch, p. 547.
9. See, however, our footnote 6.

Schizotypal Symptoms in Patients with Borderline Personality Disorders

Anselm George, M.D., and Paul H. Soloff, M.D.
(1986)

The authors assess the frequency of schizotypal symptoms in 48 criteria-defined borderline patients. In the total sample schizotypal symptoms were surprisingly common; the average patient had more than seven symptoms and every patient at least one. Even in the "pure" DSM-III borderline subgroup, 67% of the patients had perceptual symptoms, 92% had cognitive symptoms, and 87% reported other "affective" symptoms. Visual phenomena were more prevalent than auditory ones, suggesting a possible contributing role for organic factors in borderline disorders. The results also indicate a close link between borderline and schizotypal personality disorders.

The DSM-III defines two disorders in the group of borderline conditions: borderline personality disorder and schizotypal personality disorder. There has been considerable disagreement as to whether it is justified to separate these two entities or whether a unified concept should be maintained.

Spitzer et al. (1979) argued for two separate entities and defined two separate sets of diagnostic criteria. These authors found that

Supported in part by NIMH grants MH-30915 and MH-35392. Reprinted with permission from *The American Journal of Psychiatry, 143,* 212–215. Copyright © 1986 American Psychiatric Association.

"within a group of borderline patients the two item sets are independent but not mutually exclusive." Fifty-four percent of the patients in the Spitzer et al. study met the criteria for both diagnoses. In a subsequent paper (Spitzer & Endicott, 1979) they stated that "brief losses in reality testing and psychotic-like experiences" would have to be present in every borderline patient in order to demonstrate that the two disorders belong together.

In contrast, Siever and Gunderson (1979) gave reasons for a unified concept of borderline disorder including micropsychotic episodes. They wrote that "many clinicians have always viewed brief psychotic-like experiences as a central characteristic of borderline personality. Thus, examples of brief psychotic-like thinking are contained in the descriptions of borderline patients by Knight and Kernberg, and in the systematic studies by Grinker and Werble."

Two sets of diagnostic criteria for borderline disorder are widely used in the literature—the semi-structured Diagnostic Interview for Borderline Patients (DIB) (Gunderson et al., 1981) and DSM-III. The DIB includes both brief psychotic-like experiences and the group of impulsive, affective, and interpersonal disturbances. There is a heavy emphasis on the last three symptoms, since they make up three of five sections and psychotic-like symptoms make up only one. (One section measures social adaptation.) The DSM-III criteria do not list psychotic-like symptoms. Brief psychotic episodes are mentioned only as associated features.

There are four rating scales for schizotypal features in the literature—those by Meehl (1964), Spitzer et al. (1979), Khouri et al. (1980), and Baron (1981). On the basis of these available criteria and rating scales, we systematically inquired about schizotypal symptoms in 48 patients referred to the pharmacotherapy of borderline disorders study at the Western Psychiatric Institute and Clinic, University of Pittsburgh.

Method

Our sample consisted of 37 (77%) women and 11 (23%) men who were referred to our borderline disorders study from an inpatient service (N=38) or from the emergency room (N=10). The mean ±SD age was 26.7±6.8 years. After a thorough psychiatric and medical evaluation, patients gave written informed consent for this study, and the DIB was administered by one of us. A scaled score of 7 or greater on the DIB was required for inclusion in the study, as recommended by Kolb and Gunderson (1980). We used the following exclusion criteria: hospitalization for more than 2 years cumulatively over the previous 5 years, clinical evidence of CNS pathology, drug- and/or alcohol-related deficits or physical dependence, physical disorders with known psychiatric consequence (e.g., hyper- or hypothyroidism), borderline mental retardation (full-scale WAIS <70), and age less than 16 or greater than 36 years.

Patients who were classified as borderline with the DIB were then assessed according to DSM-III criteria for borderline personality disorder and schizotypal personality disorder. We used a checklist that measured the DSM-III criteria on a 5-point severity scale (0=not present, 4=markedly present). Patients were classified as schizotypal if they met four of eight criteria for this disorder, as unstable if they met five of the DSM-III criteria for borderline personality disorder, and as mixed if they fulfilled criteria for both disorders. Only items that were rated 2 or greater (e.g., mildly to markedly present) were considered clinically significant. After the patients underwent a 7-day drug-free period of observation, we independently assessed their current functioning with a number of rating instruments.

Schizotypal symptoms were measured with the specially constructed Schizotypal Symptom Inventory, a checklist incorporating all eight DSM-III items, seven items from the Khouri et al. scale (1980), and four items from the Meehl scale (1964). (A copy of the questionnaire is available from the authors.) Each item was rated by the interviewer and one observer on a 5-point scale (0=not present, 4=markedly present). Because of overlap in the scales we used 17 items, which fell into the following groups: perceptual symptoms (four items), cognitive symptoms (seven items), and other "affective" symptoms (six items).

Using 41 patients from our sample, we tested the interrater reliability of the Schizotypal Symptom Inventory. We calculated one summary score reflecting the number of symptoms present regardless of severity and another by adding the scores of all the symptoms (see Table 1). For the number of positive items the Pearson product-moment correlation was .83, and for the total severity score it was .84. Individual items had Pearson product-moment correlations ranging from .32 to .88. The two items with the lowest correlation were inadequate rapport and odd speech, both from DSM-III. Therefore, we omitted these two items from further analysis. In general, however, we concluded that schizotypal symptoms can be rated with a fair degree of interrater agreement. Subsequently, the scores of the two raters were averaged.

Table 1

Schizotypal Symptom Inventory Scores for 48 Borderline Patients and the Unstable, Schizotypal, and Mixed Subgroups

| | Total Sample (N=48) | | | Subgroup[a] | | | | | | | | |
| | | | | Unstable (N=24) | | | Schizotypal (N=4) | | | Mixed (N=18) | | |
Schizotypal Symptoms	Mean Score	N	%	Mean Score	N	%	Mean Score	N	%	Mean Score	N	%
Selected individual items[b]												
Auditory hallucinations	0.54	14	29	0.31	5	21	0.88	2	50	0.69	6	33
Visual illusions	0.93	19	40	0.69	8	33	1.75	2	50	1.03	8	44
Derealization	1.04	23	48	0.75	9	37	1.13	3	75	1.33	10	55
Muddled thinking	1.03	25	52	0.50	7	29	2.38	4	100	1.42	13	72
Micropsychotic symptoms	1.30	30	62	1.21	13	54	2.00	4	100	1.28	12	67
Hypersensitivity	1.88	35	73	2.02	20	83	1.75	3	75	1.61	10	55
Social Isolation	0.84	18	37	0.35	5	21	2.00	3	75	1.25	9	50
Pan-anxiety	0.74	17	35	0.35	5	21	1.50	4	100	1.17	9	50
Summary scores												
Perception	3.22	38	79	2.2	16	67	4.5	4	100	3.9	17	94
Cognition	6.05	46	96	4.7	22	92	8.9	4	100	7.3	18	100
Affect	5.13	45	94	4.0	21	87	7.7	4	100	5.9	18	100
Total positive items	7.43	48	100	6.0	24	100	10.2	4	100	8.6	18	100
Total severity score	15.3	48	100	11.5	24	100	22.9	4	100	18.3	18	100

[a] Two patients were not diagnosed as unstable or schizotypal.
[b] Scores for the remaining items are available from the authors.

Results

Forty-six of the 48 patients were classified as unstable or schizotypal; two patients (4%) received neither of these diagnoses. Twenty-four patients (50%) were unstable, four (8%) were schizotypal, and eighteen (38%) fulfilled diagnostic criteria for both disorders (mixed diagnosis). Table 1 lists the mean scores for selected individual items, the number of patients in whom the symptom was clearly present, and the percentage of the sample that displayed the particular symptom. These data are given for our total sample and the DSM-III subsamples for unstable, schizotypal, or both (mixed) disorders. Summary scores in the areas of perception, cognition, and affect are also given, as well as the total number of positive items and the total severity score. The average patient in our study had 7.4 positive items. All patients displayed at least one schizotypal symptom; the most prevalent symptom, undue social anxiety or hypersensitivity, was present in 73% of the patients.

Derealization, found in 48% of the patients, was the most common perceptual symptom. The most common cognitive symptom included micropsychotic episodes, brief periods of "drift-out" during the interview, and the feeling that one's mind goes blank. Visual phenomena were found more frequently than auditory ones (40% versus 29% of the patients; $t=1.76$, $df=94$, $p=.08$; two-tailed t test) (see Table 1).

When we compared the three patient subgroups (unstable, schizotypal, and mixed) on the Schizotypal Symptom Inventory with regard to the total number of positive items and total severity, the schizotypal group was highest, followed by the mixed group, with the unstable group having the lowest score (for total positive items, $F=5.6$, $df=2$, 43, p<.01; for total severity score, $F=8.1$, $df=2$, 43, p<.01). This finding was, to some extent, predicted, since eight of the inventory items were identical to the DSM-III criteria for schizotypal personality disorder. However, even in the "pure" unstable group, the mean number of positive items was six, with each patient having at least one schizotypal symptom. The differences in the mean severity scores among patient subgroups were most striking for the symptoms of muddled thinking ($F=10.3$, $df=2$, 43, p<.01), social isolation ($F=6.0$, $df=2$, 43, p<.01), and pan-anxiety ($F=3.1$, $df=2$, 43, p=.54). For the last item, pair-wise comparisons with the two-tailed t test revealed significant differences between the unstable and schizotypal subgroups ($t=3.47$, $df=24$, p<.01) and between the unstable and mixed subgroups ($t=2.61$, $df=40$, p<.02).

Discussion

Our study indicates that we were unable to reach sufficient interrater agreement on two of the 17 tested items—odd speech (Pearson r=.38) and inadequate rapport (Pearson r=.32). Both are included in the DSM-III criteria for schizotypal personality disorder. These two items are the only ones rated on the basis of direct patient observation. Such items have previously been found to have low reliability (WHO, 1973).

The individual items muddled thinking, social isolation, and pan-anxiety best separated the three patient subgroups. This lends some support to the conclusions of Gunderson et al. (1983) and the findings of Barrash et al. (1983). They suggested that more emphasis be placed on the social isolation, anxiety, and distant interpersonal relationships of schizotypal patients. We think that social anxiety and hypersensitivity to criticism, a criterion for schizotypal personality disorder in DSM-III, should be separated into its two component parts because rejection sensitivity is very frequently found in the unstable group. As it was used here, this item was the only one that was more frequently found in the unstable subgroup than in the schizotypal subgroup and, therefore, may not be a useful schizotypal symptom.

Our results also indicate that visual phenomena are more common than auditory ones. Although this difference falls short of statistical significance, the finding becomes interesting if contrasted with the prevalence of auditory and visual hallucinations in schizophrenia. Common clinical experience, textbook knowledge, and most research reports (Malitz et al., 1962; Small et al., 1966) agree that auditory hallucinations are much more common than visual ones in this disorder. Our patients were all drug free for at least 7 days before this examination and were screened for organic conditions (normal findings on physical examination, EEG, and laboratory tests). In order to further reduce the possibility of unreported drug and alcohol abuse, we repeated our analysis using only the 38 inpatients. The results were essentially the same as those reported for the combined inpatient-outpatient sample. This high frequency of visual hallucinations has been reported in other disorders in the "borderline realm." Bishop and Holt (1980) found a "relatively higher frequency of visual hallucinations" in their review of the concept of hysterical psychosis, a syndrome closely related to borderline disorders. Although no definite conclusions regarding the etiology of these phenomena can be drawn, the possibility of occult organic predisposing factors must be considered (Andrulonis et al., 1980; Andrulonis & Vogel, 1984). Further investigations of this matter using neurological soft signs, neuropsychological test batteries, EEG, and spectral analysis methods are in progress.

Our main finding is that the presence of a large number of schizotypal symptoms is confirmed when borderline patients are systematically questioned about these phenomena. This fact links schizotypal and unstable subgroups of patients who are diagnosed as borderline.

It can be argued that the diagnostic significance of these schizotypal symptoms is unclear, since their frequency in normal control subjects has not been established. However, we took care to avoid false-positive responses by asking patients to describe their experiences. We discounted phenomena that seemed clearly appropriate in the patient's life circumstances. Our data are also limited to borderline patients. Control groups of patients with near-neighbor conditions, such as schizotypal patients who do not meet DIB criteria for borderline disorder, would give a larger schizotypal sample and make our conclusions more generally applicable.

The large number of schizotypal symptoms found in this sample may reflect our patient selection procedure. The major screening device for our study was the DIB, in which certain psychotic-like features contribute to the diagnosis. In spite of this, only four patients with pure schizotypal personality disorder were admitted to the study. The sensitivity of the DIB in predicting the diagnosis of DSM-III borderline disorder was estimated by Loranger et al. (1984) to be 79% using the pooled data from three studies involving a total of 194 patients. The number of schizotypal symptoms in our sample could, therefore, be only slightly lower if we had used DSM-III as the initial screening instrument. Depending on which schizotypal items Spitzer et al. would include in their definition of "brief losses of reality testing and psychotic-like experiences," it can be stated that in our sample nearly every DSM-III borderline patient had one or more of these symptoms. Therefore, including mild perceptual and cognitive disturbances in the defining symptoms for borderline personality disorder may be justified.

Our data indicate that it is difficult to separate the schizotypal and unstable borderline syndromes using only psychotic-like symptoms. Differences between the two may lie in the areas of affect or interpersonal relationships.

Part 3

Empirical Findings

Abuses of the Borderline Diagnosis: A Clinical Problem with Teaching Opportunities

David E. Reiser, M.D., and
Hanna Levenson, Ph.D.
(1984)

The authors identify six ways in which the borderline diagnosis is commonly abused to express countertransference hate, mask imprecise thinking, excuse treatment failures, justify the therapist's acting out, defend against sexual clinical material, and avoid pharmacologic and medical treatment interventions. The paper focuses on diagnostic abuses that trainees present to clinical supervisors and educators. It attempts to show educators how to discern these abuses and turn them into teaching opportunities. These abuses are seen not only in trainees; they also occur in the professional community as a whole. Clinicians should expect the same diagnostic rigor of themselves that they expect of their students.

Few diagnoses in psychiatry currently attract more attention and controversy than the borderline conditions and narcissistic disorders. The term "borderline," popularized by Knight in 1953, filled an important theoretical gap. Knight and others recognized the existence of a group of patients whose pathology was too severe to

Reprinted with permission from *The American Journal of Psychiatry, 141,*
1528–1532. Copyright © 1984 American Psychiatric Association.

be considered neurotic, yet whose reality testing and functioning were at too high a level to be considered psychotic. Numerous other investigators (Grinker et al., 1968; Gunderson & Kolb, 1978; Spitzer et al., 1979) have continued to make important contributions to the field. It is beyond the scope of this paper to review the significant contributions to this rapidly expanding body of knowledge. Excellent reviews can be found in the reports by Gunderson and Singer (1975) and Perry and Klerman (1978). Our purpose in this presentation is to identify a troubling and, we believe, increasingly widespread trend toward significant abuse of the diagnosis in everyday clinical practice. We believe that the extent of this abuse is serious enough to put the term in danger of becoming clinically meaningless.

This paper is addressed particularly to individuals involved in the education of future psychotherapists, and we hope to do more than simply castigate abuses of the term, regrettable as these may be. We believe that when the problem is diagnosed correctly, educators can use these abuses as golden opportunities to help students learn psychotherapy more effectively. Furthermore, although we focus on abuses of the term in different training settings, we do not believe that the problem is limited to those who are still learning to do psychotherapy. Our impression has been that the same abuses are much in evidence in the professional community as a whole. Therefore, our remarks are directed not only to those who are involved directly in clinical education but to all of those who administrate or function in settings where psychiatric treatment is offered.

Distortions and misuses obviously occur with many diagnostic categories (e.g., schizophrenia, alcohol dependence). Still, it seems to us that the diagnosis of borderline personality disorder is particularly subject to such misuse for three reasons. First, the criteria for borderline personality disorder seem to depend on one's theoretical orientation (Kernberg, 1967; Klein, 1946; Kohut, 1971). Second, only relatively recently have researchers (Koenigsberg et al., 1982; Kroll et al., 1981; Perry & Klerman, 1980; Pope et al., 1983) examined the extent to which the diagnosis constitutes a clinically useful concept and a behaviorally homogeneous category. Third, patients who have a borderline personality structure often have symptoms (e.g., emotional lability, suicidal and/or homicidal ideation or behavior, serious interpersonal problems, and rage) that are difficult to tolerate, let alone treat (Maltsberger & Buie, 1974).

We have identified six ways in which the term "borderline" is commonly abused. These are use of the term 1) as an expression of countertransference hate; 2) to mask sloppy and imprecise diagnostic thinking; 3) to rationalize mistakes in the treatment or treatment failure; 4) as a justification for acting out in the countertransference; 5) to defend against sexual material, including oedipal material, in clinical work; and 6) as a rationale for avoiding medical and pharmacologic treatment interventions.

Expression of Countertransference Hate

Case 1. A senior psychiatry resident was presenting the case of a 24-year-old man whom she was treating with psychotherapy. Therapy had been difficult, punctuated by frequent suicide gestures, dangerous acting out, and rage attacks. Nevertheless, there had been considerable progress over a 3-year period. The patient was able to enter into an enduring and nondestructive relationship, and he was going back to school to complete college work. Instead of hearing his therapist's comment on the possibility of termination as well-earned praise, he became convinced that his therapist was "sick of me" and just wanted to get rid of him. As the resident presented this case for the first time to the supervisor, she said, "I've been in this residency for 3 years. I have yet to treat a real neurotic. Sometimes it feels like all I am is a professional doormat, here to get stomped on by all these borderlines."

Clinical work can be demanding, draining, frustrating, and at times thankless in the best of practices. Therapists in training are frequently young and relatively inexperienced. They are assailed by the grimmest and most tragic aspects of life—patients with no social support systems and no financial resources, people with chaotic and desperate inner and outer lives. The stresses of caring for these patients can be massive, doubly so if one is simultaneously attempting to learn psychotherapy while working with such patients. If therapists in this situation are not given adequate support, supervision, and empathy, they can and do experience despair, burnout, cynicism, a loss of empathic capacities, and therapeutic nihilism.

In our experience these often trying and demanding situations can, with skilled supervision, be understood and surmounted, turning what feels like a nightmare into an opportunity for trainees to grow professionally. Too often, however, this opportunity is not realized. Repeatedly, we have heard therapists in these institutional settings refer to a wide and markedly heterogeneous group of patients as "just a bunch of borderlines." Used this way, the term "borderline" loses all theoretical meaning and simply becomes the latest institutional epithet—another colloquial expression of contempt, like "gomer," "crock," or "turkey." When slang takes the form of pseudoscientific jargon, however, countertransference hatred becomes disguised as a technical term, making it doubly dangerous.

Finally, we have often seen the use of the term "borderline" lead to a breakdown in empathy between therapist and patient. The vignette just cited is an example of this. On the basis of the data presented, it is impossible to say whether this patient has a borderline personality organization or not. Certainly he could have. Regardless, by labeling his behavior "borderline" the resident has closed herself off from the opportunity to understand the behavior's meaning and thereby help the patient with it. In this instance the resident was helped, through supervision, to see that the patient's behavior was actually an attempt to remain with his beloved and now highly trusted therapist. Once the therapist understood this, her empathy was restored. She was able to see past his renewed threats of acting out to the fear and uncertainty that lay underneath. This, in turn, enabled the patient to work through important issues of separation and individuation during the termination phase.

Masking of Sloppy, Imprecise Diagnostic Thinking

Case 2. A beginning psychiatry resident was reviewing his caseload with a supervisor. Out of 12 active cases, two patients were diagnosed as having schizophrenia, one depression, and one marital disorder. The remaining eight were termed "borderlines."

The "borderlines" included a 30-year-old nurse who was stably employed and raising a family, a 16-year-old boy with problems of truancy and drug abuse, a homosexual woman of 48 whose lover had recently left her, a 24-year-old graduate student with anxiety attacks, and a 36-year-old woman with Crohn's disease. When challenged to defend his diagnostic formulations, the resident spoke nonchalantly of "shallow object relations," "need-gratifying as opposed to object-related behavior," "dyadic, dependent relationships," and "extensive use of splitting." This sort of jargon, unsubstantiated by any empirical observations, seemed sufficient to this resident to justify his giving eight vastly different people an identical diagnosis.

Diagnosis should lead to treatment. Equally important, it becomes an essential benchmark against which the effectiveness of therapeutic interventions should subsequently be measured. In this vignette the resident was not using a diagnosis to clarify his clinical thinking and treatment planning—he was creating an illusion, by the use of a term, that what once was confusing to him now had become clear. His patients had been "diagnosed" and therefore in his mind were now "understood." But by lumping so many divergent individuals into a wastebasket diagnosis, he had, in effect, closed off further avenues of logical diagnostic thinking and clinical inquiry.

For the typical trainee working in the typical institutional setting, the complexity of diagnosis can feel truly overwhelming. The typical patient will have complicated preoedipal pathology. Usually the patient will also suffer from major complications in all three sectors of the biopsychosocial field. Biologically, he is apt to be poorly nourished, addicted to multiple substances ranging from alcohol to nicotine, and suffering from a variety of functional and psychophysiologic disturbances. His childhood history and family relations may be characterized by chaos, instability, and tragedy. In a broader social context, he may have multiple legal, educational, and vocational deficits. Typically he may give a history of responding to such difficulties through disturbing and dangerous behavioral symptoms, ranging from self-destruction to assaultiveness.

One can understand a trainee's yearning to find an umbrella phrase, some overarching concept that creates the illusion of homogeneity and coherence. Indeed, we doubt that such a longing is to be found in trainees alone. Ultimately, however, the illusion is destructive. By treating all patients as borderline subjects and failing in the process to see their individual features, therapists soon find that none of their patients are getting any better. Such therapists are then confirmed in their opinion that borderline patients are untreatable. Not only are treatable conditions—or at least treatable parts of conditions—missed; worse still, the psychotherapist himself too often ends up with an unwarranted sense of therapeutic cynicism and prognostic despair.

Rationalization of Mistakes in the Treatment or Treatment Failure

Case 3. A 22-year-old nursing student began psychotherapy with a psychiatry resident after she went to a university health service complaining of overeating. Early in the treatment the resident discovered that she was the youngest of 13 children sired by a hypomanic sailor who had been married five times. Of all the children only the patient had remained devoted to this man, following him from city to city, often witnessing his sexual philanderings and drunken excesses. He would take her in for a month or two, tire of her, and farm her out to a foster home. By the time she was 18 she had been in 15 foster homes.

Despite her tragic history, the resident initially regarded her prognosis as optimistic. Despite her tendency to overweight, she was bright, vivacious, talented, and pretty. In addition, she admired the resident's acumen immensely and would often look at him with large, adoring brown eyes and exclaim over his brilliance, empathy, and insight. One month into the treatment, however, she threw a tantrum and adamantly insisted that he prescribe amphetamines to help her lose 10 pounds. Quite uncharacteristically, the resident had finally assented and prescribed 30 tablets of dextroamphetamine sulfate. In the subsequent months her demands escalated. She called more and more frequently, at later and later hours. She demanded more and more appointments and became inordinately jealous of the resident's other commitments, both professional and social. Initially he responded by giving in to these demands and permitting more gratification than he ordinarily would have with other patients. He justified this as necessary to treat "this borderline woman."

As months passed and her demandingness increased, he began to grow weary. She had now required two hospitalizations. She had also caused him considerable embarrassment during these bouts by complaining about his incompetence and declaring to everyone that "Dr. Smith prescribes speed." The resident, disgusted and furious beyond words, decided to transfer the case.

The woman cited in this vignette was certainly difficult to treat. She may or may not have been borderline. Regardless, in this situation we believe the resident used the term to rationalize and explain away his therapeutic mistakes. Early on, the resident had, like the patient's father, allowed himself to be seductive and overgratifying. This included prescribing amphetamines, which literally and symbolically overstimulated the patient.

In the therapy the patient soon began to relive, in a primitive and aggression-dominated transference, her rage, disappointment, and fury at the father. But the resident failed to see her behavior as a repetition compulsion. Rather, he rationalized his patient's transference as "borderline" and then felt justified in acting out the precise rejection that had traumatized his patient so repeatedly earlier in her life. As her father had done before him, the resident abandoned his patient to "foster care" after first getting her hopes up—sending her to another therapist jut when she needed him to endure her rage and stick out a tough time in the treatment. Instead, he left her, just as her father had done so many times.

This vignette is an example of how one may use the term "borderline" to rationalize mistakes in treatment. Perhaps just as common is the tendency to "downgrade" a diagnosis from neurotic to borderline simply b*ecause* the treatment has not succeeded; yet, in truth, sometimes regardless of the high quality of the therapy or the supervision, treatment failures occur. The diagnosis of borderline for these cases may represent many therapists' difficulty in accepting the limitations of the psychotherapeutic process in general, something painful for trainees who are in a developmental phase involving a positive identification with the profession. It may at times be more comfortable to ascribe treatment failures to the specific characteristics of the patient than to any inadequacy in the state of the art.

Justification for Acting Out in the Countertransference

Case 4. A strikingly beautiful 23-year-old woman who was a college senior saw a psychiatry resident in the student health service for complaints of examination anxiety. She tearfully reviewed recent losses including the following: A close girlfriend had been killed in an automobile accident; her younger brother had been arrested on a marijuana charge and required to enter a drug treatment program; her parents were stressed and on the verge of divorce. The patient tearfully asked the resident, "What should I say to my mother? She expects me to solve everything! I feel so guilty!"

The resident maintained a stony silence and asked the patient how she felt about her younger brother now and when he had been born. Initially the patient tried to respond to the request, but she kept asking, "What can I do about my mother; she expects everything from me!"

The therapist remained silent, not only refusing to answer the patient's question directly but also failing to give any indication that he appreciated the patient's weighty sense of responsibility. The resident mismarked the second appointment in his calendar and failed to appear for the patient's second appointment, to which she was on time. The patient came back for one more session, during which the resident was again distant and aloof. Subsequently the patient cancelled all further appointments. The resident stated, "I think she was probably borderline."

This vignette illustrates the common problem of countertransference acting out. The therapist held back from an unusually attractive patient and refused to be human when she requested empathy and advice.

Few relations are more intimate than the psychotherapeutic relationship. In this relationship patients typically invest tremendous power in the therapist, disclosing much about themselves and making themselves quite vulnerable in the process. Therapists can and do respond to this process with anxieties of their own. All therapists will at times feel a pull to be seductive or be seduced. It is not always easy for a therapist to be an object of adoration and occasionally of overt sexual desire.

Many therapists respond to such transference pressures by becoming excessively aloof and distant as the resident in this example did; others respond by behaving in ways that are grandiose and overseductive. The borderline diagnosis seems to be a common way for such therapists to rationalize and legitimize either countertransference behavior. The therapist who is grandiose and seductive argues that he is introducing necessary "parameters" to treat his "borderline" patients. The therapist who is rigid and unable to give offers the identical argument—invoking concepts of "limit setting" and "rigid frames" in the treatment of borderline patients to prevent "devaluation" of the therapist and "primitive aggression." Invoked in this way, these terms only obfuscate, not elucidate.

Defense Against Oedipal Clinical Material

Case 5.   A first-year psychiatry resident was presenting the case of a 27-year-old man, a performing artist, who was troubled by impotence. The patient had, in his own words, "shaken free" of a destructive marriage and was now living in San Francisco pursuing an acting career. Most recently he had been involved with a woman who was an actress approximately his age. To his shame and distress he had been impotent on the night of their first date when he had attempted to take her to bed.

The patient was the oldest of three children. His parents were intensely proud of his accomplishments and thrilled by the fact that, of all their children, this son was "the artist, the truly creative one."

As the resident presented his patient's case to the supervising psychiatrist, oedipal material seemed prominent. The patient had met earlier developmental challenges and mastered them relatively successfully. He had many friends, flexible ego defenses, and a capacity to relate warmly to others. His complaint lay primarily in his inability to enjoy his successes without guilt.

When the resident was asked for his diagnosis of the case, he stated, "No doubt, borderline." He argued that the patient's sexual inhibitions were a facade for "more serious pathology," citing his "exhibitionistic" choice of career.

While there may be truth to the argument that neurosis in our culture is declining and narcissistic character pathology increasing, it has been our experience that when a neurotic patient does appear, most trainees completely miss the diagnosis. We have observed that trainees usually tend to "pathopomorphize" neurotic patients. Confronted with an oedipally fixated patient, male or female, one whose unconscious conflicts may closely resemble the trainee's own, the trainee responds in a predictable way: He claims that such a patient is "sicker than he looks." Such patients are then banished in the trainee's mind to the hinterland of borderline pathology, where they presumably become less threatening as objects of identification.

"Borderline" becomes a way to defang the infantile neurosis by pretending that it is "pseudosexual" and therefore tame.

Rational for Avoiding Medical and Pharmacologic Treatment Interventions

Case 6.   In supervision a psychology intern was relating the evaluation of her first inpatient—a 21-year-old bright, verbal but disheveled man who was hospitalized for depression and suicidal ideation. The patient was homeless and without funds, friends, or family. The intern described the patient's turbulent past history, his dissociative and sometimes hallucinatory experiences, his unstable job history, and his isolated existence. The patient had made several suicidal gestures in the past that had resulted in short-term hospitalizations and the use of antipsychotic medication. The medication had been helpful for a brief interval until the patient discontinued it, complaining that it slowed him down.

The intern wanted to respect the patient's wishes not to be medicated. The intern agreed with the patient that medication would only be an attempt "to medicate the problem away." Her treatment decision not to medicate him seemed to be consistent with her philosophy of patients' rights and her unfamiliarity with the appropriate use of antipsychotic agents. The intern felt a professional responsibility for changing the patient's dire life circumstances during his hospitalization. She diagnosed the patient as borderline and accordingly recommended long-term, drug-free treatment.

When the supervisor began to explore the extent of the patient's pathology, the intern responded with righteous indignation about the dangers of labeling patients as schizophrenic and the need to protect patients against the often "inhumane, reductionistic medical model."

With further supervisory encouragement the intern spoke of the anger she had felt in being treated as a second-class citizen by the psychiatric residents and other physicians. She told of how she could identify with the patients whom she viewed as being degraded and made to feel powerless during their hospitalizations.

In this case the borderline diagnosis served two covert purposes. First, it was used to justify protecting this patient from receiving medication and thus reduced the medical component of his treatment. In this way, the intern was also protecting herself from the need to interact with the medical staff. Second, the borderline diagnosis appeared to give credence to the intern's desire to work with this patient in long-term therapy. The intern phrased it thus: "Borderlines need long-term therapy in which a mirroring therapist is able to withstand their rage and ambivalence over time." In supervision the therapist began to examine how her use of the borderline diagnosis actually served to justify a personal therapeutic philosophy (e.g., a belief in drug-free, long-term treatment). With help, she began to realize that more structured approaches including psychopharmacology were better suited to this patient. Such introspection and the actions it led to would have been impossible had the borderline diagnosis been accepted unquestioningly.

Conclusions

The last two decades have been a period of great interest within psychiatry regarding borderline disturbances. Major theoretical advances have been achieved, and the diagnosis clearly is here to stay. In this paper we do not question the term's value but raise the problem of its widespread abuse.

We believe that teachers involved in the education of future psychotherapists need to recognize this current tendency to abuse the diagnosis. Furthermore, we suspect that the abuses we have observed repeatedly in trainees are not solely restricted to misadventures of the young in educational settings. Rather, the abuses are ones that many psychotherapists may be prone to, at least some of the time. We have identified six common types of abuse: the diagnosis 1) as an expression of countertransference hate, 2) as a disguise for sloppy diagnostic thinking, 3) as a rationalization for mistakes made in the treatment or unavoidable treatment failures, 4) as a justification for acting out in the countertransference, 5) as a defense against sexual, including oedipal, material, and 6) as a rationale for avoiding medical and pharmacologic treatment interventions.

The following suggestions are offered:

1. The borderline diagnosis should never be accepted without critical challenge. One should always demand a logical defense of the diagnosis. The defense of the diagnosis can be descriptive, based on the Gunderson-Singer criteria (1975), or it can be psychodynamic, based on a coherent understanding of the major pertinent theoretical works on the subject. Regardless of the theoretical starting point, however, a logical and comprehensible explanation should be expected—one that points toward a suitable treatment strategy.

2. It should be recognized that many patients, by virtue of their inherently tragic plight, their complexity, and their great rage, may evoke intense feelings of countertransference fear and hate. Such emotions are understandable, but they should not be allowed to become disguised by being dressed up with pseudoscientific jargon.

3. Educators should be alert to the tendency of trainees to label all complicated material as "borderline" and should regard such lumping with great skepticism.

4. Whenever a therapist has a patient in treatment and the treatment is not going well, one should question very skeptically any use of the term "borderline" to explain the problem. Too often problems within a treatment are passed off and rationalized in this manner.

5. Educators should pay particular attention to unusual attitudes or atypical behavior displayed by therapists who are treating patients labeled "borderline." It may signal acting out in the countertransference.

6. Supervisors and educators should always have a high index of suspicion for the presence of neurotic, including oedipal, issues in patients diagnosed as borderline. Many people wonder whether the incidence of classic neurosis is declining. Some neurotic patients may not have disappeared but have been misdiagnosed.

7. Educators should apply suggestions 1–6 to themselves, in their own work, as well as expecting as much from their students. "Teacher, teach thyself."

We believe that increased attention to abuses of the borderline diagnosis will ensure its continuing theoretical and clinical utility and prevent it from becoming a wastebasket term. Supervisory skepticism about the use of the borderline diagnosis will help elucidate the complex issues involved in becoming a psychotherapist and thereby improve the educational experience.

Critical Review of the Concept of the Borderline Child

Joseph Palombo, M.S.W.
(1982)

The concept of the borderline child is reviewed in this paper. Questions are raised about the generally held assumption that a similarity exists between the dynamics of borderline children and those of borderline adults. It is suggested that no data is currently available to substantiate such a view. Further questions are raised about the assumption that the etiology of the disorder in childhood is based on poor or improper nurturance. A working definition of the concept of the borderline child is proposed that is free of preconceptions as to the etiology of the dysfunction. A hypothesis is presented for further investigation that at least some borderline children's etiology may be found in the presence of a minimal brain dysfunction or a severe learning disability.

Comparatively few publications have, in recent years, addressed the issues of the diagnosis and treatment of the borderline child (Chethic, 1980; Frijling-Schreuder, 1969; Pine, 1974; Rosenfeld, 1975; Rosenfeld & Sprince, 1965, 1963; Tooley, 1973). In contrast, an extensive literature exists on the adult versions of this disturbance. No effort has been made to explore the connection between the childhood version of the disorder and its adult counterpart, nor has the impact of adolescence on the personality's subsequent organiza-

Reprinted with permission from *Clinical Social Work, 10,* 4, 246–264. Copyright © 1982 Human Sciences Press.

tion been sufficiently explored. Only recently has Masterson (1980) published a study of the impact of treatment of borderline adolescents and the outcome of the intervention. In part, the confusion about the disorder stems from the multiplicity of points of view taken by theorists and from the absence of agreement about etiological factors. There is no general agreement as to whether the disorder represents a single entity or is a wastebasket category into which a variety of disorders that would fit nowhere else have been thrown.

In reviewing the literature on borderline children we have been struck by the similarity between the symptom picture presented by some of these children and the picture of some children suffering from severe learning disabilities or a minimal brain dysfunction. In several references, undiagnosed minimal brain dysfunctions appear in children who were in treatment and who had been diagnosed as borderline (Rosenfeld & Sprince, 1965). The knowledge about learning disabilities was not available at the time these papers were written for these factors to have been correctly identified.

There is general agreement that these children present serious difficulties for therapists who attempt to treat them. Often, heroic efforts are made to understand the nature of the disturbance. These efforts usually end up leaving the therapist feeling bewildered and defeated. The confusion about the nature of some children's disturbances has been increased by the failure to recognize the significance of the impairment in the primary autonomous ego apparatus and the impact of the deficit on the child's emotional development.

This paper undertakes a critical review of the literature on the diagnosis of borderline children and of the definition of that concept or entity. The review will highlight two major sets of problems:

A. The assumption generally made that a similarity exists between the dynamics of borderline children and borderline adults may be an erroneous one. This assumption is based on theoretical models of the symptom constellation derived from the treatment of adults, while no systematic data on children has been collected to substantiate this view.

B. The etiology of borderline disorders is generally presumed to lie in a developmental arrest at an early age. Factors of poor or improper nurturance have been implicated as contributing to the disturbance. This view may not take sufficiently into account possible biogenetic or congenital factors. A growing body of evidence is developing that begins to support the hypothesis that such factors may, indeed, play a significant role in the development of the disturbance.

As an elaboration of these two sets of problems, a definition of the concept of the borderline child is proposed as a working model that does not prejudge the issue of etiology. This definition will point the way to the research that needs to be conducted to clarify some of the issues related to this entity as it is seen in childhood.

Review of the Literature on Borderline Disorders

Initially, the term "borderline psychotic" was applied in 1921 to disorders which did not fit into the two poles of disturbances that were then more clearly understood: the neurotic or the psychotic (Stone, 1980). Knight, in 1953, suggested that a distinction be made between those disturbances which are clearly not neuroses nor psychoses, but are on the border of both. He suggested that the name "borderline" be used to characterize these disorders. This suggestion achieved wide currency and is generally accepted today.

Two divergent directions were then taken by investigators. One set of researchers attempted to develop a classificatory scheme based on the cataloging of symptoms presented by patients. These researchers attempted to derive generalizations from the empirically based data from the study of samples of these patients. To our knowledge, no similar systematic data was collected on children with this disorder; all studies conducted were on adults (Gunderson & Singer, 1975). The other direction was taken by a number of theorists whose data base was considerably narrower, but derived from the in-depth clinical study of patients. Their view of the dynamics of borderline disorders was seen in the context of the developmental perspective to which they subscribed (Shapiro, 1978). Prominent among these are: Kernberg (1975), Masterson (1978a), Giovacchini (Masterson, 1978b), Mahler (1971) and Kohut (Tolpin, 1980). With the exception of Mahler, none of these theorists had dealt with children, none discusses the condition as it prevails during childhood.

The group of studies that attempted to trace the etiology of the disorder through the medical model approach of listing the manifest symptoms demonstrates that little consensus exists even among these researchers as to what constitutes a borderline patient. Perry and Klerman (1978) summarized the findings of the major contributors. Their study divided these into four groups: Knight, Kernberg, Grinker, and Gunderson and Singer. Perry and Klerman list the various criteria spelled out by each group as defining the syndrome. They report that: (a) Knight found the presence of neurotic symptoms of macroscopic and microscopic ego weaknesses. (b) Kernberg also found nonspecific ego weaknesses, with shifts towards primary process thinking, specific defensive operations of splitting, and pathologic internalization of object relations. (c) Grinker gave some common characteristics of all borderlines, but found four subtypes: (1) the psychotic border, (2) the core borderline syndrome, (3) the adaptive affectless defended as-if personality, and (4) the border with neuroses. Finally, (d) Gunderson and Singer, who attempted to synthesize all the criteria that others use, found disturbances in affect, in behavior, in interpersonal relations, psychotic episodes, and specific findings on psychological test performance. Perry and Klerman conclude that there are three possible ways of interpreting these findings: first, it is possible that the concept of borderline is an illusion; second, it is possible that the concept may be adequately defined by the criteria given, but some criteria are nonessential; finally, it is possible that there are a number of subtypes in the group called borderline, but these subtypes are not clearly differentiated. They favor the last alternative. We will later have reason to believe that our evidence supports this suggestion.

What is of greatest interest is the common finding of general or specific ego weaknesses in all the patients studied. Whether these weaknesses were the cause of the condition or the effect of it remains an unanswered question.

A brief review of Kernberg's, Mahler's, and Kohut's contributions is offered as background for the discussion of the possible dynamics of the disorder and for its eventual redefinition in childhood. This review will be followed by a discussion of a number of authors who have discussed the syndrome as it appears specifically in childhood.

Kernberg (1975, 1976), as an object relations theorist, has suggested that the borderline personality has suffered an arrest prior to the 18th month of age, at which point the self image has remained separated from the object image, while reality testing has been established. For Kernberg, the good and bad self and object images are split. Splitting is the predominant pathological defense used in the service of keeping the affects around those images separated and in order to preserve the good feelings around the good image. The all good self and the all good object images are preserved and separated so as to prevent contamination by the bad self and object images. Rage at the object is related to the feelings of unpleasure, which are projected onto the object; envy for the object is based on the desire to possess what the object possesses but will not yield. General ego weakness, lack of impulse control, poor tolerance for anxiety, and defective superego integration result from this arrest. The external objects are devalued and the wish is to destroy them. Kernberg, while affirming that the dynamics of the disorders are related to the kind of nurturance the person received, also implicates as an etiological factor the intensity of the drives and/or the faulty nurturing superimposed upon the innate drive expression (1976, Ch. 3).

As can be seen in this scheme, which was derived exclusively from the study of adults, there is little room for the contributions of deficiencies in the primary autonomous ego apparatus or of developmental delays which often prevail in the learning disabled child. One has the clear impression, however, from reading some of Kernberg's case histories, that some of the patients he discusses may, indeed, have had such deficits. These remained undiagnosed although they must have played a central role in the formation of the personality.

Mahler's (1971, 1975) contributions are derived from inferences made from the analysis of adults and from her efforts at bridging adult psychopathology with her observations of normal children. While she has had considerable experience with psychotic children, only one reference could be found in which she directly discusses borderline and narcissistic disorders in childhood (Mahler & Kaplan, 1977). Her formulations are derived from the proposition that these conditions may be related to a developmental arrest at the rapprochement subphase of the separation and individuation phase of development. During this subphase, a number of developmental issues converge. Failure to resolve these leads to the possibility of a borderline disturbance as an outcome. The child's grandiosity is at its highest during the practicing subphase. This grandiosity begins to break up as better reality testing is established, and leads the child eventually to experience that the world is, indeed, not his oyster. Greater awareness of physical separateness intensifies separation anxiety, and a pattern of active approach behavior, seeking to become reunited with mother, emerges. This leads to the playful shadowing and darting games, which are characteristic of this phase of childhood. The wish for reunion is accompanied by the fear of reengulfment into the symbiotic shell. The father increasingly begins to play a role in fostering awareness of gender identity. The cognitive achievements of object permanence, accompanied by language development, give further impetus to the experience of separateness and to differentiation. The derailment of these developmental themes leads to failures in the integration of the good and bad self images and to an arrest at the preambivalent or ambitendent phase. Object constancy is, therefore, never fully achieved, and the possibility of phase dominance in the phallic-oedipal stage is aborted.

While the possibility of congenital factors affecting development is acknowledged, no effort is made at integrating these factors into the developmental scheme. The variations in endowment or the deficits in primary autonomous ego functions could easily and consistently be included into the theory and may, indeed, enrich it were they to be interwoven into it.

The psychology of the self (Kohut, 1971) developed out of an effort to differentiate the analyzable narcissistic personality disorders from the neurotic disturbances and the borderline and psychotic disturbances. Kohut found that some nonneurotic patients in whom there were no signs of psychosis could be best understood as suffering from problems of self-esteem. Their sense of self was deficient. These patients could be distinguished from the borderline patients by virtue of the fact that the narcissistic personality's sense of cohesion was essentially intact. Borderline patients suffered from primary deficits in their sense of cohesion and were, therefore, prone to regressive fragmentations. Their cohesion was unstable and was maintained through the use of a variety of defensive operations which serve to bind their sense of self (Tolpin, 1980). Based on this theory, Palombo (1979) conceptualized the role of perceptual deficits in the development of a troubled adolescent. It should be noted that, in this framework, either borderline or narcissistic outcomes may result from learning deficits in early childhood. The absence of cohesion may be directly related to the deficits in endowment. What is significant is that new treatment strategies become available through such an approach, while the older strategies were less successful in the treatment of these children.

Turning now to contributors who have dealt more directly with borderline children from a psychoanalytic point of view, we find that the earliest reference is in Ekstein and Wallerstein (1954, 1956). They reported on their observations of children in a residential setting, although no attempt was made to conceptualize the disturbance. Geleerd (1958) later also made reference to the disturbance. Rosenfeld and Sprince (1963) made an excellent contribution in which they raised the important question as to whether "borderline" is an entity or a specific ego dysfunction. In their formulation, they conclude that the condition probably represents an ego deviation. They feel that a deficit exists in the capacity for internalization and inner representation with a failure to maintain object cathexis. What is significant in this contribution is that their metapsychological discussion points to the presence of material relating to arrests at all levels of libidinal development, and also to deficits in ego development and specific ego functions. Thus they point to the area of perception where they found the children they observed to have difficulties in the inhibition and selection of stimuli. They saw some children as overwhelmed by external and internal stimuli. All the children they surveyed showed disturbances in the motor sphere. All showed disorders of speech and thought processes. The faulty thinking, however, was attributed to the effects of repression with primary process thinking observed, and the translation of fantasy and impulse into action being seen as primary. They did not consider that they may have been related to deficits in the cognitive apparatus itself. At the same time, they indicate that these clear failures in primary autonomous ego apparatus might be suggestive of neurological factors. However, they fail to make the connection between these and the disturbance itself.

Frijling-Schreuder (1969), in attempting to spell out "some provisional differential diagnostic criteria" between childhood borderline states and childhood psychoses and neuroses, seems to borrow heavily from the Rosenfeld and Sprince formulation. She points to ego development and its significance and finds: specific disturbances in integration, less disturbances in reality testing than in psychosis, differentiation between self and object representation, but with a tendency to regression to nondifferentiation, disturbances of the use of speech as a means of contact, often with a strong need for contact, and unrealistic ideas of grandeur, but no constant delusions; secondary process thinking is used defensively. The etiology here is presumed to be related to the deficiencies in nurturance.

More recently Pine (1974) in his discussion of borderline children distinguishes between an "upper" borderline and a "lower" borderline. The latter is closer to the psychoses while the former is closer to the neuroses. The "upper" borderline is described as suffering from: (a) chronic ego deficiencies; (b) shifting levels of ego organization; (c) incomplete internalization of psychosis; (d) ego limitations and (e) schizoid personality. Once more, one is struck by the findings of ego deficits and deviations. Pine also allows for the possibility that that the disorders may be based on neurological impairment, or minimal brain dysfunction, but that suggestion is not pursued.

Chethic (1979), in a recent comprehensive review of the concept, presents a series of descriptive characteristics common to the children with this disturbance: intense, diffuse anxiety, neurotic symptomatology, impulsivity, and a variety of character traits. These characteristics appear to be derived from clinical experiences rather than from the systematic data gathering conducted on a large sample of children. Chethic then outlines the psychodynamic factors that might be said to underlie the symptom picture. The formulations to which he arrives seem to follow Anna Freud's developmental profile (see Table 1). The significant role of the distorted object relations in these children is highlighted. Although he points to the possibility that neurological impairment may be present (p. 313), he makes no attempt to address the interrelationship between the impairment and the disorder. Thus, the ego of the borderline child is characterized as weak, helpless, and fragile. In the area of ego functions and motoric development, one sees manifestations of early distress in the form of hyperactivity, body rigidity, and peculiarities in gait and posture. In the area of perceptual development there are many associated components that are deficient. Difficulties in perception due to flooding by stimuli promote difficulties in the ability to attend and discern the origins of the stimuli. In relation to the control of drive activity, there exists an ego syntonicity with the expression of impulses during the times of eruptive behavior and a repressive quality to the lack of impulse control. The synthetic functions of the ego do not permit the unification of the libidinal and aggressive drive components of the representation of significant objects. The thought processes of the borderline child, according to Chethic, manifest a capacity to regress to prelogical thought, while on the whole, maintaining secondary thought process function. Defenses are impoverished, with failure to maintain repression, and the use of splitting as a major defense is observed. In the development of superego, difficulties also emerge. The prohibitions and standards of important love objects may be imitated, identified with, and ultimately introjected. However, these introjections are endowed with intense aggression and therefore severe. These problems in structuralization result in the building of internal prohibitions which are not well developed or markedly impaired.

Once again, the bias introduced by the perspective from which Chethic enters the viewing of the disorder leads to the impression that he too concludes that the primary etiological factor lies in the type of nurturance the child received, rather than from other factors that are contributed to the personality's development by the child's endowment.

Distinction Between Etiologic and Genetic-Dynamic Factors

A distinction may be made between etiological factors and genetic-dynamic factors as determinants of emotional disorders. The concept of "etiology" is derived from the medical model approach to disease, which attempts to define specific causal factors as contributory to a specific disease entity. The concept of "genetic-dynamic" factors is a psychological construct that attempts to link the developmental model of behavior with emotional disorders. Emotional disorders are seen as representing arrests at or regressions to specific phases of development (Kohut, 1971, pp. 254–255). The later approach explains the disorders not as being caused by specific toxic agents but rather as resulting from the convergence of a complex set of interrelated events and forces that occur in a given context and to the private meanings these events have for the person. Symptomatic behavior is understood to have meaning to each person and precludes specifying causal relations of a simplistic nature. These two differing concepts represent differing views on the nature, the onset, and the emergence of emotional disorders.

The specific determinants that contribute to the disorders of childhood continue to elude researchers. In recent years a significant shift has occurred in the areas being explored to find these determinants (Kety, 1978). Historically the psychoanalytic school began by searching for "psycho-toxic factors," as Spitz called them. The seduction hypothesis which Freud first proposed was modeled on the medical model approach which his training dictated. Factors such as specific or cumulative traumas, early loss of significant objects, or the quality of the nurturing object in early development all attempted to point the finger at a specific culprit for the disorder. These efforts failed because no event was ever found to have identical meaning for any two people. Each individual responds differently to the the context in which he or she is raised and each

Table 1
Comparative Chart of Theories of Borderline Children
(Anna Freud)

Developmental Profile	Rosenfeld & Sprince	Chethic	Frijling-Schreuder
A. Drive Development			
1. Libidinal development	a. No phase dominance. b. Material from all phases. c. The bulk of material is from oral & anal phases.		a. No phase dominance. b. Difficulties in transition from one phase to the next. c. Great dependency.
2. Distribution of libido: self-cathexis, object-cathexis	a. Merges easily, precarious self boundaries. b. On the border between object-cathexis and identification. c. Fears merger. d. Body ego problems.		a. Forms symbiotic relation-ships. b. Too much self-cathexis. c. Unrealistic feelings of grandiosity. d. Less vitality. e. Fetishistic traits.
3. Aggression	a. Poor control of aggression. It is either excessive or the opposite.	a. Aggression intense from infancy on.	a. Open aggression lacking, but impulsive outbursts are present.

Developmental Profile	Rosenfeld & Sprince	Chethic	Frijling-Schreuder
B. Ego Development			
1. Primary autonomous functions			
a. Preception	a. Deficient stimulus barrier & capacity to inhibit stimuli. b. Distractibility.	a. Difficulties in inhibiting stimuli.	
b. Memory			
c. Cognition	a. Disturbances in thinking. b. Faulty barrier between conscious & preconscious thoughts. c. Direct translation of fantasy into actions.	a. Secondary process is present, but regresses to prelogical, magical thinking.	a. Secondary process used defensively. b. Disturbances in the use of speech as a means of contact.
d. Motility	a. Disturbances in gait & posture, and body rigidity. b. Hyperactivity.	a. Body rigidities, peculiar gait & posture. b. Hyperactivity. c. Evidence from infancy on of deviant physiological functioning & of erratic patterning.	
2. Secondary autonomous functions			
a. Reality testing		a. May give way under pressure from aggressive impulses.	a. Less disturbed than in psychotics.
b. Judgment			
c. Reality sense			
d. Synthetic function		a. Ego incapable of binding & uniting the mental representation.	a. Specific disturbance in integration.

Developmental Profile	Rosenfeld & Sprince	Chethic	Frijling-Schreuder
e. Drive control & regulation	a. Faulty relationship between ego & drives.	a. Capacity for neutralization underdeveloped. b. Problems with impulse control.	
f. Frustration tolerance	a. Operates at level of pleasure principle. Postponement of gratification impossible.	a. Unable to wait or tolerate tension.	a. May be high except in specific traumatic situations.
3. Defenses	a. Projection plays a large role. b. Denial is used. c. Displacement, introjection and regression. d. Repression is defective. e. Uses withdrawal into fantasy.	a. Defenses not effective in binding anxiety. b. Denial & projection are used. c. Overcompensates through their overuse. d. They are inflexible. e. Uses splitting. f. Uses idealization & devaluation.	a. All kinds of defenses used. b. Projection & identification are more primitive than in neurosis. c. Defenses are very ineffective.
4. Object relations	a. On the border between identification and object-cathexis. b. Precarious self boundaries lead to regression and merging. c. Disturbance in distinguishing between self & object representation.	a. Separation of self & non-self has been achieved. But a search for an all giving & gratifying object is present. b. Projection of all gratifying images onto objects. c. Difficulties in object constancy lead to clinging to object & to act coersively towards it.	a. Differentiation between self and object representation exists, but with a tendency to regress to nondifferentiation.

Developmental Profile	Rosenfeld & Sprince	Chethic	Frijling-Schreuder
		d. Lack of empathy for others. e. Unintegrated self-other bond. f. Wish for control over others.	
5. Affects a. Anxiety	a. Intense, diffuse, paniclike, disintegrative, annihilative. b. Signal anxiety is overwhelming.	a. Chronic, diffuse, free-floating. b. Absence of signal anxiety function. c. Fear of annihilation. d. Fear of separation. e. Fear of disorganization. f. Fear of the strength of impulses, wishes, or affects.	a. Pan anxiety. b. Much anxiety at every developmental step. c. Danger of psychosis if pushed to develop.
b. Mood c. Quality	a. Subdued. a. Flat.		
C. Superego Development	a. Capacity for internalization impaired. b. Dependent on external objects as reinforcers.	a. Problems in structuralization lead to failures in internalization, introjection, and identification. b. Functions are preautonomous. c. Its characteristics are: severe, hypercritical, self-deprecating, inconsistent, and endowed with intense aggression.	a. Primitive structures are very dependent on outer objects. b. Some internalization with a tendency to reexternalization.

takes something different from that context. Psychic reality does not parallel physical reality. Psychoanalytic psychology has therefore moved away from an attempt at finding a close correlation between external events and internal responses to these events. It has had to enlarge its purview to include such factors as "the intensity of the drives" (Kernberg, 1976, Ch. 3) or central nervous system dysfunctions (cf. Mahler, 1968, in regard to autism). Other contributors, such as Kohut, have given up altogether trying to make such linkages. A hermeneutic point of view which essentially says that psychology is the study of meanings rather than of causal relationships has developed as a separate school of psychoanalytic thought in France (Ricoeur, 1970).

To date no consensus has been established as to which of these two explanatory models is appropriate to the understanding of the borderline disorders, much less to these disorders as manifest in childhood. Given, furthermore, that no systematic data has been collected on children, the application of either model to the observed dysfunction would only represent the expression of a particular bias. However, a growing body of evidence is emerging that can be brought to bear in support of a position that suggests that at least for some children the disturbance is explainable through an understanding of the specific etiological factors that appear to determine the course of the dysfunction.

In any case, even if agreement could be reached on a definition of the borderline syndrome in childhood, it appears clear at this time that the entity is far from a unitary one and that it encompasses perhaps a broad variety of disorders. Some children's chaotic backgrounds appear to be major determinants for the disorder. This would seem to implicate genetic-dynamic factors as contributory to the symptomatic picture. Other children from the same family, however, will seem to emerge much more intact than their less fortunate siblings or than one would be led to anticipate given the absence of nurturance. This raises some serious questions as to the correlations between the symptom picture and causal factors or genetic-dynamic factors.

While this discussion seems to dichotomize etiologic and genetic-dynamic factors, in reality it is simplistic to think in these polarized terms. Most developmental theorists (Weil, 1973, 1978) concede that a child's endowment contributes in a major way to his or her interaction with the environment and the individual's adaptive or maladaptive capabilities. What is not clearly explicated is the extent to which congenital givens impose limits on the child's

ability to utilize the available nurturance. Mahler (1968) hypothesized precisely such factors in the case of infantile autism but she did
not generalize that perspective in her work on other children. The
environment, by being responsive or nonresponsive, can mitigate or
maximize the impact of a child's limitation upon the course of the
development of the personality. However, there are limits beyond
which no environment, no matter how therapeutic and benign, can
eradicate the devastating effects of certain developmental deficits.

It may be that the more balanced view to take is one in which
borderline disorders are seen as a residual category composed of a
variety of disorders and within these disorders some are clearly
reflective of poor endowment while others are clearly reflective of
poor nurturance and a continuum between the two may be seen to
exist. The diagnostic issue presented would be that of determining
which of the two sets of factors may play a more dominant role in the
pathological outcome.

Discussion

These considerations and those made above in the discussion of
the literature clearly demonstrate that there is at present no basis
for assuming that the adult borderline conditions are necessarily
similar in etiology or in dynamic structure to the childhood form of
the disorder. Furthermore, it is far from established that a connection between the two forms of the disturbances exists. Studies of
adult borderlines have not demonstrated that those patients
suffered from borderline disorders as children. In fact, the evidence
from the clinical case descriptions would support a view that
indicates that many of those patients functioned at much higher
levels as children than as adults and that the crisis in their lives may
have occurred either at adolescence or at a later point in time. For
those borderline personalities who do not develop the disorder until
early adulthood it is hard to see how it could be maintained that the
disturbance is traceable to an arrest at the rapprochement phase of
development. One would at least have to maintain that the disorder
reflects a regression back to that phase. Such a suggestion, however,
runs counter to the general formulations that the disorder is
reflective of an arrest in development.

The converse of this is equally true. Children who have been
diagnosed as borderline in childhood may or may not mature into
borderline adults. It seems clear from the small sample seen in my
clinical practice and in consultation to social agencies that some of

these children negotiate adolescence sufficiently successfully as to make a reasonable adaptation to young adulthood. They do not seem to manifest the signs and symptoms of borderlines. Other of these children suffer psychotic breakdowns and deteriorate in adolescence and young adulthood into chronic psychosis. The factors that determine either outcome remain unknown at this point.

While Masterson (1980) has studied adolescents who were diagnosed as borderline and has followed them at least into young adulthood, his data lead him to suggest that with intensive treatment the outcome for these patients is variable. Some make a good adaptation while others do not.

To complete this picture there is some limited clinical evidence to suggest that some children who are diagnosed as schizophrenic or psychotic and who received intensive milieu and individual treatment grow to resemble the "as-if" personalities that Grinker describes. Other of these children who have been medicated and receive only special education services appear to grow to be more like the classic borderline that Gunderson and Singer describe.

At best what may be concluded from all of this is that there is no simple dynamic that can explain either the childhood or the adult borderline disorders in their totality. The etiological considerations are multiple as are the genetic-dynamic factors. We are far from being able to understand the range and nature of this disorder.

In view of all this the following strategy is being proposed for further research in this entire confused area. It is suggested that a consensus definition of the concept be taken as a starting point and that this definition be sufficiently inclusive to encompass a variety of points of view. In line with the suggestions made by DSM III (APA, 1980) one might then study the condition without prejudging the issue of etiology and presumably arrive at some classificatory and clarificatory ways of looking at the disorder.

Proposed Consensus Definition of the Concept of Borderline Children

The consensus definition of the condition is arrived at through an amalgamation of the major contributors to the fields. (See Table 2.) Those that have contributed to the literature on the childhood form of the disorder are exclusively considered in order to avoid the biases of the definition that includes aspects of the adult form of the condition. The definition is composed of two major parts. The first part limits itself to a listing of the symptomatic behavior commonly manifest in the condition as described by these contributors. The second part is also descriptive but is organized along the lines of the developmental profile of Anna Freud. Table 1 attempts to corrolate some of the contributors' major findings.

Symptomatic Behavior

The following (Chethic, 1979) is a summary of the symptomatic behavior manifested by these children.

1. They suffer from neuroticlike behaviors which include their being polysymptomatic, having rituals, obsessions, phobias, and inhibitions.
2. They are generally impulsive, suffering from temper tantrums, aggressive outbursts, and affective constriction, and are commonly involved in fantasy.
3. Their anxiety manifests itself as chronic, often diffuse, with separation anxiety and fear of fragmentation being present.
4. Their character traits manifest grandiosity, low self-esteem, self destructiveness, overdependence, and ease of regression, and have paranoid aspects to them.
5. Socially the children are isolates, seeming not to be able to form peer relationships.

The second major component of the definition includes the following typical development profile of the borderline child.

Drive Development

Libidinally the children manifest no phase dominance with material from all phases seeming to be present. They seem to merge or form symbiotic relationships easily and have precarious self boundaries. They are more self-cathected than cathecting others. They fear mergers while wishing to merge. They suffer from unrealistic feelings of grandiosity. They commonly have body ego image problems. In the area of aggression, their self control is poor and is either excessive restraint or aggressiveness or open and intense expression of it.

Ego Development

There are two major areas to consider regarding the state of the ego. The first is the area of the primary autonomous functions. With regard to the primary autonomous functions, the area of perception is deficient with difficulties in the capacity to inhibit stimuli or to screen out the reception of stimuli. Distractibility is also a problem. Interestingly, none of the contributors mentioned memory problems, although these should not be excluded. In the area of cognition there are disturbances in thinking, with secondary process being present or used defensively but regression to prelogical and magical thinking occurring. There are faulty barriers between conscious and preconscious thinking with disturbances in the use of speech as a means for making contact, and the direct expression of fantasy in action. With regard to motility there are disturbances in gait and posture with body rigidities being present and generally hyperactivity being noticed, with evidence from infancy on of deviant physiological functioning or patterning.

With regard to the secondary autonomous functions reality testing is present but is less disturbed than in psychotics and may give way under the pressure of aggressive impulses. The synthetic functions of the ego are faulty with disturbances in integration but some capacity is present to bind and unite mental representations. Drive control and regulation is faulty with capacity for neutralizations of drives underdeveloped and there are problems with impulse control. The child operates at the level of the pleasure principle with frustration tolerance not being present and the postponement of gratification often impossible.

The defenses manifested are often projection, denial, displacement, introjection, and regression. The use of the splitting is noted, and the use of idealization and devaluation as well as withdrawal into fantasy. The defenses, however, are often ineffective in achieving repression.

The area of object relations is disturbed, with self-cathexis predominating over object-cathexis. There are difficulties in the establishment of object constancy with coercive clinging towards objects, lack of empathy for objects, and wish for control over objects being present.

In the area of affects, anxiety is intense, diffuse, chronic, free-floating, disintegrative. The signal function of anxiety is ineffectual; fears of separation, of disorganization, and of the impulses are present. The child's mood is subdued and the quality of the affect is flat.

Superego Development

The capacity to internalize controls and prohibitions is impaired. The child is dependent on outer objects for restraint and control, and when functional, the superego is characterized as being severe, hypercritical, self-deprecating, inconsistent, and endowed with intense aggression.

Based on this consensus definition of the syndrome, it will perhaps be possible to formulate some hypotheses to begin to clarify the nature of some of the disorders. For example, some of the children who fit the consensus picture of a borderline child also suffer from minimal brain dysfunctions and learning disabilities. It would be interesting to investigate the correlation between these specific deficits with the syndrome itself and to clarify whether or not a relationship exists between the occurrence of those deficits and the borderline syndrome. Other hypotheses might be generated that could point in a different direction.

Conclusions

The detailed review of the literature on borderline disorders in children raises serious questions as to whether or not this disorder is the same as that discussed by investigators who have studied the adult forms of the disturbance. There are also questions as to whether a continuity existed between the disorder that is manifest in childhood as it exists in adulthood. Furthermore, a distinction may be made between etiology and genetic-dynamic formulations about the disturbances. If the distinction is valid it suggests that there are two frames of reference through which the disorder may be viewed and that while no systematic research exists to date to substantiate which frame of reference best explains to disorder, a consensus definition of the disturbance may be of help as a beginning for clarification of the distinctions. It is possible that one can then formulate hypotheses and collect data to unravel some of the confusion that this syndrome presents.

Disturbances in Sex and Love in Borderline Patients

Michael H. Stone, M.D.
(1985)

Once more he had found her out, got through the barrier and seen her for what she was, a beautiful woman who could not believe in her own beauty or accept love without casting every conceivable doubt upon it. Now and every other time that they quarreled, she was merely seeing how far she could go, leading him to the edge of the pit and making him look down, threatening their common happiness in order to convince herself of its reality.
William Maxwell, Time Will Darken It

Since borderline conditions are situated either expressly (within the broad definitions of Kernberg, 1977, Vanggaard, 1979, or Bergeret, 1975) or indirectly (within the syndromal definitions of Gunderson and Singer, 1975, or DSM-III, APA, 1980) in between the neuroses and the psychoses, it should not be surprising that, alongside the characteristic disturbances in identity, impulse control, and mood regulation, disturbances in intimate relationships are encountered with some regularity. Within the borderline domain, Freud's bipartite division of life into *Liebe* and *Arbeit* finds partial expression under the heading "poor sublimatory channeling" (Kernberg, 1967) or "work below capacity" (Gunderson & Singer, 1975). Less attention has been paid to the other half of life in borderline patients, though some authors have alluded to their chaotic sexuality. Hoch and Polatin (1949), for example, spoke of "pan-sexuality" in their pseudoneurotic schizophrenics, many of whom would be considered borderline by contemporary diagnostic standards. Included in that no longer popular term were such manifestations as promiscuity, "polymorphous perverse practices," and rapid fluctuations between homosexuality and heterosexuality.

Our examination of the problems experienced in this realm of life by borderline patients will be facilitated if we divide Freud's *Liebe* once again into sexuality and love. Such a division is all the more relevant when speaking of borderline patients, insofar as these attributes are less often integrated in this group than in normal or "neurotic" persons. Feelings of love (including the components mentioned by Erich Fromm: tenderness, concern about the welfare and personal growth of the beloved, etc.) regularly coexist with lustful feelings in those that have the capacity to integrate these strong emotions. In those whom we call "borderline" this integrative capacity is, for a variety of reasons, either lacking or seriously enfeebled. The borderline's general disturbance in identity-sense may contribute to this lack, or the borderline person may have been reared in an environment where striking inconsistencies and deficiencies in the parents' ability to love simply left their children with no template, no pattern, for mature, integrated loving with which to identify and utilize later. As a result, when one examines the intimate relationships of borderlines, one may find sex unaccompanied by love, compulsively and throughout the life cycle (even in long-term partnerships, where ideally these elements are blended), or else sex and love combined, but in a way that seems immature, a grotesque caricature of the ideal state: a stifling possessiveness within the context of a symbiotic partnership, rather than a sexual love between two people who respect and foster each other's needs for continued individuation and evolution.

The sources from which my impressions are derived consist of borderline patients seen over the past 17 years in private practice and less methodically studied samples of inpatient borderlines seen, over a 20-year period, at the three hospitals where I have been affiliated (New York State Psychiatric Institute, New York Hospital/ Westchester Division, and the University of Connecticut Health Center). In the office sample there are, as of this writing, 54 patients, all "borderline" by Kernberg criteria (1967) (poor identity integration, yet with adequate capacity for reality testing), of whom 39 are female and 15 are male. Homosexuality has not been particularly common in this group, having been noted only in one male and in three of the female patients. Among the latter, one was exclusively homosexual, one was predominantly homosexual, and one was episodically homosexual. These figures did not differ significantly from the equally low incidence of homosexuality among the neurotic patients seen in private practice for psychotherapy over the same period of time.

We would like to be able to answer such questions as whether homosexuality is more common in borderline patients than in better-integrated patients, and whether female borderlines would be any more prone to develop along homosexual lines than female neurotics. One is tempted to ask these questions, partly in relation to the popular theories concerning the psychodynamics of borderline development (Kernberg, 1967; Mahler, 1971; Masterson, 1981; Rinsley, 1982), stressing, as they do, serious problems in effecting emotional separation from the maternal figure (which could, speculatively, predispose borderline-to-be females to remain excessively attached to or yearning for closeness with motherly females) and also problems that are conducive to narcissistic object-choice (which might predispose future borderlines of either sex to remain fixated at the "homosexual level," as the latter is envisioned by psychoanalysts who espouse a linear model of psychosexual evolution).

The homosexual community is a large one, and granted that within it males considerably outnumber females, there is little convincing evidence that its emotional health is appreciably lower than what one finds in the heterosexual population. Psychiatrists and psychoanalysts see a skewed sample, naturally: those who suffer and seek help (Friedman, 1983). It is for the epidemiologists, not for us, to say whether a systematic survey of male or of female homosexuals, where those not seeking psychiatric help were also included, would turn up a higher proportion of emotionally ill persons than would be expected in the general population. I am not acquainted with any such survey, let alone one measuring the prevalence of "borderline" conditions according to some commonly accepted criteria.

One's impressions about the relative mental health of homosexuals would be influenced by the particular system one chose for arriving at a borderline diagnosis. Psychoanalysts, for example, tend to regard human nature with normative lenses, according to which homosexuality is *eo ipso* a deviation (some analysts do not share this view; Judd Marmor, for example, or Robert Stoller or Richard Friedman). Those who exhibit homosexuality tend to be regarded as manifesting a problem in gender identity more often than might be the case if viewed by a clinician without psychoanalytic training. But "identity disturbances" is the hallmark of borderline personality organization in Kernberg's (psychoanalytic) schema. I know of some homosexual patients who, despite their not being impulsive, angry, or given to suicidal gestures, get labeled "borderline" by Kernberg criteria, even while they would not be considered Gunderson, or DSM-III, borderlines. In the absence of hard data, I am inclined to adopt the more conservative position—that borderlines, at least as defined by the narrower criteria of Gunderson, may not be overrepresented in a population of homosexuals.

In my private practice series, among 39 female borderlines there were 3 who were homosexuals (7.7%); of the 15 males, 1 was homosexual (6.6%). The incidence in the female subgroup may be higher than what is found in the general population, but from a small, nonrandom sample of that sort one is not entitled to draw conclusions. Among the 29 inpatient DSM borderlines at the University of Connecticut Health Center who were part of our diagnostic research project, there were no homosexuals.

In general, it is difficult to create a representative sample of borderlines within a particular community, in order, for example, to evaluate the incidence of homosexuality. It is likewise difficult to select a "random" sample of homosexuals within which to study the incidence of borderline psychopathology. Both tasks would require a broad epidemiological survey.

Promiscuity

By *promiscuity,* I refer not so much to the number of sexual partners, to the brevity of relationships, or to the rapidity with which partners are exchanged in favor of others as to the drivenness and dehumanization, or impersonality, that characterizes the sexual patterns of those whom we may meaningfully regard as "promiscuous." One sees not only compulsive seeking of one partner after another but also the joylessness accompanying this process, along with a general handicap in forming a deep and integrated relationship with another person.

The correlation between borderline psychopathology and sexual promiscuity seems impressive in contrast to the situation with homosexuality. More than 25% of my office-practice borderline patients exhibited this trait: 2 of the 15 males, 12 of the 39 females. Promiscuity was rare among their neurotic counterparts. I recall only one analysand within my experience to whom this label could be said to apply. She was a lonely, narcissistic graduate student given to seducing men met casually in the elevator of her apartment building or at work or at the musical events she was fond of attending, and inviting them to enjoy with her what she called, adopting the phrase from Erica Jong's *Fear of Flying,* a "zipless fuck." But this combination of loneliness, hunger for attention, indifference to social convention, and impulsivity was common among the borderline women especially. Other manifestations of their drivenness and affect hunger included alcoholism and abuse of various drugs. A significant difference, for example, emerges when the borderlines with promiscuity and those without are compared with respect to substance abuse. In the nonpromiscuous group, 8 out of 40 abused drugs or alcohol (20%), while substance abuse and promiscuity were found in common in 9 of 14 instances (64%).

A number of factors appear to converge in creating the emotional environment in which promiscuity is likely to occur. This "overdetermined" system is found in patients, most of whom are female, who show a particularly low and self-denigrated self-image. Often they have been called "tramps" by fathers who, unable to deal more maturely with their daughters' burgeoning sexuality during adolescence, protect themselves from their own incestuous impulses toward the latter by a projective mechanism, where the girl rather than the father is seen as the tramp. Subjected to this interaction long enough, the daughters often live out their fathers' unconscious yearnings and become "whores."

In another subgroup of borderline women, incest has indeed been acted out and not merely defended against (Stone, 1981). This was so in 16% of my female office-practice borderlines, and in over 50% of a sample of inpatient borderline women at New York Hospital/ Westchester Division. Probably the majority of the nonpsychotic hospitalized girls with a history of incest, as described by Emslie and Rosenfeld (1983), were functionally borderline. One may compare these figures with those noted for the general population, where about 1 woman in 20 in the United States has had incestuous experiences with a brother or an older male relative.

Side by side with a low self-image, and especially in those who have either experienced incest or been raised by overtly seductive fathers, is a morbid fascination with sex as well as a pronounced tendency toward "sensation-seeking." Ambivalence toward men is marked: idealization is intertwined with contempt and hatred for having been misused. In the casual sexual encounters with strangers, there is opportunity to live out these contradictory attitudes. The stranger is viewed as mysterious, powerful, protecting, loving (as with Mr. Goodbar), but he is also viewed (perhaps more accurately) as inconstant and unfaithful, as exploitative but paradoxically easily exploitable, by the woman who lures him with the promise of sexual favors.

Inability to postpone gratification is characteristic of the promiscuous group, almost by identification; their capacity for sublimatory activities is almost invariably impaired (Kernberg, 1967). The sexual drive in borderlines is often intense to start out with, owing to constitutional factors, of which the most important is predisposition to hypomania (where all the drives are intensified— hence the pacing, rapid speech, overspending, impulsive planning, and so on). Add to this the extra measure of intensification through sexual overstimulation by family members during childhood or adolescence, and one can appreciate how the trait of promiscuity becomes an all-but-inescapable outcome.

In many borderlines with this trait, rapid alterations in attitude are often discernible in relation to their sexual partners. These oscillations, taken together, can be seen as a manifestation of the "splitting," both in self-image and in the internalized representations of others, that is characteristic of the borderline patient (Kernberg, 1967). The following vignette is illustrative:

Promiscuity as Paradoxical Fidelity

A woman in her late 20s entered psychotherapy following hospitalization for suicide gestures and abuse of alcohol following a romantic disappointment. She came from an upper-class New England family, consisting, besides two siblings, of a father whom she idealized and a mother whom she experienced as perfectionistic, hypercritical, and intrusive. Though of average appearance and refined manners, she saw herself as ugly. Longing for acceptance and approval by men, she would, especially when lonely, either place herself in situations where she could get "picked up" by strangers or would accept dates with men who, though they had been "properly introduced," did not really appeal to her. In either case, she could not say no to either advances and invariably ended up in bed. During the beginning moments of sexual play, she would feel

exhilarated, basking in the admittedly illusory enthusiasm
of her partner, feeling for these few minutes that she was
pretty, desirable, and as capable as the next woman of
"getting a man." But this euphoric mood would dissipate
shortly before orgasm, to be replaced by a mood of self-
denigration and hostility. She would vilify her partner (not
usually out loud) as a manipulative cad who was just out
to "get laid" and who would scarcely remember her name
the next morning. Herself she would vilify as a pathetic
tramp, a stain on the family escutcheon, and so forth.

Much more hidden from her view was another set of
attitudes toward these one-night stands, which emerged
only from prolonged and meticulous work with her
dreams—wherein the men were prized never for themselves but only to the extent they could become symbols
to her of the cherished father. She could not love a man for
himself without relinquishing something of the excessive
attachment to her father, and that she was unwilling to do.
In this sense, *promiscuity* with unimportant strangers was,
as is so often true with borderline women, the reverse side
of the coin, on whose obverse was a pathological *fidelity*
to the all-important father.

In this case, the father had not behaved in a particularly
seductive manner, nor had the woman experienced incestuous
advances or play. Perhaps because of this her sexuality, although
disturbed, was not as grotesque or chaotic as what one often
observes in those who have experienced incest (see below). Her
quasi-delusional conviction of being ugly is something one encounters often among borderline women. The psychodynamics are not
always the same. This symptom, which has received some attention
in the literature under the disarming rubric "dysmorphobia,"
deserves a closer look and will be discussed in detail later.

Hypersexuality

Despite the frequency of promiscuity in borderline women and
in some borderline men, it is less common to see hypersexuality, if
by this term we refer to a morbid and incessant craving for sex and a
preoccupation with this topic throughout almost all one's waking
moments. The three patients in this category, with whom I have
worked, consist of two females and a male. All had incestuous
relationships throughout much of their childhood (through adolescence). The male, a homosexual, was masturbated by his mother,

who presided over his nightly bath until he was 15. He became "obsessed" with sex; as a young adult, he would supplement what he could not get in the context of a relationship with encounters with strangers in subway men's rooms. One of the women, who thought about sex all day long and would never "get enough," despite intercourse with her husband three or four times a day, had had an incestuous relationship (involving oral sex) with her father from the time she was 6 until she was 16. The other woman, a divorced schoolteacher, would be desolated if her fiancé failed to make love to her in the morning, even if they had had sex two or three times the evening before and if he were exhausted or else worried because he was late for some important business meeting. She would become convinced he no longer loved her. During her younger years, she had incestuous involvements with both parents—the only patient I have heard of so far where this was true—the mother masturbating her under the pretext of checking to see if her organs were "all right," her father engaging in intercourse from about the time she was 11.

It is perhaps relevant that in these three patients there had been no physical cruelty in the parent-child relationship (instead, the psychological cruelty of so grossly misusing one's child in the first place). The balance between sexual excitement and hostility toward the older person was tipped much in favor of the former, at least in the women: overstimulated as youngsters, they became hypersexual as adults, but always with the view of sex as something natural and joyful. The male patient reacted against his seductive mother in repudiating his heterosexual impulses (which were still a part of his fantasy life until his late 20s), reaching out instead to men, though with the same compulsive and insatiable quality noted in the two female patients.

That there could be a constitutional component to hypersexuality (nymphomania), of a sort similar to what we speculated could be operative in certain promiscuous patients, seems likely in some instances. Here again a predisposition to hypomania seems the most probable factor. Isolated cases of this sort have been described in the earlier literature, the most noteworthy example being that of Voisin (1826), a portion of which (concerning a 3-year-old girl who grew up to become a nymphomaniac) I have translated elsewhere (Stone, 1973).

Kraepelin (1921) was aware of hypersexuality as one possible accompaniment of "manic temperament," by which he referred to the constellation of personality traits one sees often either in true bipolar patients or in their close relatives. In fact, it is the hallmark of manic psychopathology that one is excessive in everything: besides hypersexuality, common manifestations are verbosity, overspending, a diminished need for sleep, hyperactivity, and aggressiveness. Some nymphomaniacs are, so to speak, nympho*manics* (and responsive to lithium).

Incest: Its Impact on Psychosexual Development

We have already alluded to several instances of incestuous involvement among borderline patients with specific sexual problems. The topic deserves further mention, not only because of the profound effects on psychosexual development that incest regularly brings about but also because of the unusual frequency with which a history of incest will be elicited in a borderline population. Although I have encountered isolated instances of father-son incest in borderline men, the overwhelming majority of cases concern young women who have had some form of sexual involvement with a male relative. Even if the latter were a stepfather or some other non-blood-related male living within the close family circle, the example should be counted as incestuous, if for no other reason than that the *emotional* impact would approximate the traumatic level engendered by incest with an actual blood relative. Estimates of incest frequency in women, chosen randomly from the normal population, converge around the 5% level (Finkelhor, 1979). The frequency noted among my private practice borderline women was three times this figure (16%); in a hospitalized sample of 39 borderlines at New York Hospital/Westchester Division, over half the females had experienced incestuous relations either occasionally or over protracted periods of time throughout childhood (Stone, 1981). When I have presented this material at symposiums on borderlines, in various communities throughout the United States or in Europe (chiefly the Scandinavian countries and France), therapists who do any considerable work in this diagnostic domain have shared with me their perceptions, namely, that incest is remarkably common in the sameness of their female borderlines also.

If one thinks about the characteristics of borderline organization as Kernberg (1977) has described it, and compares these features with the typical attitudes engendered in young persons who have participated in incestuous relations, it will not be difficult to see the close correspondence between them. The defense pattern in borderlines consists largely of primitive mechanisms such as denial, disavowal (refusal to acknowledge verbally what one is already consciously aware of), splitting (coexisting contradictory attitudes, only one of which is conscious at any given moment), devaluation, idealization, and omnipotent control. But the actualization of sexual feeling toward a parent, or submission to the incestuous impulses of an older, more powerful family member, leads quite predictably to excitement by, idealization toward, and passionate infatuation with the older relative-turned-sex-object, but at the same time contempt, revulsion, and hatred toward this same person as having taken unfair advantage, as having betrayed a trust, violated a taboo, interfered with one's development, and so on. The ambivalence, in other words, that is inherent in all human relations, and certainly in the oedipal situation, becomes unavoidably magnified and intensified to levels far in excess of what the average young person has to cope with. Because daughters are far more apt to become incest victims than sons, the theme of incest is mostly relevant to women, whose image of men is often distorted beyond the powers of psychotherapy to rectify. As the incest victim grows up, men become for her cherished persecutors to be alternately adored and vilified. To make matters worse, the early fixation of sexual interest on the father or other male relative renders all newcomers ultimately less fascinating, less appealing—such that even the most suitable man (judged by realistic standards) will after a time be scrapped as the woman returns emotionally to the original figure. To a far greater and grossly pathological extent (compared with what is true of normal women) her heart belongs to Daddy—forever. But it is just this tendency to oscillate between adoration and vilification that the clinician recognizes as a form of "borderline" splitting. Likewise, the incest victim sees her own self in conflicting and sharply drawn images: She is at once outraged victim and, to the extent that she found the forbidden experiences exciting and gratifying, perfidious whore. Particularly in instances of father-daughter incest, the girl sees herself as having mocked and betrayed her mother; the ensuing guilt is often overpowering. As she matures, she fears inordinately the tables being turned on her—by her own daughter.

Her attitude about motherhood is vitiated by this anticipation of betrayal and abandonment, as life finally exacts its vengeance for having betrayed her mother. Vengefulness and scorn may become extreme in relation to men. It appears common for incest victims (at least those who come to the attention of psychotherapists) to become borderline, and not only that but to develop the character traits of spitefulness and jealousy to extreme degrees. This is all the more true when the sexual relations with the family member were highly sadomasochistic in nature, where hatred of men would become in inevitable outgrowth.

The aftereffects of incest are often shattering with respect to psychosexual development. Incest can, I believe, create "borderline" psychopathology, even in the absence of constitutional predisposition to psychosis (a factor otherwise important, in many other borderlines, as I have underlined elsewhere, 1980, 1981), and probably helps account in no small measure for the lopsided female preponderance (2:1 to 4:1) in most borderline patient samples.

In the following clinical example, the "splitting" and storminess are particularly striking:

Chaotic Marital Relationship in a
Borderline Woman with a History of Incest

A 36-year-old woman had been married for 15 years to a man of conventional habits and placid temperament. She kept the emotional atmosphere tense, however, and at times explosive, owing to rapid shifts in mood (from adoration to hostility and vindictiveness toward her husband, from possessiveness to indifference toward her children). Throughout the marriage she made repeated suicidal gestures, always staged to coerce her husband into gratifying some impulse of the moment. When in a happy frame of mind, she would be sexy and loving, but suddenly and with no or only slight provocation, she could become verbally abusive, humiliating him in front of family friends, with such remarks as "I'd like to cut off your dick!"

While growing up, from age 7 to 17, she had sexual relations with her four brothers, who forced themselves on her at first in a kind of gang rape. She developed, and maintained on into adult life, intensely ambivalent relationships with her brothers as well as intensely sadomasochistic relations with men in general.

As her daughter entered puberty, the woman became convinced that her husband "had designs" on their daughter in the same way her brothers had taken advantage of her. For weeks at a time she would take her daughter and go into hiding. When they returned, she would taunt her husband with innuendos about her having developed a sexual interest in various women; their own sexual relationship deteriorated. Finally, she sued for divorce and tried to prevent him from having any access to his daughter, who she was still convinced was the object of his "incestuous desires." Even toward her daughter, however, her behavior was inconsistent, fluctuating between the inappropriate protectiveness just described and aloofness or cruelty. Once when her daughter tearfully complained to her mother, "You don't love me," she slapped the girl's face. But the next night, confronted with a similar complaint, she would console the girl with hugs.

As a final comment on this issue, it is worth noting that borderline incest victims were reared without adherence to the ordinary boundaries—between blood relatives, between the generations—that are respected and that create the foundation for social integration by the vast majority of people. They become, and almost invariably view themselves as, pariahs. They expect the worst from all human relationships (particularly that marital bonds will not be honored) and are quite prepared to extract revenge at any price for wrongs done them either in fact or in fancy. Some avoid intimacy altogether (in a few cases known to me vows of celibacy have been taken in connection with a religious order). But others may live out a pattern of seduction, betrayal, cruelty, and abandonment, inflicting on relatively innocuous men the hurt inflicted on them by their not so innocuous relatives. As a result, their love relationships fail. Worse still, the expectation of betrayal is so ingrained, having been engendered by a breach of trust within the home itself, that therapeutic relationships are also undermined. Trust either never develops or, in the rare instances where the doctor-patient relationship is satisfactory, the problems in everyday living remain insurmountable. Most borderline women with this history find it impossible to adapt to a world where the majority of people (men included) are acknowledged as fundamentally wholesome and fair. Their psychic machinery has been too distorted to permit this view, and in addition their deviant assumptions and behavior patterns would not allow them to become comfortably integrated into conventional society. It remains easier to see everyone as corrupt and despicable, which conforms with life as the incest victim "knows" it. Besides, if everyone is basically corrupt, then father (or whoever) was not really so bad after all. In other words, the gloomy world-view becomes, paradoxically, a view compatible with the incest victim's loyalty and continuing love toward her original sexual object.

Unusual Avoidance of Sex

Unlike the patients described in the preceding sections, some borderline patients avoid sex altogether. In the absence of studies bearing directly on this issue, the precise frequency of this phenomenon is difficult to estimate. Among my borderline patients in private practice, about 1 in 8 (7 out of 54), ranging in age from 20 to 45, had never had a sexual experience progressing to orgasm with another person. One instance concerned a man in his late 20s who had been used sexually by his father; this schizotypal borderline man showed pronounced paranoid features, mistrusting people of either sex (as wanting only to "hurt" him in some way) and eschewing the company of others almost entirely. The oldest patient in this group had been reared in a wealthy home where the parents were often away for long periods; several family members, including her mother, were schizophrenic. The patient formed fantasy relationships with homosexual men, for whom she would bake cookies and send cards but who showed no interest in her even as a friend. Dynamically, these homosexual acquaintances served as mother surrogates, whom she hoped would compensate for the extreme deprivation she experienced from her own mother. But as one might expect, all that happened was that she reduplicated the early deprivation through her choice of men who returned none of her affection. Another woman was a hostile and infantilizing woman who made clear her intolerance of any moves toward independence on the part of her daughter. The younger woman complied to the extent of avoiding romantic involvements of any kind; her negative feelings toward her mother were acted out against her own person, however, in the form of self-induced illnesses (culminating in her putting out one of her eyes with a pencil). Several other asexual patients had been brutalized by a parent throughout their childhood, so that they now choose to live more or less as hermits rather than risk further humiliation and hurt from other people.

"Sins of commission" (incest, child abuse) involving quite real pain or humiliation are probably harder for a child to overcome than "sins of omission" (neglect), unless the latter are extreme. Many of these asexual borderlines, having been abused (beaten, locked in closets, tortured) as children, were just as overwhelmed, and rendered to the same extent outcasts from society, as were the victims of incest. Their improvement in psychotherapy was meager or negligible, as with the incest group. Only a few established a close friendship, and none has thus far formed a sexual relationship with anyone.

Dysmorphophobia

Originally used to denote, in persons of average appearance, a delusion of ugliness (Koupernik, 1982; Morselli, 1866), the false conviction usually centering on the face or the breasts, the term *dysmorphophobia* has also come to be used in reference to certain even more paradoxical situations where an unusually attractive woman imagines herself ugly (Hay, 1970). Some of the patients in the original descriptions were presumably schizophrenic, but it seems that this phenomenon is quite common in borderline patients, more so in women but occasionally in males as well. Recent authors have emphasized only the exaggerated nature of the patient's perception, taking at face value the supposition that the patient would wish if at all possible to be rid of the ugly self-image. At times that may be so, but in my experience at least, the "dysmorphophobia" is a rank misnomer (to say nothing of the fact that ugliness is not an external object of which one could have a true phobia). The patient is often a beautiful woman who clings paradoxically but desperately to the notion of being "ugly" by way of minimizing what is to her way of thinking murderous envy on the part of other women—or else the conviction of ugliness serves dynamically to "protect" her from the emotionally unmanageable advances of men. I have noted this surprising dynamic particularly in beautiful women who have had incestuous relations with a father or older brother: to be "pretty" means to be the target of illicit desire, to be "ugly" means to be safe. Their complaint of being ugly acquires the force of delusion, masking the far worse fear of being (what they actually are) beautiful. I have even encountered one male patient, extraordinarily handsome, who imagined himself to be of insect-like repugnance to others. As a child of 8 or 9, he had been sodomized by his father. To think of himself as ugly was his way of neutralizing the leering stares of homosexual men or the envious glances of heterosexual men whom he would pass in the street.

In the more common cases where women of average appearance feel ugly, there is often another paradoxical dynamic related to the father. These women complain as if their ugliness disqualifies them for romantic attachment to a potential lover or husband. They feel "condemned" never to marry, but underneath they are extraordinarily closely attached to their fathers, not because of incestuous involvement but because their mothers were rejecting and their fathers were warm and accepting. Through their distorted self-image they remain permanently unattached to any new men and permanently close to the one safe object of their earlier years.

Recently I worked with two borderline women, each of a markedly "infantile" personality (Kernberg, 1967), where their attempts to achieve any closeness in a love relationship were frustrated not only by a "father fixation" of the sort just described but also by an emptiness, an impoverishment of personality. Both tended to be critical, intolerant, and impatient of any shortcomings in the men who courted them. They had no real interests in life (and were therefore boring) and no real interests in the men as individuals. As a result, each woman, despite her pleasing appearance, was unattractive as a long-range prospect for any man. The patients spoke as though they had some inchoate awareness of where the real trouble lay, but to recognize that one is undesirable because of having "no personality" (and because of one's contemptuousness) is terrifying: these are not qualities one can easily modify or control. Instead, each dwelt to a morbid degree on her looks, becoming "dysmorphophobic." This was, to be sure, an unpleasant symptom, but one that seemed amenable to ordinary measures: the hairdresser, the gym, the plastic surgeon. To remedy the real problem—the *inner* ugliness—was, as each patient intuitively recognized, an almost insuperable and much less well defined task.

Occasionally, one will discover a somewhat different dynamic theme in a borderline woman with "dysmorphophobia." I have worked with a few, for example, where their attractiveness was denied and their appearance chronically derogated by their fathers, all throughout adolescence. In these instances it emerged during the course of psychotherapy that the father was struggling with incestuous impulses toward a very attractive daughter, sometimes within the context of a deteriorating marriage. The defense the father utilized was that of denying his impulse and then criticizing the daughter's looks, as though she were the last woman on earth who could stir up in him a sexual feeling. The advantage in these cases was that no incest occurred; the disadvantage was that it gave a shattered self-image to a young woman, who began to feel not only unattractive but also unlovable and worthless. As they enter adult life, these women, if handicapped further by functioning at the borderline level, are extremely sensitive to the mildest disappointments, let alone criticisms, in a love relationship. It is impossible to reassure them sufficiently to keep the relationship afloat and smooth-sailing. Their lives are characterized by one broken romance after the other, until in their late 30s or early 40s they give up on men entirely. This gloomy prospect is sometimes reversible with psychotherapy, but the task requires many years.

As a final comment on this intriguing condition, it is worth mentioning that one will encounter from time to time a borderline "dysmorphophobic" woman whose conviction of ugliness stems mainly from an inchoate realization of having an "ugly" nature. Their conviction of this becomes the concrete expression ("my face is ugly") of a figurative turn of phrase ("my personality is ugly"). Sometimes the personality will have become deformed owing to external circumstances—incest, sadistic treatment, verbal humiliation—of which the future borderline woman started out as a victim. Or constitutional aberrations, including perinatal brain damage, may even in the absence of adverse parental influences predispose her to insatiable drives, affect hunger, uncontrollable rage, and a grotesque abrasiveness of personality, noticeable from earliest childhood. In either event, a true ugliness of personality develops (with contemptuousness, mendacity, manipulativeness, hostility, and other socially offensive qualities), which causes alienation and loss of friends, as well as the dysmorphophobia—here consisting of a secret ugliness that corrodes the attractive exterior until the latter, too, is experienced as "ugly."

Jealousy

Freud (1922) spoke of three varieties of jealousy: The *competitive* or "normal" type; the *projected* type, where one's own impulses toward infidelity are projected onto one's partner, as though the latter is untrustworthy rather than oneself; and the *delusional* type, where unresolved homosexual feelings are dealt with via a mechanism where (to take the case of a male patient) the subject claims, "*I* do not love him; *she* loves him," and consciously experiences jealousy toward the often nonexistent other male. Freud adds that in the delusional cases jealousy is not restricted to this last type but involves all three mechanisms.

Considering the frequency with which serious disturbances in psychosexual development and in interpersonal relations are encountered in borderline patients, one might expect to find in them the more severe forms of jealousy also. Delusional jealousy remains, nevertheless, an uncommon phenomenon, at least in the borderline patients whom I have treated or seen in consultation. Nor has the theme of homosexuality been prominent in every case. Granted that many of Freud's so-called neurotic analysands would be considered *borderline* today (namely, the Wolf-Man, Freud, 1914), with his strong latent homosexuality, seduction by a sister, dysmorphophobia regarding ths nose, etc.), his clinical experience seldom included the near-psychotic end of the borderline spectrum. It may also be that in our day less stigma attaches to homosexuality impulses than in Freud's era. At any rate, some cases of pathological jealousy known to me involve intense fear of betrayal and separation and only secondarily, if at all, homosexuality. One such patient, a man of 22, was preoccupied with the fear that his fiancée would take up with another man. Though domineering, athletic, and free of any difficulties in sexual performance, he would become enraged by the most trivial sign of friendliness on the part of his fiancée toward another man, even though she was never seductive or flirtatious with other men and was totally devoted to the patient. His mother had been intrusive, infantilizing, and extremely seductive toward him for many years, barging into his room when he, or even she, would be undressed, ostensibly to chat or to lay out his clothes for the next day. He found his mother's behavior at once repugnant and exciting. He began to develop a view of women according to which they were all whorish Jezebels whom God condemned men to fall in love with, even though they were destined to desert their men just as surely as his mother deserted, at least emotionally, his father in favor of her son.

Another borderline man of 23, married with two children, had been given up at age 4 to foster care by his parents, who were unable financially to support their three sons. His foster parents, their demonic sadism subsequently corroborated by the courts, subjected him and his brothers to grotesque brutalities under the pretext of teaching them obedience. He was forced to kneel on rice for hours at a time, whipped to the point of bleeding, knocked unconscious, and so on. In response to this systematic torture, he developed a paranoid personality; his extreme touchiness about his personal "space" was a reaction not to fear of homosexual assault but to fear of purely physical assault. Wary of people in general, he had few friends and was extremely dependent on and possessive of his wife, whom he suspected of infidelity from time to time, not on account of any proclivities in that direction on her part but simply because he expected the worst from everybody, including her.

Jealousy, in a hospitalized borderline woman named Donna, took the form of extreme overattachment to her therapist (a woman) and violent reactions to the inevitable interest shown by the latter in relation to other patients in her case load. Once, when her therapist was assigned a new female patient, Donna ran off the hospital grounds and made deep gashes in both wrists, creating an emergency that she hoped would preempt her therapist's time, rendering her unavailable for the new "sister." As with the preceding patient, maternal deprivation and possessive love were the wellsprings of the pathological jealousy, to a much greater extent than any repressed homosexual longings. But Donna did express some homosexual interest in her therapist, and it may be that maternal deprivation in a *female* patient predisposes, via subsequent erotization (in adolescence) of the yearning for closeness, to a homosexual interest such as might *not* develop in a male patient with a similar dynamic constellation. In a few instances known to me, borderline women with delusional jealousy have been bisexual, their homosexual tendencies not repressed at all. In any event, it is easy to appreciate how the more severe forms of jealousy interfere with romantic relationships, disrupt marriages, and so forth, since (a) the jealous person is incapable of distinguishing between a trustworthy partner and one whose behavior would truly merit his suspiciousness; (b) the jealous person will tend to torment the partner with unfair accusations until the latter is driven away, and (c) partners are usually chosen, albeit unconsciously, for conformity to the jealous person's unrealistic anxieties—meaning that the partner with whom one falls in love *really is* unfaithful, so of course the relationship is stormy and ultimately unworkable.

This last point relates to a curious facet of the "assortative mating" that brings one possessive person together with another. Naively, one might guess that the best antidote to pathological jealousy is extreme trustworthiness and devotion in the partner, but this is not so. Those qualities are the attributes of fairly integrated, emotionally healthy persons, but healthy people have friends, even nonsexual friendships with the opposite sex. They live in the world. Their emotional organization is not symbiotic. All this is immensely threatening to a jealous borderline person, for whom anything less than exclusive round-the-clock possession of the "important other" causes unbearable anguish. If the borderline person has also been an incest victim, he (or, as is more often the case, she) will assume that all human relationships end up in bed, so that innocent friendships become resented not only as sources of inattention, which is bad enough, but as potential sources of infidelity, which is intolerable. Hence, it more often happens that a possessive, jealous, symbiotically organized borderline will fall in love with someone who is quite similar and equally friendless, whose own inordinate need for an exclusive relationship is in harmony with that of the borderline person. But the latter, having avoided the Scylla of a partner's friendships, now turns into the Charybdis of the partner's immaturity, irascibility, and so forth. The comfort of choosing someone as ill as oneself endures only a short time and then collapses. Particularly with the delusionally jealous, whose hidden agenda is not to forge a harmonious relationship with another person but primarily to seek revenge for wrongs (real or imaginary) once suffered, inflicting similar torment on the partner, relationships are doomed from the beginning. Worse still, the tendency to externalize and distort, and the generally poor capacity for reality-testing about people, render psychotherapy with jealous borderlines unrewarding. The success rate is low.

It may be that some of the confusion and controversy surrounding the theme of homosexuality in delusional jealousy stems from the failure to distinguish between latent and conscious homosexuality. This is the point raised and later resolved by Frosch (1983) in his lucid discussion of the issue as it relates to patients (some of them "borderline") who partake of what he terms the *psychotic process*. The delusionally jealous are only occasionally overt homosexuals; not many are even latently so, in the sense that "latent" refers to a tendency not yet lived out in behavior but about to be, or one that could eventually be acted on. These patients, instead, are (like Schreber) heterosexuals who are preoccupied nonetheless by uncertainty regarding gender or by repressed yearnings for closeness with the same sex, not accompanied, however, by sexual excitement in relation to persons of the same sex (as would characterize the true homosexual). Frosch notes that the delusionally jealous, as with other markedly paranoid patients, have often been victims, as children, of one or another sort of humiliation. Frosch's comments are not directed to the borderline case specifically but are strikingly exemplified in the jealousy of a borderline "hysteroid dysphoric" woman whose unconscious homosexuality manifested itself in several unusual ways.

This woman, recently divorced and in the midst of a new relationship, would frequently manipulate the old and the new lover so that they would encounter each other. After sex with her new partner, she would sometimes submit to oral sex with her ex-husband, who was eager to suck out the semen of his rival. She thus made herself the instrument of a homosexual act. Having been abandoned by her mother as an infant, she was left with an inordinate (though repressed) longing for physical closeness with a woman, and it was this that expressed itself indirectly in her delusional jealousy. Another form taken by her preoccupation with women was her encouragement of her lovers—as if that is what they wanted—to engage in a *ménage à trois* with herself and another woman. She thus served, sandwich fashion, as the pretext for two men to indulge their "homosexuality," or made of her male partner the pretext to indulge hers. Psychotherapy was able to unearth these themes, but it had only a minimal effect on attenuating the force of her jealousy.

Sadomasochism

Here we speak of a clinical phenomenon that needs some separate discussion, as though it were an entity entirely apart, despite the close interrelationships that often exist between sadomasochism and, say, jealousy, promiscuity, homosexuality, or incest. There is a difference, however, between the psychological sadomasochism implied when a borderline person subjects a love partner to mental cruelty, as it is aptly known in the courts, via jealous taunts or promiscuous behavior, and the more direct forms of this perversion, where sexual excitement is intertwined with the literal infliction or suffering of bodily pain.

My clinical experience in this area is not broad enough to permit me to make even an educated guess as to whether couples given to whipping or bondage necessarily contain at least one member who is "borderline" by one or another definition. Since extremism—all-or-none thinking, all-or-none behavior—is of the essence of borderline pathology, it stands to reason that, almost by definition, people whose sexual excitement depended on whips, ropes, and chains, to say nothing of more bizarre or sophisticated instruments of torture, would tend to be acting out very primitive, "pregenital" fantasies and often turn out to be "borderline." Similarly, borderlines might be overrepresented among people who subject their sexual partners to acts whose social meanings signify something disgraceful—eating feces, for example—or among those who actively crave submission to such practices. In my practice I know of no neurotics, and only two borderlines, in this category.

By the same token, my clinical experience with the physically painful forms of sadomasochism is confined to borderlines, whereas I have seen some of the less exaggerated or painful forms of "unusual" sexual practices (voyeurism, exhibitionism) in my neurotic patients. A homosexual borderline man of 21, admitted to New York Hospital because of a suicide gesture, was involved in a sadomasochistic relationship with a man who used to beat him with whips as a prelude to sex. At a certain point the patient's lover abandoned him, whereupon the patient strangled to death his lover's pet German Shepherd (how this was effected without suffering further bodily injury was never made clear). When his rage subsided, giving way to loneliness and despair, he made a suicide gesture, cutting his wrists superficially with a razor.

The one instance of bondage known to me involved an obsessive and somewhat sadistic but reasonably well integrated man and his fiancée, a delusionally jealous and frequently promiscuous border-line woman of 20, who abused marijuana and who subjected her lover to humiliating arguments in public. His retaliation consisted of tying her to the bedposts with ropes, whipping her, engaging in intercourse, and then leaving for a number of hours without telling her when, or whether, he would return.

Masochism: Moral vs. Self-Mutilative Aspects

Even within the realm of borderline conditions it is not common to find sexual arousal dependent primarily on physical pain. Much more common is the pattern of "moral masochism," when intimacy and, particularly, sexual pleasure are purchased at a price of displeasure, often at the level of mental anguish, within the context of a self-defeating relationship. Several paths are open to the "moral masochist" with respect to self-defeat. One could choose a partner with whom a lifetime relationship is possible but where the lifetime of togetherness is punctuated by episodes of extreme unfairness, unfounded accusations, humiliation, and psychological cruelties of every sort. The partner, alternatingly loving and cruel, brings about oscillations in the relationship as a whole, such that each period of intense pleasure is "paid for" by the anguish that unaccountably but predictably follows, each period of anguish made tolerable by a happy reconciliation. Characteristics of the partner who creates this kind of roller-coaster existence include extreme jealousy and perfectionism, but one may also encounter a markedly ambivalent attitude toward closeness. For example, one borderline patient, a female homosexual in her early 20s, became enamored of a somewhat older woman who, though not taunting her with the wish to seek other partners, would nevertheless torment the patient by suddenly disappearing for hours, days, or a week without provocation or reason. The patient, running the gamut of painful emotion from frenzy to despair, would be near the point of making a suicide gesture when, with equal suddenness, her lover would turn up again, as loving and seemingly devoted as before. The lover, herself borderline, had suffered the rejection and disappearance of her mother on multiple occasions throughout her childhood. The patient saw in her lover the embodiment of her parents' own stormy relationship: her "long-suffering" (read "masochistic") mother and her alcoholic, alternately passionate and sadistic (and chronically unfaithful) father. Despite, or perhaps because of, these episodes of abandonment and reunion, the patient felt completely "at home" with her lover, as the two busied themselves with the unconscious living out of the only patterns of intimacy either had ever witnessed or experienced.

Another self-defeating pattern involves the choice of partners, one after the other, with whom only a brief relationship is possible—and that stormy and ultimately ungratifying. Sometimes the partners are selected, unconsciously of course, for some cruel or menacing quality, which has the effect of expiating the guilt engendered by the borderline's sexual activity. Typifying this pattern was an attractive 22-year-old college student who had been admitted to New York State Psychiatric Institute for globus hystericus, depressive symptoms, and two superficial wrist-cuttings. This woman had a series of brief involvements with older men, many of whom were crude, abusive, and from the wrong side of the tracks socially, in contrast to her aristocratic background. All these elements—the cruelty, the brevity, the indifference—were of special significance when viewed against the backdrop of her own family history: her father had abandoned her mother when she was 3½ and had not spoken to her since. Attracted only to cruel and inconstant men, she was cruel and inconstant herself to the "nice" men who fell in love with her.

Overlapping with the already mentioned themes of dysmorphophobia, jealousy, and masochism is another form of painful relationship encountered frequently among borderlines, though it is hardly unknown within the broader realm of neurotic individuals. I speak of a sadomasochistic trend, directed ostensibly at the sexual life, whose primary purpose centers around the "pregenital" concern over separation. This trend manifests itself as an unending, outrageous testing of the partner's continuing devotion. A typical example concerns a borderline woman with chronic worries about her attractiveness and a tendency to disbelieve compliments about her beauty, who will subject her spouse or partner to unnecessary separations, social humiliations (such as spoiling a dinner party by suddenly absenting herself from her guests without any explanation), sexual rebuffs, and the like—all by way of seeing whether her partner "still loves her." If a husband imploringly professes his undying adoration after his wife made an embarrassing scene in front of his boss, the case is much more "convincing" than if similar remarks were as pillow talk after a lovely day. Many of the acts and assertions of the borderline caught up in this pattern have a half-conscious and therefore gamelike quality, as with the taunt "You never really loved me." The beautiful woman who acknowledges her own attractiveness "loses" (to the extent that she may be borderline and woefully lacking in self-esteem) a valuable weapon with which to extract reassurances from the men in her life. The mechanism I allude to is well known, and more tellingly described, by literary authors than by psychiatric authors: Murray Shisgal in his play *Luv* stages a hilarious battle between the two lover-protagonists, each of whom torments the other with a series of escalating insults (she kicks him in the shins, he slaps her in the face, she breaks his glasses, he throws her mink coat over the bridge . . .)—each insult followed by the urgent question, "Ya still *luv* me?!"

Recently I became aware of still another unusual masochistic dynamic. Pain is endured not so much as expiation for sexual guilt but rather as a necessary by-product of a relationship whose main effect is to shore up a negative self-image (through the choice of a partner who is truly inferior in some important way). Thus a schizotypal borderline woman who was herself markedly gauche and irritating in social situations began to date a man who was considerably more disrespectful of social convention than she was. For example, he was crude, his hygiene was poor, and he would flaunt his interest in other women in front of her. All this she complained of as immensely annoying, yet she clung to the relationship. At first this seemed inexplicable, but gradually it emerged that she felt for the first time a kind of social and moral superiority over someone, whereas in relation to just about everyone else she had become used to the uncomfortable image of being the obnoxious one, the less poised one, and so on. According to the calculus of her particular psychic economy, this feeling of moral superiority, along with the surcease from loneliness and the mild sexual pleasure he afforded, weighed heavier in the balance than the suffering she endured on account of his shabby treatment.

Self-damaging acts constitute one of the diagnostic items for the DSM-III diagnosis of borderline and are important in the Gunderson schema as well. Though such acts are neither necessary nor sufficient for the diagnosis, many borderlines exhibit them from time to time, often flamboyantly. Whereas only one in six of my office-practice borderlines indulged in wrist-cutting, burning, or other self-mutilative acts, these acts figure almost invariably among the precipitants of hospitalization, such that any sample of inpatient borderlines (particularly of the affective variety) will contain very few who have *not* engaged in self-mutilative acts just prior to admission. In female borderlines these acts will often be found to have taken place premenstrually (Stone, 1983), especially if there had been a recent disruption in a romantic relationship. Psychodynamically, these self-damaging acts are frequently intertwined with sexual themes, or else are part and parcel of an exploitative attitude toward the loved one, as manifestations of a desperate, not to say outrageous, effort to control the latter's psychological freedom.

Pregenital themes may be fused with strictly genital themes, but to such an extent that the various motifs that underlie the self-mutilative act cannot easily be pried apart. For example, a 22-year-old depressed and hospitalized borderline woman, having heard of her therapist's impending vacation, broke a light bulb and scratched her wrists. The more obvious meaning of her act concerned anxiety about separation, but she also experienced herself as in love with her therapist, whose vacation she interpreted as personal rejection. Implicit in her act was the taunt "If you really loved me, you'd drop what you're doing and minister to my wounds."

Adoration and Hatred, as the Borderline Falls—and Fails—in Love

As we hinted above, if one is borderline the extremes are "average," and average behavior, average attitudes, are almost unknown. Falling in love has been compared by such diverse groups as poets and psychiatrists to psychosis. This is a bit unfair to love, because even though love draws its strength from unconscious and irrational forces, it is too common an experience and is too often conducive to stable, gratifying relationships lasting years to qualify truly as a brand of madness. The early stage of most love relationships is characterized by "infatuation," two of whose characteristics are idealization and uncritical acceptance of the loved one. Everything is "perfect," or what imperfections the lover permits himself to notice—a tooth out of line, a few hairs where they shouldn't be—only add to the individuality and charm of the beloved. This reverential attitude toward the beloved is often accompanied by the spontaneous assertion "I adore you." The adoration resembles the adoration of the religious ecstatic and indeed may constitute one's sole experience of this intense and blissful emotion—especially in our era, when for most people, religious fervor has become unfamiliar and passé.

But adoration may also be seen as the counterpart to the symbiotic mode of interrelatedness—whether encountered, under quite normal circumstances, in the mother-infant relationship (Mahler, 1971) or in abnormal situations, such as the attitudes prevailing in the early transference relationship between a schizophrenic patient and his therapist. Borderlines too, with their intolerance of separation and their predilection for possessive, symbiotic attachments, are also more prone than better integrated people to fall into and remain in the state of adoration. If they love at all, they adore.

If borderlines were able to sustain feelings of adoration for long periods, or if their reactions to the inevitable shortcomings, negative qualities, social gaffes, and so on—of which their loved ones will sooner or later be "guilty"—were less drastic, all would be well. But precisely because borderlines cannot construct an integrated and blended view of other people (no more than they can of themselves), the first recognition of an unpleasant trait in the loved one, the first glimpse of the hair under the nose, as it were, tends to be shattering. Minor blemishes that ordinary folk would scarcely notice may provoke a disappointment so keen as to be insuperable, leading in turn to dissolution of the relationship. The beloved has indeed been placed on a pedestal, but the pedestal was balanced on a pin. I think in this regard of a couple I once worked with, where both members were borderlines, a plastic surgeon and his wife, who was "Miss—" in the Miss America contest. Despite her being unusually attractive, her husband had a catalog of objections; her jawline was not straight enough, her incisors jutted down too far, her nose "needed a little work" (all of which he himself was eager to perform on her until I forbade it), and so forth. Whenever he would castigate her for these anatomical deficiencies, she would burst into tears, then rage, and would lock herself in the bathroom to scarify her wrists with a razor. The situation did not right itself until I prescribed for her a therapist of her own and for him the reading of Hawthorne's "The Birthmark." Fortunately this powerful tale of a man who destroys his beloved wife in the process of trying to extract her insignificant birthmark struck home, and he was able to understand the grotesqueness of his perfectionistic standards. Behind these standards were the important dynamic layers having to do with a hostile symbiotic attachment to his own ambivalently loved mother, compared with whom every other woman, even a beauty queen, had to be rejected. This marriage happened to succeed, since both partners were amenable to therapy and were motivated to remain together. But the more typical story involves a partnership that is severed, when the phase of adoration is abruptly replaced, on recognition of the first "fault," by an equally intense and irrational hatred—either that, or the borderline person begins to oscillate between adoration and hatred, with the inevitable consequence of wearing down the patience of the loved one until he or she finally breaks off the relationship.

Identity Disturbance and the Love Relationship, with a Note on Don Juanism

A serious disturbance in the sense of a self, in "identity," is a necessary element in the Kernberg (1977) definition of borderline and an almost universal feature of borderlines diagnosed by checklist criteria (Spitzer et al., 1979; Stone, 1980). What are the implications for such a disturbance with respect to the capacity for love? the implications are profound, and they affect the love life in at least two important ways.

The extremely low self-esteem routinely encountered in border-line patients contributes to their suspicion that the love others may claim to feel toward them cannot be genuine (along the lines of Groucho Marx's famous quip that he would not wish to be a member of any club that was willing to accept him). This conviction, analogous to dysmorphophobia, may contribute to pathological jealousy inasmuch as a cripplingly low self-esteem robs one of the feeling of lovability: in comparison to oneself, *any* outsider would "therefore" be preferable in the eyes of one's beloved. The borderline patient with an esteem problem of such dimensions requires inordinate reassurance, which vitiates the love relationship, exhaust-ing, worrying, and ultimately offending the partner (who cannot help but wonder, "Why is my sweetheart so down on himself? Maybe he knows something I don't know").

In the more restrictive situation where gender identity is grossly disturbed, as it is in a fairly large subgroup of borderlines, there may be another source of impairment in a love relationship, stemming from uncertainty about the very sex of one's potential partners. It is unclear to me whether bisexuals are apt to be borderline or whether borderlines contain more than their share of bisexuals, but where these situations coexist it is easy to see how one cold never be happy in a relationship of long duration with either a man or a woman. This plight was portrayed with considerable effectiveness in Harvey Fierstein's recent play *The Torch-Song Trilogy* (in which a bisexual man cannot at first make up his mind between a transvestite and his "straight" wife). Even bisexual borderline patients who feel relatively unconflicted and comfortable (I have only worked with one) often have troubled relationships: if they marry, they still maintain their homosexual interests, and partners, discovery of which is usually impossible for the spouse to accept with nonchalance.

Not unrelated to the foregoing is the phenomenon of Don Juanism (Pfister, 1931; Robbins, 1956), somewhat related to promiscuity and seen usually in males, whose dynamics have been ascribed to unconscious homosexual impulses defended against by a compulsive display of heterosexuality.

Actually, conventional usage makes subtle distinctions between promiscuity and Don Juanism, based partly on sociocultural differences between the sexes, partly on biological differences. Some men engage compulsively in making sexual conquests. Mozart's Don Giovanni racked up just over a thousand in Spain alone, if we are to believe his valet, Leporello. These conquests do not represent the warding off of intolerable loneliness, as is the usual dynamic underlying promiscuity, so much as the less primitive dynamic concerning a reaffirmation of one's gender identity and sexual prowess. For a man to pick up a woman in a bar and have sex with her is still (in his eyes) a bit of a conquest; for the women it is more often than not an act of desperation. However, a woman can be a Don Juan if she uses her attractiveness (an unprepossessing woman could never be a Don Juan) to make repeated conquests of men whom she views as ordinarily out of her reach, not the anonymous fellow on the adjoining bar stool but men of prominence, power, and fame. Most borderline women are intensely lonely, and if inclined toward driven sexuality, they tend to be promiscuous (rather than female Don Juans). The character of Blanche in *Streetcar Named Desire* is a prototype of the latter. Nevertheless, a few borderline women flaunt their beauty in an effort to "conquer" men of social prominence, often by way of seeking revenge against hurts suffered earlier at the hands of an important male figure from early life. One may correctly consider these women female Don Juans. Numerically there is good reason to suppose there are more males than females who exemplify this phenomenon. Not all Don Juans are borderline, but the more extreme cases probably are, especially where the component of contemptuousness toward women is disproportionately great. The highly narcissistic Don Juan who murdered his wife and daughters, as described in McGinniss' recent book (1983), is a case in point and was very likely borderline by Kernberg criteria. Since it is not in the nature of the Don Juan type to admit faults of any kind, let alone worries over sexual prowess, he seldom seeks psychotherapy. I have worked, briefly and unsuccessfully, with only one, a man in his mid-30s forced by his wife to get help, alongside the treatment she was in the midst of, because of his compulsive womanizing. Far from feeling any guilt over subjecting his wife to the details of his escapades, he was proud of being able to juggle so many women at once. He was asymptomatic and quit therapy after seven or eight sessions. Another instance I am familiar with concerns a clearly borderline graduate student in his late 20s who exhibited, in addition to his promiscuity, pseudologia fantastica—making up the most preposterous stories about his sexual exploits. One New Year's Eve he announced to his buddies at school that he was about to go to his engagement party, his fiancée allegedly being the daughter of a famous European nobleman. Dressed in tuxedo, tails, and top hat, he waved ta-ta to his friends, cradling a box with 12 American Beauty roses ostensibly for the delight of his betrothed. Followed surreptitiously by a fellow student, he was observed dumping the roses in a trash bin at the end of the street and then entering a nearby pool-hall to while away the evening with the local hustlers. His roommate noted that he did not once use their bathroom during the entire year, performing his ablutions in some other locale, presumably to preserve the illusion that he was somehow above the smells and noises to which the remainder of humankind is prone. Unusually handsome and dapper, he was adept at getting dependent girls to fall in love with him, only to humiliate them shortly thereafter, often with exquisite cruelty. Don Juans of this type are borderline in personality organization, but they are also largely psychopathic and as such incapable of warm and mutual relationships with anyone: sex is compulsive, love is nonexistent.

Disturbances in Empathy and Compassion in Borderlines

If one thinks in normative terms of the "narcissistic path of development," in contrast to the object-relational path, then every borderline person must exhibit some narcissistic abnormalities, for this path concerns, ideally, awareness and realistic appraisal of one's personality traits, of the impression one makes on others, and of one's potential, self-worth, self-regard, and the like. Borderlines, by virtue of their impaired sense of identity, represent one kind of failure, of deviation, in this path, since their self-image is full of contradictions and distortions. In addition, many but not all borderlines show a constellation of abnormal personality traits that we also call "narcissistic," no longer in the normative but in the pathological sense. Kernberg (1967, 1974) has outlined the salient features: excessive self-absorption, superficially smooth social adaptation, intense ambition and envy, grandiosity , feelings of inferiority, craving for acclaim, a sense of emptiness, deficiency in empathic capacity, an incapacity to love, and exploitativeness, even ruthlessness, toward others. The presence of this pathological narcissism in a borderline patient augurs poorly for social recovery, let alone for success in love relationships. It should not be difficult to grasp why this is so, since psychotherapists have ample opportunity to discover how easy it is to dispel various (egodystonic) symptoms, yet how hard it is to bring about constructive changes in character formation. Empathy and compassion, if they are seriously lacking, cannot be taught even by the most skilled and patient therapist, although in some persons a rudimentary compassion may be "released" when certain neurotic traits have been modified through analysis. The Wolf-Man (Gardner, 1971), in fact, spoke of how his analyses with Freud and Mack Brunswick freed him up to become, in his later years, much more sympathetic and kind to those around him than he had been at the height of his neurosis.

If I divide the borderline patients with whom I have worked in private practice into three groups—those with dramatic recoveries, 11; those with modest improvement, 19; and treatment failures, 21— I notice that empathy and compassion were well developed in all but one of the highly successful cases and in three-fourths of the middle group, but only in half the treatment failures.

How seriously self-absorption and lack of compassion may interfere with love and intimacy can be surmised from the following vignette:

> An unmarried borderline woman of 34 was referred for therapy because of an eating disorder. Two subjects preoccupied her mind to the exclusion of all else: her food and her figure. She hungered for testimonials to her beauty, eschewed the company of her (few) friends unless her weight and shape were "perfect," and even then was in a state of high anxiety lest a waiter, a passerby, or some other stranger in a restaurant appear to be more in awe of her girlfriend's looks than of her own looks. Sex frightened her; she had had only a few brief affairs. Though she craved the attention of men (actually only of handsome

men), she had no interest in them as individuals; they were simply machines from which she could, under the right circumstances, extract an approving stare. The idea of having to *relate* to one, to express genuine concern as to how his day went, what his insecurities and worries were, and so on, was incomprehensible to her. When she did accept a date, she would spruce up for hours and emerge as a "fashion plate," to *stun* him (literally) with her attractiveness. Once he shook off the effects of being stunned in this way and began to talk to her, she was out of her element. After it became clear to the man, two or three dates later, that she did not care much about him as a person, his enthusiasm cooled. It is interesting that she came from a family where hardly any attention was focused on this or that family member's humanity, but rather on how each one looked. Her own lack of compassion may have come about as a result of her hostility at being so neglected, except as a "package," as well as out of her general lack of practice, coming from such a family, in learning and enjoying learning what makes other people tick.

Empathy and compassion do not travel on quite the same tracks; it is possible to read others' feelings correctly (i.e., to possess *empathy*) but yet to lack compassion. Many borderlines who are also (pathologically) narcissistic lack both and, to the extent that mature love depends on genuine concern for the beloved, are capable at most of lust but not of love. Some schizotypal borderlines have a measure of compassion but so woefully misread the feelings of others as to render lasting relationships impossible. Because of their lack of empathy, they are constantly misconstruing the intentions of others, incorrectly estimating their affections, and so on. Worse still, they cannot easily understand why someone considered their responses off the wall, so they tend to pursue, without self-correction, a jarring and inappropriate attitude (e.g., cracking a joke at a funeral to cheer up the bereaved). Unempathic but compassionate schizotypes of this sort can sometimes maintain a relationship with someone else of a similar nature, whose emotional insensitivity renders the schizotype's out-of-tune comments less irritating.

Where compassion and empathy are both in short supply, relationships could endure only to the extent that the partner could tolerate sex without affection. But here one is usually dealing with a coldly exploitative borderline who is not only incapable of love but scarcely able to gratify the sexual needs of another person.

Final Comment

I am aware, as I complete this catalog relevant to the borderline domain of impediments to love and gratifying sexuality, that I have painted a dreary picture. Happily, however, there is more to the picture than the masochism, jealousy, narcissism, and so forth, on which I have dwelt. Among my borderline patients with the more successful outcomes, half were able to form quite satisfactory love relationships of a lasting nature. Two female homosexuals were in this group. These patients had predominantly affective rather than schizotypal traits, although several schizotypal borderlines also functioned at this high level. All were orgastic without difficulty (several began treatment with complaints of unresponsiveness, but they grew less inhibited as treatment progressed). In a few instances, hypomanic personality features were present, including a marked degree of intensity in all their behavior. In the same way manic patients tend to be "augmenters" in their response to stimuli of whatever kind, the borderlines with these traits sometimes reacted to orgasm with exhilaration rather than postcoital drowsiness, such that while their partners would be trying to sleep they would spring out of bed and engage in exercise and all sorts of activities, including another round of lovemaking. Apart from dyssynchronies of this sort, their relationships were for the most part harmonious.

It is also worth noting that, despite the prevalence of empathic difficulties in this category of patients, some borderlines are unusually capable of reasoning with those around them, including their love partners, as though whatever combination of constitutional and experiential factors rendered them overly sensitive to the actions of others, left them, as a compensatory advantage, so to speak, better able than average to sense the hidden feelings of those with whom they are close. Their knowledge of what it is to suffer, and the lengths they go to in order to put their love partners at ease, helps to solidify their intimate relationships. The gratitude and love inspired by their attentions make it much easier for their loved ones to endure and to remain supportive during the emotional crises to which these borderline persons are periodically subject.

Among borderline patients in general, based on my private practice experience, I have the impression that adequate sexual performance and enjoyment are more common than the capacity for mature love. The patients with the best outcomes did well in at least one of these two areas. Half functioned well in both sex and love. In the intermediate- and poor-outcome groups, adequate sexual performance was present in half, the capacity for love in only a few. One-third of the patients in these two groups demonstrated serious deficiencies in both.

The inability to love was often related to chronic mistrustfulness. This is very much in line with a personal communication from a well-known analyst, Henriette Klein: "Where there is no trust, there is no love." We have already examined one form that this mistrust takes, namely, jealousy. But some borderline patients, even without being particularly prone to jealousy, were mistrustful of and angry at their sexual partners. They were often hypercritical, in a manner suggesting that they foisted onto their partners (via "projective identification") the harsh criticisms with which they, consciously or otherwise, regarded themselves. This issue of *basic trust,* though of fundamental importance in understanding borderline pathology (especially in the realm under discussion here), has its elusive aspects. For example, the patient who has incestuous experiences with both parents, though hypersexual and schizotypal, was orgastic and had the capacity to love, even though her life story at first glance would have led one to suppose she had no reason to develop trust. Some favorable if less dramatic elements in her relationship with her parents must have offset the effects of the sexual abuse. In another instance, a schizotypal borderline woman had unusually warm and supportive parents and seven normal siblings. There was no history of physical or sexual abuse, yet she became hostile, paranoid, referential, and irascible as she entered her 20s. Could these traits be the reflection of her (apparent) constitutional defect alone?

While there is much that is blatant and simple—as we attempt to understand the borderline's difficulties in sex and love—there is still much that is subtle and puzzling. In the meantime, one can summarize the borderline's plight by stating that, among border-lines, one often sees sex without love, or love without sex, or else both sex and love—but with a partner that is unsuitable. In other words, sex and love remain unintegrated.

Excerpts from

The Prediction of Outcome in Borderline Personality Disorder: Part V of the Chestnut Lodge Follow-up Study

Thomas H. McGlashan, M.D.
(1985)

Predictors aim at providing some notion about subsequent course in various psychosyndromes. In nature they may be factors predisposing to illness (etiologic), factors affecting course of illness (environmental and treatment), or factors otherwise associated with the various outcomes (prognostic). To date, virtually all investigations of predictor phenomena have been limited to schizophrenic samples. The reasons for such an exclusive diagnostic focus are obscure, especially since heterogeneity is not the exclusive province of schizophrenia. This paper, however, studies the existence and nature of outcome predictors in a group of nonschizophrenic (and non-Axis I) patients, specifically patients defined by recent diagnostic criteria as suffering from borderline personality disorder (BPD).

This study has been supported in part by grant MH 35174-02 from the National Institute of Mental Health and by the fund for Psychoanalytic Research of the American Psychoanalytic Association. Reprinted with permission from *The Borderline: Current Empirical Research,* edited by Thomas H. McGlashan, Chapter 4, pp. 63, 82–86, 1985, American Psychiatric Association. Copyright © 1985 by Thomas H. McGlashan.

Strongest Predictors Across All Outcome Dimensions

A strong predictor here was arbitrarily defined as one emerging at least once among the three analyses for two or more of the six outcome dimensions. Sixteen such predictor variables qualified. Four of them have already been encountered as the strongest predictors of global outcome: IQ, affective instability, distractability, and length of prior hospitalizations. The remaining 12 were: 1) gender; 2) family history of substance abuse; 3) premorbid heterosexual functioning; 4) severity of stressor at onset; 5) magical thinking; 6) inadequate affect; 7) dysphoria; 8) elation; 9) devaluation, manipulation, and hostility in relationships; 10) meeting the Gunderson and Kolb (1978) criteria for borderline; 11) length of index hospitalization; and 12) transfer rather than discharge from Chestnut Lodge.

The association of male gender with better outcome may represent sampling artifact deriving from differential hospital admission policies for male versus female patients with BPD. More severely ill male patients with borderline character disorders often present with serious antisocial/criminal behaviors and are not accepted for admission. As such, the male BPD patients who were admitted may derive from a healthier sector of the borderline spectrum. This bias then carried through into long-term outcome functioning.

Less frequently, family history of substance abuse was associated with better outcomes. Although this variable included any and all forms of chemical abuse, alcohol was the identified substance in the vast majority of cases. Substance abuse was the only personality disorder criterion that could be rated reliably from the family history records, making it the only variable reflecting character pathology in the family. Loranger et al. (1982) noted an increased rate of personality disorders in the family members of patients identified with BPD. The present finding may further suggest that the presence of familial character pathology predicts a poorer prognosis for the borderline proband. An important negative finding in the family dimension for BPD patients was the absence of a relationship between family history of schizophrenia or affective disorder and outcome. That is, if a familial predictive relationship exists (genetic or otherwise), it may be specific to personality disorder.

Superior outcomes were associated with "better" premorbid heterosexual functioning, that is, regular (not promiscuous) dating, marriage, or living with a sexual partner for an extended time. Although not unexpected, it was surprising that only this variable (and IQ) among the premorbid component variables emerged as a strong predictor. This contrasts with the literature on schizophrenics and with the findings from our own schizophrenic cohort (McGlashan, 1983) where premorbid social, sexual, and instrumental functioning were strongly related to outcome, especially in the realms of relationships and work.

The variable severity of stressor associated with illness onset derives from Axis IV of DSM-III. Our results demonstrated a correlation between lower levels of psychosocial stress and better long-term outcomes. This was an unexpected finding and contrasts with the literature on schizophrenics, where the presence of clear precipitating stress augurs a better prognosis. In BPD external stress may arrest the development or obscure the expression of maladaptive behavior, thus preventing or masking signs of illness. That is, external stress may serve paradoxically as an antidote to personality disorder (like war for the antisocial character). Therefore, the development of a disorder despite the presence of high titers of external stress may constitute a poor prognostic sign.

Under the dimension of psychopathology, magical thinking (superstitiousness, clairvoyance, telepathy, sixth sense, "others can feel my feelings") emerged as important. It constitutes one of the DSM-III symptom criteria for SPD. Its presence in patients with BPD, therefore, suggests concomitant schizotypal traits. Since pilot work (McGlashan, 1983) on this sample demonstrated an overall poorer outcome in patients with SPD compared to patients with BPD, it was not surprising that the presence of a criterion symptom for SPD carried negative prognostic valence.

Three variables relating to affective symptoms in the manifest illness proved predictive: dysphoria and elation were predictive of good outcome and inadequate affect was predictive of poor outcome. Dysphoria was defined as chronic feelings of dysphoria and ahedonia, emptiness or loneliness (i.e., clearly distressing subjective affects). Elation meant essentially the opposite, that is, the presence of euphoria or pleasurable affects. Both may be related to good outcome insofar as they reflect the presence of an intact capacity for hedonic experience, discrimination, and motivation. This was further suggested by the association of poorer outcomes with inadequate affect, which may represent the absence of hedonic capacity. That is, inadequate affect was defined in this study as an emotional life that is rigid, dull, and minimally reactive to stimulations of any strength. This triad of predictive symptoms suggests that the ability to experience pleasure and to tolerate psychological pain (unpleasure) may be as important to health and strength in patients with BPD as it is in patients with schizophrenia (McGlashan, 1984).

Devaluation, manipulation, and hostility refer to the nature of the patient's object relations. The variable derives from the Gunderson and Kolb (1978) criteria for BPD and was defined as follows: the patient has recurrent problems with devaluation (discredits or ignores other's strengths and personal significance) or manipulation (uses covert ways to control and gain support from others) or hostility (repeatedly and knowingly hurts others) in close relationships. In essence, the dimension rated the borderline patient's ability to contain ambivalence in attachments or to control aggression in significant relationships. The more this could be done, the better the outcome and vice versa.

Good outcomes were found more frequently in patients meeting the Gunderson and Kolb (1978) criteria for borderlines. A similar finding was reported on a pilot sample (McGlashan, 1983). As discussed there, such a result was expected because the Gunderson and Kolb system includes items relating to premorbid functioning and specifically excludes patients with symptoms strongly suggestive of schizophrenia.

The final two strong predictors relate to illness course. Greater length of index hospitalization and transfer to another institution rather than discharge from Chestnut Lodge were both associated with poorer outcomes. Again, this should hold no surprise and these findings basically extend the earlier discussed (similar) predictive value of length of previous hospitalization.

Findings by Individual Outcome Dimension

Hospitalization

As expected, BPD patients spent more time hospitalized after Chestnut Lodge if they were transferred rather than discharged and if they had been hospitalized more frequently prior to their index admission. The other hospitalization outcome dimension (not shown in the tables) was the number (as opposed to length) of hospitalizations in the follow-up period. This dimension was highly correlated with length of prior hospitalizations ($R = .38$, $p<.0001$) and with transfer to another institution from Chestnut Lodge ($R = .37$, $p<.0001$). That is, number of postdischarge hospitalizations much more so than the length of hospitalizations was related to prior experiences with institutions. For most of our BPD patients, subsequent hospitalizations were relatively brief and crisis-oriented, even when numerous. As such, prior hospitalization appears to determine greater hospital-seeking behavior during later stress. In contrast to our schizophrenic patients, however, prior hospitalization was not associated with the chronic use of institutions in a custodial fashion.

Several other rather widely scattered variables also emerged as predictors of hospitalization. They are difficult to integrate into any meaningful or recognizable profile.

Work Time

Time employed postdischarge was also associated with a motley set of predictors. Consistently absent, however, was any relation between "postmorbid" work time and premorbid work functioning (both qualitatively and quantitatively). This contrasts strikingly with schizophrenics (McGlashan, 1983). For BPD patients, the predictors most consistently associated with good work outcome involve the absence of extreme affective dysregulation (mania, depression, affective instability, and inappropriate affect).

Social Functioning

Social functioning in the follow-up period appeared unrelated to premorbid social functioning, again in contrast to our findings with schizophrenics (McGlashan, 1983). The two most powerful predictors of this dimension relate to manifest illness: distractability (which, as discussed, is probably spurious) and dysphoria. The latter is understandably related to social functioning insofar as dysphoric feelings of loneliness and emptiness motivate object seeking.

Intimacy

Intimacy after discharge seemed less associated with unexpected predictor variables. Greater intimacy, for example, was predicted by better premorbid heterosexual functioning and by fewer conflicts around issues of giving and receiving care. At the same time, as with work and social functioning, the intensity of association between pre- and postmorbid intimate functioning was attenuated for BPD patients in contrast to the schizophrenic patients (McGlashan, 1983).

The strong connection between intimacy and length of index hospitalization may represent an interaction effect. That is, BPD patients with established intimate relationships (or who develop such during their hospitalization) are less likely to remain hospitalized because of greater availability of alternative living arrangements.

The close association of better follow-up intimate relationships with higher levels of psychopathology in the families of origin was unexpected, especially because another family variable (history of substance abuse) predicted in the other direction. Perhaps it represents some form of psychologically reparative regression toward the mean. BPD patients who came from highly deviant families may have "resolved" to develop less chaotic and more stable interpersonal relationships as a result. Before further speculation is offered, however, the replicability of this finding requires testing.

Symptomatology

Length of symptom expression in the follow-up period was most closely correlated with length of index hospitalization and the Elgin 10 Scale total score. Neither relationship held any surprise. Longer periods of hospitalization were likely to result from more chronic conditions with greater symptomatic compromise. The Elgin 10 Scale (Wittman, 1941) consists of 10 subscales which together estimate both degree of chronicity (institutionalization, deficit syndrome) and length of symptomatology (mostly of a schizophrenic nature). The association of better symptomatic outcome with poorer levels of work premorbidly was unexpected and offers no ready explanation.

Borderline Defenses and Countertransference: Research Findings and Implications

Les R. Greene, Ph.D., Judith Rosenkrantz, and Deborah Y. Muth, M.S.W.
(1986)

Among Main's (1957) several cogent insights about the nature of defensive and countertransferential reactions to those so-called special patients who ungraciously refuse to improve—patients who in today's parlance would most assuredly be diagnosed as borderline—is his hypothesis that some of us may flee some of the time into research activities to avoid the frustrations and disappointments of clinical work. Writing from the dual perspectives of researchers and psychotherapists, and with the interest of furthering the integration of these often split-off enterprises, we offer some observations on the amassing body of empirical data about the borderline patient, observations which bear upon and lend support for Main's speculation regarding the detachment of researchers from the emotionally charged dilemmas facing the therapist in working with the borderline patient. We also present some findings from our ongoing investigations of borderline dynamics in groups and organizations, which underscore the role of defensive and countertransferential processes in the psychotherapeutic treatment of borderlines. Finally, based upon our observations of the extant data as well as our own findings, we offer a

---

suggestion about the direction of future research on borderline pathology, proposing a shift away from the largely descriptive-level diagnostic studies and toward the investigation of the therapeutic relationship, with a particular focus on countertransferential dynamics.

With respect to our analysis of the research to date, our first impression has to do with the sheer mass of the findings (Gunderson, 1982, 1984; McGlashan, 1985a). There has been an enormous undertaking to investigate and elucidate borderline phenomena over the past five years, by far overshadowing studies on other personality disorders introduced into the psychiatric nomenclature in DSM-III. Scores of analyses, from sociological, psychological and biological perspectives, have been offered to clarify the apparent conceptual ambiguities surrounding this term and its multiple meanings and usages, as reflected in such phrases as borderline personality disorder, borderline schizophrenia, borderline syndrome, and so on (Aronson, 1985; Nuetzel, 1985). Paralleling this conceptual work have been numerous empirical efforts designed to establish the construct, discriminant and convergent validity of this diagnostic entity, to demonstrate its meaningfulness, sensitivity and specificity as a discrete nosological category. Unresolved diagnostic controversies seem to abound and preoccupy the attentions of the clinical researcher: Do borderlines, as descriptively defined in DSM-III, indeed exist or are they really variants of schizophrenic or depressive conditions? If the borderline concept is valid as a unique, differentiable diagnostic entity, what are its etiological and dynamic links to psychotic-level conditions and to other personality disorders? Is the borderline concept internally consistent or are there qualitatively distinct levels or subtypes of borderline pathology? Virtually all of the empirical work thus far has focused on these diagnostic uncertainties, all aimed, in essence, at clarifying the boundaries of this term.

As detailed elsewhere (Gunderson, 1984; Greene et al., 1985), the almost exclusive methodological goal to date seems to have been the development of the most reliable and valid operational definition of the borderline concept. At our last count, for example, we have collected 10 published studies attempting to discover a borderline-specific patterning of responses on the MMPI and at least as many investigations identifying Rorschach correlates of borderline psychopathology. Beyond the analyses of these kinds of standardized psychological tests, a host of ad hoc self-report and clinician-report questionnaires and checklists have been devised, all basically variants of Gunderson's Diagnostic Interview for Borderlines (Gunderson et al., 1981). This methodological array has, in turn, spawned a burgeoning number of second-generation studies examining empirical overlap and convergence among these measures (Hurt et al., 1984; McGlashan, 1983; Nelson et al., 1985).

What substantive conclusions can be drawn from this abundant data base regarding the borderline diagnosis? Unfortunately, interpretations of the accumulated findings run the gamut from not-so-cautious optimism to outright skepticism. At one end of this continuum are those researchers who argue that considerable validation has been mustered for the borderline concept and its several methodologically diverse operational definitions (cf. Barasch et al., 1985). At the other end of the spectrum are critics (Raifman, 1984; Widiger, 1982) who refute the supportive empirical evidence by pointing out the shortcomings in experimental design, flaws in methodology and fallacies in data interpretation in the research that has generated the data at hand. Some have gone so far as to suggest that the term itself be dropped from the nomenclature (cf. Aronson, 1985). Our second impression, then, is that the research on the borderline diagnosis seems largely to have intensified, rather than lessened, the surrounding clinical controversies.

Finally, we note the disproportionality in diagnosis-related versus treatment-oriented research. The empirical investigation of the psychotherapy of the borderline patient is extremely rare. While such an imbalance in the literature could be understood in light of the medical dictum to diagnose first, other—and deeper—interpretations cannot be ruled out. The few preliminary retrospective and follow-up studies that have been published are quite telling, primarily in demonstrating how difficult and unrewarding the therapeutic work is (McGlashan, 1986; Pope et al., 1983; Skodal et al., 1983; Waldinger & Gunderson, 1984). In one of these recent archival studies conducted within the context of an outpatient clinic, the authors report that the more the patients manifest borderline symptoms, the less likely it is that they will actually receive treatment in that setting, either because of the increased probability of referral elsewhere or because of premature, abrupt endings of therapy (Skodal et al, 1983). Even in private practice settings, where it might be expected that the patients are higher functioning and/or the therapists have a greater investment in effective psychotherapy, therapists' assessment of successful treatment for borderlines is rare (Waldinger & Gunderson, 1984).

Reiser and Levenson (1984) have recently speculated that therapists may act out their countertransferential reactions to difficult patients by name-calling, that is, by inappropriately or pejoratively applying the borderline diagnosis in order to serve such esteem-protecting purposes as blaming and avoiding. We would extend this hypothesis to the research sphere. Our observations regarding the preoccupation with the borderline label among clinical investigators, particularly in terms of their apparent need to find the most valid set of descriptors, and the meager research on treatment issues may themselves similarly be thought to reflect a defensive process. More specifically, the research efforts to date suggest that when it comes to dealing with borderline patients it may feel more rewarding, for the researcher as sell as psychotherapist, to name them than to tame them. What we are suggesting, in an admittedly speculative fashion, is a defensive response in the form of avoidance of treatment-related research on borderlines, a reaction that involves intellectualized controls over and emotional distancing from borderline psychopathology. To whatever extent such a process is operating and unacknowledged, it seems that the value of this research either to the practitioner or the borderline patient will likely be limited. As the central thesis of this paper, we propose that quantitative empirical work on borderline psychopathology would prove more productive at this point by shifting its focus away from the descriptive diagnostic area and toward the therapeutic enterprise, with a particular emphasis precisely on those defensive and countertransferential processes thought to arise in the psychotherapy of borderline patients.

Borderline Pathology and Countertransference

In his integrative volume on borderline pathology, Gunderson (1984), a pioneer in the empirical study of borderline phenomena, begins his chapters on psychotherapy with a section on countertransference. In similar fashion, Kernberg (1975), in the first of his highly influential volumes on borderline conditions, devotes the second chapter to a discussion of countertransference, preceding several chapters on other theoretical and technical aspects of the psychotherapeutic enterprise. How is the prominence given this topic by acknowledged experts in this field to be understood?

To answer this, we turn to theory and specifically to contributions from a psychoanalytic object relations perspective, contributions which have so significantly shaped current thinking about borderline pathology and its treatment. Just as the whole corpus of modern psychoanalytic theorizing, increasingly influenced by the British object relations school (cf. Sutherland, 1983), has shifted and expanded from a metapsychological, impersonal and primarily intrapsychic framework to a more clinically rooted, "experiential-near," and interpersonal perspective, so the concept of countertransference has evolved. While still appreciated in its classic sense, as a neurotically determined inappropriateness located primarily or exclusively within the intrapsychic world of the psychotherapist, an increasingly acknowledged object-relations position views this phenomenon as rooted in the interaction and dynamics between therapist and patient. The Kleinian concept of splitting and projective identification (Grotstein, 1981; Horwitz, 1983; Segal, 1964), Racker's notion of complementary identification (1968), and Grinberg's projective counteridentification (1979) have all contributed significantly to this revised view of countertransference by underscoring the forceful, evershifting and mutually reciprocal projective and introjective processes arising in the patient-therapist dyad.

Specifically with regard to the borderline patient, theory posits, and psychoanalytic research tends to confirm, that malevolence and primitive aggression are central features of the internal world (Greene et al., 1985; Lerner & St. Peter, 1984). A libidinal, trusting core that in normal development serves to neutralize aggression has not been attained (Blatt & Shichman, 1983); a host of persecutory and abandoning fantasy objects continuously threaten whatever fragile sense of goodness does exist in the internal world. Consequently, enormous defensive efforts must be exerted in keeping these malevolent objects at arm's length. As formulated by Kernberg (1975, 1976), the borderline's chief defensive strategies are thought to be splitting and projective identification, processes aimed at maintaining some distance from and control over the destructive, potentially overwhelming and contaminating contents of the internal world.

By means of splitting operations, good and bad, idealized and devalued internal objects are forcefully dissociated from each other; the borderline's internalized social schemata are thought to consist of rigidly dichotomized and polarized categories—pleasing and need-satisfying versus threatening and need-thwarting—of interpersonal experiences. To reinforce these emotionally crude distinctions, loved and hated internalized objects are continuously and massively projected onto and into different segments of the current social field. As we have proposed elsewhere, the borderline scrutinizes any and every actual social setting in terms of its offering suitable containers for the safekeeping of externalized mental contents (Greene, 1983; Greene et al., 1985). To say that the borderline patient cannot distinguish transference from social reality may be theoretically correct in terms of identifying the pathognomonic boundary deficit in this form of pathology (Lerner et al., 1985), but it is partly misleading. The borderline basically is not invested in the painstaking work of discovering the reality of actual social objects; the paramount need is to find external figures capable of being transformed magically and immediately, via projective endowment, into the good and bad, protective and haunting objects of the borderline's internal world. Through the externalization and control involved in the process of projective identification, the borderline feels a greater sense of mastery over both disturbing and desired fantasied objects. Projective identification enables borderlines to know with reassuring conviction and certainty who and where their friends and enemies are.[1]

The recipient of any projective identification, as Bion (1959) has so aptly stated it, is asked to play a role in somebody else's fantasy. To be asked to play the roles offered by the borderline patient is usually more than we as psychotherapists bargain for; and the asking, or perhaps more accurately, the coercing seems to be the major kind of transaction initiated by the borderline patient in the psychotherapeutic relationship. Pines (1978) describes the therapist's experience thusly: "one of the greatest stresses that we undergo in our work is the feeling of being dragged, unwillingly but inevitably, as if by a great force, into the pattern imposed by the patient so that we begin to feel provoked, hostile, persecuted and to behave exactly as the patients need us to, becoming rejecting and hostile. . . . What is real for them are our impulses and our primitive superego contents: for them, these are what are genuine and real; our ego activities are regarded with suspicion as 'phoney,' as malicious, as tricks" (pp. 115–116). Being on the receiving end of borderline-level idealizing transferences, while perhaps less damaging in the sort run, is ultimately no less disconcerting and disruptive to the therapist's familiar sense of self.

From an object-relations perspective, empathic connection, and indeed the essence of therapeutic action, requires the therapist's tolerance for experiencing the distortions to his or her conception of self induced by the patient's primitive projections (Burke & Tansey, 1985; Loewald, 1960; Sandler, 1976; Tansey & Burke, 1985). Temporary regression to and activation of the therapist's own more archaic introjects and an identification of these with the projected contents from the patient are deemed vital to the full emotional understanding of the patient's inner experience. Theoretically, the countertransferential obstacles to empathy are twofold. On the one hand, there is the danger of flight from the internal experiences induced by the patient's projective identifications. Prematurely pulling away from the emotional experience is frequently due to the therapist's anxieties over the raw aggressive impulses and/or the loss of clear self-other boundaries arising as part of these regressive experiences. In these situations the therapist cannot accept, even temporarily, becoming the tormentor or masochist or any other highly charged role found in the borderline's internalized repertoire. The opposite countertransferential danger is the acting-out of these internal experiences, in essence becoming transformed by the patient's projections and enacting a collusive, complementary and primitive object tie. Frequently in these instances, the patient's projections strike a chord with early characterological features of the therapist, such that the therapist's sense of self becomes more chronically and pervasively altered.

Ideally, the therapist negotiates a delicate balance between these two extremes, being sufficiently receptive to the primitive material from both outside and within and yet capable of maintaining enough psychological distance and control to contain and organize the material. To understate the point, we suspect that in the work with borderlines this ideal is not achieved with any frequency, especially as the intensity of the patients' projective identifications increases. Clinician and researcher too often may flee or rely upon previously renounced characterological defenses in response to the borderline's powerful projective tugs.

Borderline Defenses and Countertransference Acting-Out in Group Co-therapy: A Preliminary Empirical Investigation

It would be useful to be able to document empirically some of these propositions regarding borderline pathology and counter-transference. Unfortunately, the previous research on countertransference (Singer & Luborsky, 1977) offers little help: The research tradition in this area is too limited, the work has primarily focused on the more narrow, classic definition of this term, and no attention has been paid to specific borderline phenomena. As a stimulus toward more research activity in this area, we report findings from our ongoing studies of borderlines in groups and organizations (Greene et al., 1985), findings that bear on the relationship between borderline defenses and countertransferential reactions.

Our data were generated within the context of an intermediate-term day-treatment program specifically geared for the borderline patient. As described in greater detail elsewhere (Greene, 1983; Greene et al., 1985), this program treats approximately 20 borderline adults through a series of integrated group modalities, all informed by a psychoanalytic object-relations theoretical perspective. Of central importance are the thrice weekly, co-led therapy groups that aim at examining and interpreting here-and-now transference distortions. In our earlier papers, we presented a conceptual rationale about the goodness of fit between borderline defenses of splitting and projective identification and the co-therapy situation. Briefly, we posited that the simultaneous presence of two therapists serves to highlight borderline-specific defensive operations to the extent that the co-therapists become repositories for the borderline patient's externalized, contradictory and dissociated experiences of early maternal authority. Based on ideas and procedures from research with the Interpersonal Repertory Grid (Bannister, 1965; Watson, 1970), we employed a semantic differential methodology to assess the borderline patient's perceptions of each co-therapist and took the divergence in these perceptions as an index of the patient's enactment of split-off transferences. The greater the polarity in characteristics ascribed to the two therapists, the stronger the presumed reliance upon splitting and projective identification. We then examined associations between this index and other borderline-specific signs and symptoms. Correlations, calculated over 42 patients from five different therapy groups, showed significant relationships between our index and specific conceptions of self, object representations and boundary disturbances. These findings offered preliminary validation of our measures of borderline defenses as well as support for the intrapsychic structures and processes thought to underlie this pathology.

In the present study, we analyzed additional data from the same sample to examine empirical associations between the patients' views of their co-therapists and these therapists' clinical judgments about their patients. More specifically, we wanted to assess whether the magnitude of the patients' polarizing of their co-therapists would correspond with the degree of divergence of the co-therapists' ratings of pathology. Would co-therapists' disagreements with each other about a patient parallel that patient's splitting of the co-therapists? To the extent that such an association was obtained, the findings would be consistent with and supportive of the idea that countertransference acting-out is more problematic as borderline defenses intensify.

As part of the extensive initial evaluation of patients in this day-treatment program, a battery of tests is administered 1 to 2 weeks following admission. The two measures of interest in the present analysis are: 1) a semantic differential form and 2) a target complaint inventory. A 4-part semantic differential was designed to tap patients' current perceptions of themselves, each of their group co-therapists (who serve as their primary clinicians), and their small therapy group as a whole on 15 7-point adjective rating scales; adjectives were selected to reflect Osgood et al.'s (1957) factorially derived dimensions of evaluation, potency and activity. Following our earlier studies, we developed indices of borderline defenses by calculating absolute differences in patients' perceptions of their co-therapists along each of the three semantic dimensions. In addition, we arithmetically combined these dimensions as in our earlier work to examine patients' splitting of their co-therapists by idealizing one and devaluing the other.[2]

The second measure of interest in the present study, the target complaint form, was designed to record three presenting complaints and their degree of severity on 7-point rating scales. Following the completion of this inventory by the patient, the co-therapists, blind to the patient's ratings, were asked to rate independently the same complaints listed by the patient. The absolute difference in co-therapists' ratings of severity of pathology was calculated as an index of their being split-off from each other and, consequently, of an enactment of countertransferential reactions. The greater the divergence in co-therapists' ratings, the more the presumed counter-transferential distortion.

Completed data sets, including the co-therapists' ratings of severity of presenting problems, were collected from 35 of the 42 subjects in the original cohort. As in our earlier study, these data were gathered across five different therapy groups, with the aim of thereby increasing the generalizability of the obtained findings. Each group was led by a unique pair of co-therapists, all of whom were either beginning-level therapists or students training in psychiatry, clinical psychology and psychiatric social work; with the exception of one pair of female therapists, the co-therapy teams were composed of male-female pairs.

The distributions of scores from all of the indices described above were subjected to median splits to form dichotomous variables; four chi-square analyses were then performed to test the hypothesized associations. Looking first at the relationship between the patient's tendency to split the co-therapists along an idealization-devaluation dimension and the co-therapists' divergence in ratings, we found a marginally significant association, displayed in Table 1 (corrected $\chi^2=2.95$; $p<.10$). In line with our hypothesis, co-therapists' tendencies to make either similar or discrepant ratings of patients' complaints mirrored the degree of patients' reliance on splitting and externalization, as operationally defined by the semantic differential. Co-therapists' discordance occurred more than twice as often as their agreements when patients tended to cast them into idealized-devalued dichotomies. On the other hand, the co-therapists were much more likely to make the same clinical judgments when their patients viewed them in similar ways.

Of the three additional chi-square analyses performed on the separate components of the semantic differential, statistically significant association (corrected $\chi^2=4.71$; $p<.05$) obtained on the evaluation dimensions, also shown in Table 1. Again, in line with our hypothesis, we found that therapists' divergence in their clinical judgments paralleled patients' polarizing of their co-therapists into good versus bad evaluative categories. Discrepant clinical judgments occurred much more frequently than similar ratings, almost three times as often, when patients split their co-therapists; conversely, therapists agreed more frequently when their patients' opinions of them were consonant.

Taken together, these findings lend some preliminary empirical support to the idea that countertransferential reactions, manifested as distortions in perceiving the here-and-now situation, will intensify as patients' use of borderline-level defenses increases. Of course, our statistical analyses do not imply specific causation and other, competing interpretations of the data cannot be ruled out. One viable alternative is that both variables under investigation—borderline splitting and co-therapist disagreement—may be related to some third, mediating variable. For example, patients who depend more heavily on borderline-level defenses may be more difficult to

Table 1
Associations Between Patients' Reliance on Borderline Defenses
and Co-therapists' Disagreements in Clinical Ratings

	Co-therapists' Disagreement in Overall Clinical Ratings	
	High	Low
Patients' splitting of co-therapists into idealized and devalued categories ($p<.10$)		
High	35%	15%
Low	18%	32%
Patients' splitting of co-therapists into good and bad evaluative categories ($p<.05$)		
High	40%	14%
Low	14%	32%

assess accurately because of their comparatively stronger need to conceal aspects of self—the true self in object-relations terms—thus forcing the therapist to use only partial and misleading data and/or to make deeper inferences in making clinical judgments. From this perspective, greater therapist disagreement can be understood not in terms of the dynamic notion of countertransference, but as a direct consequence of the more complex cognitive task involved.

Another plausible explanation of our obtained association posits a causal connection in the directions opposite from our hypothesized relationship. For example, therapists may have either comparable or dissimilar personality traits which predispose them to respond in similar or divergent ways to the same patient; the borderline patient, keenly aware of such personality characteristics, may, in turn, react identically or differentially to the two therapists. Such a chicken-and-egg dilemma cannot be definitively sorted out by the data at hand. Given our provocative findings, however, we did conduct a number of ancillary analyses to shed further light on the underlying dynamics accounting for the present associations.

First, in the significant chi-square analysis reported above, we looked at the cell composed of those patients who made extremely dichotomous evaluations of their co-therapists and whose therapists strongly disagreed in their ratings of pathology. The observations here deal only with absolute differences; we wanted to examine whether or not there was a specific and unique directionality associated with these divergences. Our reasoning concerning this analysis went as follows. If personality traits of the therapists, such as relative comfort with fusion experiences (cf. Horwitz, 1985), were the primary determinant of the associations reported above, then we might theoretically expect the absolute differences in this cell all to be in the same direction. Given that borderline patients are thought to be arrested at approximately the same level of development, they should respond in similar fashion to salient personality features of their therapists. Those co-therapists who have comparatively less discomfort with symbiotic-like relationships, for example, might typically elicit positive reactions from the borderline patient, while those therapists who prefer greater interpersonal distance and aloofness might regularly become the externalized abandoning object. On the other hand, if the associations reported above were caused by the patients' splitting, less clear-cut directionality could be expected. In this situation, a patient's choices of transference objects can be based on relatively minor and inconsequential features of the therapists. One casual or humorous remark by a therapist, for example, can become the entire basis for massive projective embellishment.

What, then, is the directionality of the absolute differences in this cell? Of the 14 cases, 10 showed the same directionality: the co-therapist who received the more positive evaluation (i.e., the "good" therapist) rated the patient's problems as less severe than the "bad" therapist did. In the four remaining cases, the reverse pattern obtained: the "good" co-therapist judged the patient's problems as more severe than the "bad" therapist. These findings fail to lend unequivocal support for either our working hypothesis or the competing interpretation elaborated above; more generally, they seem to point out the complexity of the underlying processes involved in our empirical association. It may well by that both borderline defenses and therapist personality, including characterological traits and defensive styles, co-determine our empirical findings. The notion of patient-therapist "fit" (Gunderson, 1984; Singer & Luborsky, 1977), which discards the idea of simplistic antecedent-consequence relationships in favor of the view of collusive and/or reciprocal interactional processes, may ultimately prove to be a more important conceptual tool in guiding the kind of clinical process research reflected by the present study.

Our second kind of ancillary analysis focused on the nature of the patients' problems reported on the target complaint form. We wanted to examine whether our obtained significant relationship between splitting along a good-bad dichotomy and co-therapist divergence was dependent upon the content of the complaints being rated. Content specificity, if found, would seem to lend greater credence to our empirical associations. As a first step, we attempted to classify the range of patients' presenting complaints by using Masterson's (1981) formulations about the underlying abandonment depression in borderline pathology and the pathognomonic defensive strategies manifested either as excessive clinging and compliance or as defiance, hypervigilance and counterdependence. We used these notions to develop three categories of complaints: 1) depression (including feelings of worthlessness, despair and suicidality), 2) complaints based on the need to cling (including lack of assertiveness and feelings of helplessness, dependence, and insecurity), and 3) complaints based on the need to defy (including anger and blame toward others, paranoid tendencies and withdrawal). Using this classification schema, the first author rated the three complaints of each patient; to assess reliability, the second author independently categorized the complaints of a random sample of 10 patients.

Descriptively, this scoring system proved satisfactory. Interrater agreement in categorizing the complaints was 90%; kappa, an index of agreement correcting for chance, was .85. With respect to comprehensiveness, at least one of the three complaints per patient could be scored; overall, 70% of the total number of presenting problems were classified within this system. Not surprisingly, more patients in this intensive treatment setting reported problems having to do with both depressive experiences (N=21) and concerns over anger and distrust (N=20) than reported concerns about excessive dependence and overcompliance (N=14), considered expressions of higher-level defenses.

Of the three chi-square analyses we then performed using this classification system of presenting complaints, one significant association was revealed. As shown in Table 2, a relationship obtained between patients' dichotomizing of their co-therapists into good and bad evaluative categories and the corresponding therapists' divergence in ratings of depression. Co-therapists' differences of opinion about the severity of depressive symptomatology directly paralleled the extent to which they were polarized by their patients (corrected χ^2=6.40, p<.01). Because the last finding is based on a small sample (N=21), it must be viewed most cautiously. Nevertheless, it does match clinical studies of staff countertransference in working with borderlines (Book et al., 1978; Brown, 1980), impressions which suggest that intrastaff conflicts frequently revolve around concerns over the seriousness of patients' suicidal behaviors

Table 2
Association Between Patients' Reliance on Borderline Defenses and
Co-therapists' Rating of Depression

	Patients' Splitting of Co-therapists into Good and Bad Evaluative Categories	
	High	Low
Co-therapists' disagreements in ratings of depression		
High	48%	14%
Low	0%	38%

and depressive symptoms. In these circumstances, opinions often become sharply divided as to whether the borderline patient is genuinely depressed or merely manipulative and exploitative. Tentatively, the present findings suggest that staff, in general, and co-therapists, in particular, may have an easier time in realistically assessing the severity of borderline defensive styles than in accurately judging a patient's underlying depression. Again, it needs to be stressed that our data do not indicate whether these differences in clinical opinions of depression are manifestations of countertransferential dynamics or are, more simply, cognitive errors in judging aspects of patients' hidden, true selves.

Implications for Future Research on Borderline Pathology

Taken together, then, the findings from this admittedly small-scale investigation seem to offer some empirical support for a hypothesized linkage between borderline patients' use of splitting and externalization and therapists' countertransferential responses. While causal connections cannot be determined from the present data, our findings are consistent with the view that the more that the borderline patient simplistically dichotomizes therapists into positive or negative evaluative categories, the more likely it is that these therapists will manifest distortions in clinical judgments, particularly involving critical calls about depression and suicidality. These findings dovetail with the recent results reported by McGlashan (1985b), who has found that both of these variables—borderline-level defenses and therapist countertransference—are significant predictors of outcome of treatment for borderlines.[3] On the basis of such empirical discoveries and in conjunction with analysis of the extant data base on borderline psychopathology, we propose that it is time to shift the direction of research on this clinical population. Interpretations of the cumulative findings from the primarily descriptive-level diagnostic studies have been conflicting, and it is unclear whether additional studies in this genre will eventually elucidate or merely perpetuate the controversies surrounding this nosological category. What does seem apparent is that such research has been of little help in assessing or improving the treatment strategies in working with borderlines. Precisely because defensive and countertransferential processes are weighed so heavily in both the theoretical and clinical writings on the treatment of borderlines, we suggest that their study by systematic empirical investigation will prove fruitful and, dare we say, helpful to the therapist and ultimately to the borderline patient.

If nothing else, our present investigation reveals how a relatively simple and economical methodology, but one guided by dynamic formulations of the therapeutic relationship, can be productively applied to the study of countertransference. In an excellent integrative review of recent experimental work from cognitive and social psychological laboratories, Singer (1985) has demonstrated how such concepts as personal constructs, scripts, prototypes, and schemata have major and direct implications for the systematic study of transference dynamics in psychotherapy; in a compelling argument, he asserts that transference, defined as the idiosyncratic ways in which individuals construe new social situations based on engrained assumptions, expectations and beliefs about themselves and others, can be brought under rigorous scrutiny by borrowing from these experimental research domains. In a similar vein, what seems needed now, in terms of research geared toward the treatment of borderlines, are measures and procedures that assess such theoretically important relational concepts as the therapeutic alliance (Frieswyk et al., 1986; Hartley & Strupp, 1983), the therapeutic enterprise as a holding environment, and therapist-patient "fit," mentioned earlier. Such terms are not mere extensions of the static, acontextual, and relatively unproductive "patient variables" and "therapist variables" of earlier process research, but notions that attempt to capture the current experiences of the patient and therapist within the therapeutic interaction.

We offer a final note in the way of a caveat. There is a renewed effort at hand in conducting psychotherapy research, motivated to a large degree by increasing demands for accountability. Under such pressure, psychotherapy research, both outcome and process, seems to be gaining greater sophistication and calibration, as manifested through the mushrooming development and use of training manuals. Unfortunately, the danger with this trend is that clinically meaningful constructs will be sacrificed for precision and reliability. In particular, we can cite a recently constructed psychotherapy manual geared specifically for measuring therapists' techniques in working with borderlines (Koenigsberg et al., 1985); we note the omission of more inferentially based categories for assessing the more subtle aspects of the clinical exchange, including defensive and countertransferential responses of the therapist. Process researchers such as Mahl (Kasl & Mahl, 1965) and Dahl (Dahl et al., 1978), in their indices of speech parapraxes, remind us that measuring what is said is not enough in understanding the therapeutic relationship.[4] Assessment of the intentionality of the therapist, including defensive needs during turbulent transferential storms as well as technical aims, seems critical in validating and expanding our current psychodynamic formulations about working with the borderline patient.

Notes

1. A recent clinical encounter on an inpatient psychiatric ward illustrates the relief, albeit tenuous, afforded by projective identification. A patient approached me as the director of the therapeutic milieu and said, "I want to thank you, Dr. Greene. I think this is a very good program here; I didn't always feel that way, but I certainly do now that I understand it."
    "How is that?" I asked.
    With an air of confidence and pleasure, the patient answered, "Well you and Dr. L. [the ward chief] are the good guy and the bad guy. Of course, you keep alternating roles and you want us to learn who is who and how to cope with your changing roles. I think it's very clever of you."
2. The arithmetic combination for idealizing is calculated as: Evaluation+Potency/2+Activity/2. By applying this formula to each therapist and taking the absolute difference, we have an index of idealization-devaluation.
3. In a personal communication, McGlashan reports finding no empirical association between these two variables. This apparent contradiction to the present data may be due, however, to differences in methodology between his study and ours. McGlashan's operational definitions of variables were based upon and his data were gleaned from hospital records. Because these records are subject to inspection by hospital administrators and others, it seems reasonable to assume that the

documentation of staff countertransference might be downplayed. Indeed, in only 30% of his sample of borderline patients were instances of countertransference noted, suggesting a tendency to underreport this phenomenon. However, in the 25 cases where countertransference reactions were recorded, borderline defensive behavior co-occurred 88% of the time.

4. In one staff meeting on the psychiatric ward referred to earlier, two slips of the tongue were noted in discussions of the dispositions of two very taxing borderline patients. With regard to one of the patients, one staff member asked, "How can we help him to go to the Hawkins Funeral Home, I mean Hawkins Nursing Home?" In reviewing the second patient, another staff member suggested that the best way to find him a permanent living arrangement would be to contact "all the boarding facilities throughout the Northwest, uh, Northeast." The wishes to be rid of these patients contained in these slips seem self-evident.

Part 4

Case Presentations

Borderline and Narcissistic Fusional Attachment: Psychotherapeutic and Theoretical Considerations

Introduction to Symposium

Michael B. Sperling, Ph.D.
(1986)

Developmental theorists have begun to elucidate the sequences of early attachment, separation and object constancy, with occasional prospective speculation regarding the form of later attachment and love relations. Psychoanalytic theorists have invested much in speculating about early psychic mechanisms and structural development (particularly oedipally determined processes) based upon inference from patients' material. But clinicians and theorists are just beginning to focus more exclusively on the pre-oedipal developmental antecedents of fusional attachment and love relations in adulthood, as informed by work such as that of Ainsworth (1978) and Mahler (1975).

In attempting to outline the salient normative developmental antecedents of adult love relations, Kernberg (1976) has proposed a continuum of configurations regarding the capacity for falling in love and remaining in love, which focuses in addition on borderline and narcissistic relational pathology. This symposium, too, focuses on borderline and narcissistic love and attachment, particularly the

Presented at the annual convention of the American Psychological Association, August 23–26, 1986, Washington, DC.

ubiquitous desire for symbiotic fusion (whether indirectly or directly enacted), in order to better understand any patient's early attachment style and consequent adult desire for and experience of fusional attachment and love.

The three papers to be presented examine various manifestations of the early dynamics and adult desire for fusional attachment, as organized around Kernberg's (1976) continuum. This continuum suggests five levels of intimate relational pathology, from the almost total incapacity of severe narcissistic personalities for genital or tender relations, to a second level of sexual promiscuity in moderately ill narcissistic personalities, to a third level of clinging dependency and primitive idealization characteristic of borderline personalities, to a fourth level of the neurotic capacity for tenderness and stability without full genital gratification, and lastly, to the integrated capacity for genitality in stable, tender love relations.

The papers constituting this symposium are derived from our clinical work and research interests with borderline and narcissistic character disorders in both outpatient and long-term inpatient settings. In the first paper, Robert B. Handley will use empirical data and case material around therapist-patient separations to highlight indirect manifestations of fusional dynamics at the earlier narcissistic and borderline positions on Kernberg's continuum. The second paper, by James W. Hull and Robert C. Lane, will examine fusional imagery in borderline patients as represented by concerns about body intactness. In the third paper I will elaborate theory and present case material around the borderline and normative enactment of fusional love relations. Characterized as desperate love, this style of relation is based in the third and fourth, or borderline and neurotic, positions on Kernberg's continuum. Finally, Charles R. Swenson will suggest some of the emergent themes, and discuss the rationale for including the diverse clinical phenomena presented in these papers within a symposium on fusional attachment.

Therapist-Patient Separations: Fusional Attachment Phenomena in a Borderline Personality

Robert B. Handley, Ph.D.
(1986)

Attainment of libidinal object constancy is viewed as an essential task of the first three years of life, while failure to attain object constancy is regarded as central to narcissistic character disturbance (Roiphe & Galenson, 1986). The importance of achieving libidinal object constancy is implicit in Rebecca Behrends and Sidney Blatt's (1985) views on internalization. They write, "The individual's major existential task throughout the life cycle is one of continued separation-individuation, which is accomplished through progressive internalizations of need-gratifying aspects of relationships with significant others" (pp. 34–35). The failure to internalize these need-gratifying aspects of the other leads to the tenuous self-other differentiation that may be seen in the pathological fusional states of some narcissistic personalities at points of regression. In addition, it can lead to the drying up of libidinal sources and the excessive development of aggressive drives in severe borderline psychopathology.

In my view, the study of the quality of libidinal object constancy and fusional relations can be dramatically explored at points of separation from key attachment figures. Mary Ainsworth's observa-

Presented at the annual convention of the American Psychological Association, August 22–26, 1986, Washington, DC. The case material and quantitative analyses were previously published in the article: Handley, R. B. & Swenson, C. (1989), Acting Out of Separation Conflicts in Borderline Pathology: An Empirical Case Study, *Bulletin of the Menninger Clinics*, 53, 18–30.

tional studies of mother-infant separations (Ainsworth et al., 1978) and Margaret Mahler's (Mahler et al., 1975) prospective work on separation-individuation both provide precedents for the study of separation reactions. Ainsworth's experimental paradigm the "strange situation" has provided a method for classifying the quality of mother-infant attachments in 1-year-old infants into secure versus insecure ones, based on the infant's response to the mother following a brief separation period. Infants who can utilize the mother to quickly soothe their distress in a reunion phase are characterized as securely attached while those who either avoid, ignore, or aggressively react to the mother on reunion are classified as insecure. These characteristic reunion responses to separation are, I believe, behavioral manifestations of the current internalized object relations of the child.

In this paper, I employ an analogous observational method to the study of a patient's reactions to separations by recording the naturalistic observations of nursing staff organized around separations from her therapist. I will build a picture of this patient's internalized object world by presenting case material drawn from therapy sessions and combining these intrapsychic data with observations of her behavior on the hospital unit. My aim is to reveal the internal and external manifestations of her fusional relations with significant others.

The patient is a 27-year-old, single, female college graduate whom I shall refer to as Elaine. She voluntarily admitted herself to a long-term inpatient hospitalization on a unit which specializes in the treatment of severe personality disturbances. Her treatment consisted of three sessions per week of psychoanalytically oriented psychotherapy and participation in a highly structured hospital milieu. Elaine had a long history of self-destructive behavior including self-cutting, chronic suicidal gestures, substance abuse, periods of depersonalization, social withdrawal, manipulative interpersonal relationships, and brief episodes of auditory hallucinations. At the point of this hospitalization she was unable to function independently and was viewed as being a serious suicide risk. She was seen as having severe borderline and narcissistic pathology.

In the interest of brevity, I will move directly to the observational data and forgo a more complete case history. To highlight Elaine's behavioral reactions to separation I attempted to code and quantify all clearly observable instances of expressed aggressive behavior and heightened instances of anxiety documented by nursing staff. The observational data covers the first 8 months of her treatment

Table 1
Events Coded for Indication of Anxiety and Provocative Behavior as Clearly Documented in the Chart or Communication Log

Restrictions
  Given for behaviors such as: failing to sign in after appointments, missing medications, late on pass

As-Needed Medication
  Given for increased anxiety

Requesting Quiet Room

Refusing Treatment
  Includes refusing therapy session, walking out of groups, refusing medication

Destroying Property

Bulimic Episode

Elopement Risk

Requires Quiet Room
  Staff views patient needing seclusion for emotional control

Submits 72 hour notice

Psychotic Episode

Self-mutilating

Requires Restraints

Elopement

AMA Discharge

Suicide Attempt

Suicide

and is coded from her medical record and the unit communication log. The relevant behaviors are shown in Table 1.

During these 245 days, there were eight separations from her therapist of varying lengths. A separation period was divided into three phases, an anticipatory phase, preceding the separation (maximum of 5 days), the separation phase, per se, and the reunion phase (maximum of 5 days).

During the 245 days, 73 days had an entry involving one or more of the targeted behaviors. Table 2 presents the proportion of these behaviors in relation to different phases of separation. You will note that there is a rate of provocative behavior averaging almost once

Table 2
Days in Which Events are Recorded by
Phase of Separation from Therapist

| Status of Separation | Days | | Proportion |
	Occurrences	Nonoccurrences	of Events
Nonseparation Phase	38	104	.27
Anticipatory Phase	6	23	.21
Separation Phase	13	33	.28
Reunion Phase	16	12	.57

every three days, and this is practically doubled during the reunion days.

I next sought to capture the intensity of the provocative behavior by attempting to rank order and scale the different forms of behavior. The ranking of intensity was completed by staff who were asked to consider the seriousness of the behaviors and make judgments on every comparison of two separate behaviors, e.g., self-mutilation compared with as-needed restrictions for missing her medications. The paired comparison method was originally used in early psychometric studies. I took the average of the rank ordering and transformed the ranks to z-scores and employed a 0–100 point ordinal scale. The behaviors and point values for each behavior are shown in Table 3. If we calculate our ratings of severity of expressed behavior for each day, average this for the different phases, and present it as a function of the amount of time in a phase, the pattern shown in Figure 1 results, and the intensity of her behavior on reunion becomes strikingly apparent.

Case Material

I would like now to focus on one of these separation periods and provide a sense of the clinical material involved. This episode begins at the time I announced an upcoming vacation, approximately 3 weeks before the actual separation. In this session, Elaine began to focus on my leaving at the end of the academic year: "I am thinking about the time when you leave. Do you think I will be ready to leave then?" I responded, "That's unclear. It depends upon your progress." She said, "I think of Denise [another patient] not coming to your session. I wouldn't do that—I want what you've got. I want your head—I mean, your head up there, not down there." Later in the

Table 3
Scale Ratings for Severity of Anxiety or Provocative Behavior

Events	Point Values
Restrictions	2
PRN Medications	7
Requesting Quiet Room	11
Refusing Treatment	28
Property Damage	30
Bulimic Episode	36
Elopement Risk	42
Requires Quiet Room	48
72 Hour Notice	50
Psychotic Episode	62
Self-Mutilating	64
Requires Restraints	67
Elopement	72
AMA Discharge	82
Suicide Attempt	93
Suicide	100

session she described a fantasy of being chased by two staff members and of being subdued. That evening she came to the nurses' station and reported in a provocative manner that she had been lightly banging her head. That next evening she called her former therapist saying that she missed him. In addition, she approached a male staff member in the dining room and said with a sarcastic tone while holding a plastic knife, "I would like to cut you up with this knife." The staff member confronted her with the sadistic quality of her humor.

Ten days later in session, she began, "I hate you. I feel like putting my fist in your face." "What makes you so angry?" "I'm angry about your vacation. You set me up, talking about closeness, and then you leave." "So, in your eyes, I am someone who seduces you into dependence and then drops you." She appeared to be ignoring me and withdrawing at that moment. I commented, "You act as though I am not even in the room now, as if I don't exist." She responded, "Why shouldn't I? I've been wiped out by you!"

Three days later, she began a session with a dream. "I dreamt that Charles [a patient on the unit] came after me with a razor, he sliced me up, and I went to the nurses' station for help. Stan [a staff member] wasn't there, but someone bandaged me up, and then I shot Charles. But then things changed. It wasn't me who shot

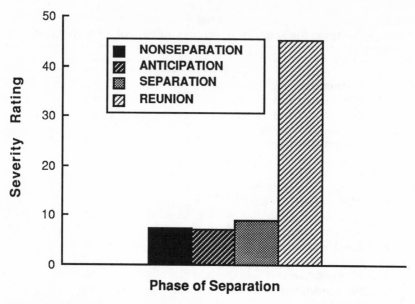

Phase of Separation

Figure 1. Mean severity of provocativeness as a function of the phase of separation

Charles; it was Sara [a nurse] who did it." On a pass that weekend, she had actually been wrestling with the patient mentioned in the dream. The day before my vacation, she was very anxious and described having racing thoughts, and her speech was pressured. She stated that she wanted to hold on to the positive feelings she had toward me. But her anger erupted in statements like "I want to rip something off of yours." I pointed out both the angry and positive feelings she felt toward me.

The separation phase which followed generated an escalating series of events. On the first day, she approached the nurses' station and, in an angry accusatory manner, she blamed the nursing staff for causing her menstrual period to come a week early. Staff were puzzled by her reaction, particularly because she didn't recognize the irrationality of this accusation. Later in the day, staff informed her that she would not be getting a Thanksgiving pass due to her recent provocativeness and potential for impulsivity. She went into her room and broke a statue and was escorted to the quiet room. She was tense, sullen, and angry during most of the separation. In the last few days she began to threaten elopement. She would run down the hall or try to go out the door. Staff responded but said that she really didn't seem to be going anywhere. They held her by the arm. She didn't struggle as if she were afraid or wanted to escape, but instead passively collapsed to the ground, sometimes bruising herself. Staff felt that it was extremely provocative and controlling, and they felt forced into using physical means to contain her because she was denying and minimizing all verbal interventions. She did say to the nursing staff that she felt better in the quiet room, and that she felt "soothed" when she heard a particular staff member's voice. This staff member was also the target of many of her elopement attempts. She also reported that she was trying to fantasize her conversations with Dr. H. and wasn't sure what she had told me.

On my first day back she brought in a dream: "I dreamt I was being raped by an older man, who turns into a monster, and later it turns into Jill [her nurse administrator] who wanted to kill me." On reflecting on her provocative behavior on the unit, she said, "I feel very powerful, almost like Hitler." She felt she was stirring up the males on the unit and really being a "cocktease." The behavioral enactments intensified, and she became more overtly paranoid, stating that she felt staff wished to punish her. Yet she continued to act in a sadistic way toward them. In session, I confronted these contradictions between her sadistic behavior and the victimized fears she was expressing, but I too felt de-skilled and helpless. Neuroleptic medication was again started at this point and the extreme provocativeness gradually subsided. On the Monday following the weekend, she described a dream: "I dreamt again it was Charles [a patient] who was trying to rape me, not staff."

In the following sessions, she became less resistant in therapy and began holding on to a pillow which was on my couch. She would abruptly hold it in a comforting manner and poke her finger through it. I pointed out her behavior as a metaphor from which we talked about the positive and negative feelings she felt toward me.

A final dream she brought in during this time represents a condensation of her experiences around loss. She said, "I dreamt last night that my teeth were falling out and that my mouth was all bloody. I went up to the nurses' station and they told me I would have to go sit in the observation area and wait for the doctor on call. I sat there waiting and the blood just kept flowing out, then finally Dr. W came up to examine me and he said I had gonorrhea."

Discussion

The behavioral observations and the dream and fantasy material combine to portray the essence of this patient's internal object world. We do not know what the intrapsychic world of the infants in Ainsworth et al.'s (1978) study is like when the mother returns to them. But in the material of my patient we can begin to sort out her subjective experiences to loss. I wish to focus on her vulnerable self-object differentiation, her impoverished capacity for libidinal object constancy, and her omnipotent aggressive effort to refuse with the object on reunion.

The separations highlight this patient's tenuous self-object differentiation. The early menstrual period, the head banging, the dream of her teeth falling out, and the dreams of rape each convey the unconscious threat to the body ego posed by object loss. At a primitive, unconscious level, the therapist does not have an existence of his own, but is instead a narcissistic extension of the patient. Disruption of this fused selfobject entity is threatening and leads to an ensuing cycle of projection and reintrojection of pathogenic introjects. Loss is experienced, and the destructiveness is attributed to the nursing staff in the forms of having caused the menstrual period, shot the patient, and failed to attend to her adequately while her teeth were falling out. Thus, a hostile destructive object emerges, which fuels a paranoid process. Blum (1986) writes that "the constant, hostile persecution is the reciprocal of libidinal object constancy and may be regarded as a desparate effort to preserve an illusory constant object while constantly fearing betrayal and loss" (p. 265).

In the absence of libidinal constancy, the predominant aggressive drives emerge unneutralized and overwhelm libidinal aspects. Efforts to recapture a soothing object are attempted as she calls her former therapist, listens to a staff member's voice, and rehearses conversations with her doctor, but these efforts are insufficient. Without the internalization of need-gratifying aspects of significant others, important libidinal resources are unavailable. The libidinal stream instead appears contaminated by the predominant aggressive drives. I should add that she revealed that sexual intimacy was seen only in terms of a sadomasochistic act. She further reported that she had never had sexual intercourse outside of a single drunken experience because of her fears, and that she had given up masturbation several years earlier. Thus, not only had she lost the capacity to experience tender, gentle feeling toward others, but this attitude toward herself was lost as well. This drying up of important libidinal sources is strikingly similar to Roiphe and Galenson's (1986) account of a 2-year-old girl who likewise failed to develop object constancy. In ths child, separation experiences triggered, on reunion, vicious physical attacks on her mother and a disturbing trend in which kissing and hugging would suddenly transform into pinching and biting attacks. In addition, normal masturbatory stimulation of the genitals was replaced first by self-injurious rubbing of her navel and ultimately total constriction of masturbation.

Finally, I wish to turn to the heightened level of "acting out" on reunion. Here, I think one can see the omnipotent attempts to control the object. Aggressive, self-destructive behavior was evident at different phases of the separation, but the intensification of her efforts on reunion point to the therapist as being the primary target of her rage. There is an economy to her actions, she can't directly punish her therapist while he is gone, but in addition, it speaks to the attachment she has to this key figure. Her attachment to the object is dominated by aggression and painful feelings. Thus, as described by Vallenstein (1973), we can speculate that early affects associated with the self and self-object had, primarily, a painful valence. Now upon reunion, this patient in her own way attempts to restore a fused selfobject entity. Unfortunately, this patient's gross deficits in libidinal object constancy, and the contamination and deficits in libidinal drives, make this patient's efforts of fusion overwhelmingly aggressive and destructive.

Bodily Representation of Conflicts Around Fusion and Individuation in Borderlines

James W. Hull, Ph.D., and Robert C. Lane, Ph.D.
(1986)

In 1938 Otto Isakower described a type of experience which had been reported by a number of his patients. At the moment of falling asleep these patients experienced amorphous physical sensations involving different regions of the body, principally the mouth, skin and hand. The experience often involved a blurring of different body areas and an uncertainty about what was internal and what was external. There was an accompanying visual impression of something round, shadowy and indefinite coming nearer and larger, then receding. Auditory impressions of humming, murmuring or some other indiscriminable sound were frequent, as well as a tactile sensation of something crumpled, sandy or dry, experienced in the mouth and, at the same time, on the skin as a whole. The person felt as if there were a soft, yielding mass in his or her mouth, yet knew this was something outside the self. A sensation of floating, giddiness or depersonalization was common. Isakower hypothesized that these phenomena represented an archaic ego state temporarily reactivated as the external world was decathected during the process of falling asleep. Such moments were characterized by increased cathexis of the body ego, which reverted to an early undifferentiated state associated with experiences of hunger and

Presented at the annual convention of the American Psychological Association, August 23–26, 1986, Washington, DC.

satiation at the mother's breast, with oral sensations diffused over the whole skin.

Psychoanalytic investigators since Isakower have further documented perceptual and body ego experiences connected with the symbiotic and presymbiotic states. Spitz (1955) investigated the infant's experience during the earliest state of nondifferentiation, before discriminations between self and object, psyche and soma, and various ego faculties had been achieved. He described such experience as coenesthetic, involving total fused experiences. These consist largely of contact sensations from the oral cavity, the hand, the labyrinth and the outer skin surface, but also involve other sensory impressions including sight and hearing. Later when the sensorium has been more fully cathected, focused distance perception involving audition and vision becomes prominent. Spitz highlighted the importance of early sensations in the oral cavity, which he referred to as the "primal cavity," and saw in these experiences the origins of all perception. Hoffer's (1950) discussion of early body ego formations based on sensations of the mouth and the hand is consistent with these formulations. Woodbury (1966) has described different levels of body ego experience in adult patients, with the most primitive referred to as the visceral body ego, where "tongue-in-mouth" sensations predominate.

Kafka (1971) has discussed how the body is experienced at a stage just after the tongue-in-mouth organization. At this point the body is felt to be a fragile container which has openings that allow substance to pass in and out. The container has no features and no differentiation in itself, and similarly the contents are unknown and undifferentiated, with thoughts, feelings and physical contents such as organs and food all experienced similarly. Attached to this primitive body concept are a number of fantasies, including the idea that the container could easily be ruptured, that dangerous material might intrude from without, or that the unknown material within is dangerous and could leak or spill out, damaging others. Kafka gives a number of clinical examples illustrating how this type of primitive body concept is manifested at points when unresolved separation issues are activated in the patient. Experiencing the body in this way is seen as an attempt to recontact the mother at a very primitive level, while still maintaining some degree of separateness. Kafka argues that such symptomatology stems from archaic ego states which predate the splitting mechanism. This concept of the body as a fragile container has also been discussed by Rosenfeld (1984).

We feel that these conceptualizations of early perception and body ego experience have relevance to some aspects of borderline symptomatology. In particular, these concepts detail aspects of symbiotic and presymbiotic relatedness to which borderlines frequently regress during transient psychotic episodes. Kernberg (1975) has described the breakdown in ego structures that occurs in such patients under the impact of primitive aggressive impulses and wishes to fuse or merge with the object. We feel that formulations of the infant's earliest modes of perception and experience of the body, particularly tongue-in-mouth sensations that are diffused across the surface of the skin and the experience of the body as a fragile container of fluid which is easily ruptured, can elucidate the experience of the borderline patient at such moments of regression. We will review clinical material from two patients who illustrate a number of these points, and then offer further speculations regarding the role of such symptoms in the borderline picture.

Case Examples

A young borderline woman sought treatment as a result of school failure, increased disorganization, isolation and severe impulsivity involving recurring episodes of wrist cutting and bulimia. Her difficulties began after the end of an incestuous relationship with a relative which had lasted through her latency years.

Early in treatment this patient described how no one could really understand her inner experience. She felt that it could never be expressed in words; words would never do it justice. What she experienced was more fused and total; there were no boundaries inside her; it was like some kinds of music, or a movement of colors and lines. She did not feel these things all the time, but occasionally they built up to an intensity that was unbearable. At those moments she began to feel depersonalized, as if her body and the objects around her were not real, and she was not sure what was internal and what was external. Eventually the tension built to the point where the only way she could obtain relief was by binging and vomiting, or cutting herself. While binging she was conscious only of the physical sensation of food in her mouth and stomach, which gradually became intolerable. She had fantasies that the food would become alive and control her. When she vomited she regained a sense of the reality of her own body and the world around her.

Episodes of wrist cutting also began with experiences of depersonalization, but as the tension built up her skin became acutely sensitive, so much so that it was painful to feel the warm sun on her exposed arm. Eventually this tension could be relieved only by slashing. When she saw the blood flow she felt more real, and her perception of objects around her became clearer. Also she felt a great sense of relief, and described cutting as one of the only ways she could comfort and soothe herself. After cutting she usually went to sleep, and she described the experience as "orgasmic." She connected cutting to a longing to be held by her mother, and said the prohibition to cut was "like losing your mother."

This patient had a number of fantasies which illustrate Kafka's hypothesis that in such early ego states, the body may be experienced as a fragile container. Throughout her analysis she had the phobic fear that something would leak out of her during sessions, which led her to repeatedly change chairs and to check the seat as she got up to leave. She also was afraid to cry, because this would mean she was leaking. She said her insides were a mass of filthy, evil, horrible material, and that she was "poisoned by blood that has nowhere to go and never drains or spills." Cutting was one way of letting the slime drain out. She was afraid that if she got close to her analyst, the filth would begin to leak out. As she discussed whether or not to use the couch during her sessions, she said that if she lay down on the couch she would regurgitate her entire past. At one moment when she did allow herself close contact with the analyst, she had the fantasy of leaking into him, then feared this would poison him, because he would be unable to digest her poison and would vomit.

This patient produced repeated references to skin and skin sensations. Early in her sessions she reported a repetitive dream of being skinned alive, and when her conflicts around attachment were mobilized in a particularly strong manner, the feelings from this dream returned during waking hours and were so real that she felt as if it were actually happening. Fantasies about either annihilating or merging with the object were also most frequently expressed in terms of the skin metaphor. In moments of brutal self-attack she wrote that she wanted to be mutilated, maimed, tortured, ripped open, torn, slashed, to have her skin lacerated and burned from her. Later when these aggressive impulses began to be worked through, she moved toward experimentation with her body and skin sensations. A healthier form of autoerotism emerged, and on one occasion she told of her experience in the shower. Normally she took only ice cold showers and enjoyed the feeling of having her skin "etched" by the cold water. On this particular day she decided to take a warm shower to see what it would feel like. At first it was luxurious and sensual, as if she were being enveloped by the warm water, but suddenly she became intensely anxious at the thought that the skin boundary between herself and the water had disappeared, and she did not know where she stopped and the water began.

At the end of her first year of analysis she shared the following fantasy, which she described as a favorite daydream, a story in which she could become involved again and again and completely lose herself. This daydream represents one version of this patient's central masturbation fantasy (Laufer, 1976). In this fantasy the patient was attacked by someone who was grotesque and mutilated. He tied her up and began to cut and lacerate her skin, leaving her "a bloody pulp." Eventually she got away from him and met another man who had the same name as her older brother. He cradled her in his arms, and took off his shirt to cover her and soothe her wounds. After this either one or both of them attacked the mutant and destroyed it.

In this clinical material one sees numerous examples of sensations and experiences which could be related to early ego states from the symbiotic and presymbiotic periods. The description of her inner experience as unable to be expressed in words, like music and color, is reminiscent of Spitz' discussion of preverbal coenesthetic experience. Her sense of unreality and the blurring of internal-external boundaries, as well as her acute consciousness of mouth, stomach and skin sensations, bear resemblance to the Isakower phenomenon. Cutting clearly had an autoerotic quality related to early soothing by the mother. Primitive fantasies about the body as a fragile container of dangerous substance were abundant. In her central masturbation fantasy this patient portrayed her inner experience of the good and the bad object. She had to protect herself against a sadistic object that wished to deprive her of skin, in this way making it impossible for her to be a separate and autonomous person. The good object covered and soothed her wounds, providing her with a second skin.

A young man sought out treatment at the suggestion of his girlfriend, to learn to control his violent temper. He explained in the first hour that sometimes she would say or do something that made him hate her intensely. At those moments, her face changed in front of his eyes, it became ugly and he wanted to tear the skin off. In such rages he felt that he could murder her.

He was an only child and described a very troubled early history. His mother was overprotective, doing everything for him even to the present day, but at the same time she was fanatically obsessive and critical. She flew into a rage if he walked across the newly vacuumed carpet because his footprints spoiled the smooth appearance of the rug. She was intrusive and repeatedly conveyed how miserable he made her life. His father was described as coarse, prone to abuse his mother verbally and physically, and quick to ridicule any display of emotion on the patient's part. During childhood the patient had been a loner and had enjoyed torturing and killing small animals. Even as an adult, at moments of intense rage he would kill frogs by kicking them across the street. He had always been afraid of the dark and could not stand being alone in the house. In adolescence he had become heavily involved in alcohol and drugs, which he used to calm himself. His friends had been his drinking and drug pals, and he felt he had never had any real relationships.

Eventually this man found his girlfriend and gravitated to her in an intense way. He stopped acting out through alcohol and sexual promiscuity and tried to better himself in order to make their relationship more secure. He got a new and better-paying factory job and began to save money. And he entered therapy in order to control his rage. Many times he said that all of the changes he made were for her, that she was his world and she had given him a life worth living. In her family, with whom he became involved, he found the nurturant environment which he had never experienced.

After a year and a half of weekly therapy, this man's girlfriend suddenly and unexpectedly left him. He became frantic, was obsessed with her, and feared he was going crazy. He needed to see her, would watch her house with binoculars, and wait along her route to work to have a chance of waving at her. He could not do his own work and felt that all of his abilities, all the progress he had made, really belonged to her and had been taken away when she left. As his distress mounted, he began to have fantasies of killing himself by cutting his wrists. He also reported that he could no longer eat. He imagined blowing out his brains in such a way that they would splatter into her face.

One evening at the height of this crisis, he came to his therapy session and said he was so depressed he was afraid he was losing his mind. Recently he was experiencing things that had never happened to him and scared him. That day in work he could not get his girlfriend off his mind. Everything anyone did or said reminded him of her. The tension built up so much that finally he couldn't stand the physical sensations. He was aware of his skin and an intense feeling in his stomach, not pain but more like an empty feeling or nausea. His senses began to blur; what people were saying no longer made sense. He could hear them, but the speech was unintelligible. Needing to get away, he went into a small room, turned out the lights, and curled up in the dark. He began banging his head rhythmically against the wall, in an attempt to obtain relief. He was acutely aware of his body, feeling as if there was something horrible and black inside of him, which needed to get out. He began to claw and scratch at his skin, wanting to break through so that this material could come out. Even when he hit himself to the point of causing bruises, he felt no sensation, could not feel his skin. Eventually he lay down, put his head in the crook of his arm, and put himself into a trance while listening to the rhythmic noise of the machine in the next room. When he came out of this trance he was calm, felt his body was once again real and familiar, and was able to go back to work.

This vignette, describing the inner experience of one man trying to cope with profound object loss, contains a number of elements which appear to be echoes of earlier ego states. In his fantasies about his girlfriend's face, wanting to tear the skin off or cover it with his own splattered brains, one can see primitive aggression directed at what Spitz has referred to as the first visual percept, the mother's face. The sensations he described during his moments of distress, including acute awareness of the skin and stomach, blurred senses, and an inability to comprehend language, are reminiscent of that type of preverbal experience described by Isakower. The man also experienced his body as a container of dangerous material which needed to be ruptured, as discussed by Kafka. In his attempts to soothe himself, he first resorted to an autistic mechanism, head-banging. Later, by recreating the physical sensation of his head resting in the crook of an arm and focusing on a rhythmic sound, he was more successful at creating a transitional experience which eventually left him feeling soothed and more alive.

Discussion

This case material illustrates the relevance of psychoanalytic theorizing about early infant development to the transient psychotic episodes experienced by borderlines. At moments of intense regression, when ego structures break down under the impact of primitive aggressive and fusional impulses, the patient's experience appears to be an echo of that which is hypothesized for the infant first becoming aware of the object. Prominent elements in the ego states which get recreated at those moments include oral sensations and the diffusion of these across the skin, and a concept of the body as a fragile container.

We strongly agree with Kafka's assertion that these experiences represent attempts to recontact the mother at a primitive level, while at the same time maintaining some sense of separateness. In recreating such ego states, there is a reliving of early experiences of contact. At the same time, these experiences have an autoerotic aspect. They are attempts at self-soothing, and substitute for an object relationship. This provides a good illustration of Anna Freud's (1963) point that autoerotic gratification, which from the beginning is under the child's control, provides a first step away from the maternal object.

This understanding of borderline regression as at least one implication for the management of such regressive acting out in psychotherapy. While severe destructiveness obviously needs to be controlled, it should be kept in mind that these patients may need to act in order to work through early conflict. Just as the child originally learns to think only through the development of sensory-motor and action schemes, these patients may be able to gain access to such preverbal experience only through the medium of action. A tempered approach on the part of the analyst, consisting of attempts to limit extreme destructiveness while at the same time placing the greatest emphasis on exploration of inner meaning, may eventually help the patient raise such experience to the level of meaningful verbal discourse.

Fusional Relations in the Borderline and Normative Realm: Desperate Love

Michael B. Sperling, Ph.D.
(1986)

The experience of a fusional quality to a love relation can, in extreme, be considered pathologic, as is frequently the case with borderline personality organization, yet it can also be a normative aspect of healthy love relations. This symposium is focusing on the manifestations of underlying fusional and aggressive dynamics in relationships. This paper is concerned with the conditions under which fusion becomes directly enacted relationally, and both the process and outcomes of such enactment.

Discriminating healthy from pathologic fusion in love relations is a formidable task. As almost everyone knows from personal experience, a feeling of fusion can offer enormous gratifications— sexual and emotional. Yet direct fusional experiences are infrequent in most cases, occurring in adult life largely in the context of sexual union and psychotic states. The positive feelings associated with fusion of self and object world (what Freud, 1930, referred to as the oceanic feeling) can occur more indirectly in such diverse solitary and dyadic activities as religion, drug-induced states, creative activity, and special moments of sharing in friendships and intimate relations. Paradoxically, the pursuit of fusion, or the enactment of fusional desires, can also engender terrible loneliness at the reification of one's inevitable separateness from others, or produce

Presented at the annual convention of the American Psychological Association, August 22–26, 1986, Washington, DC.

sustained fusional feelings which weaken one's boundaries and self-identity.

In the service of trying to distinguish the dynamics of healthy versus pathologic fusion in love relations, I would suggest that three mediating developmental factors are crucial: 1) the quality of the early maternal symbiotic relationship; 2) the resolution, particularly in response to the frustrations and gratifications of rapprochement, of the regressive pull for reinstatement of fusion in the face of separation; and 3) the path chosen, or necessitated, for oedipal and adolescent enactment of fusional desires. Relevant contributions of each of these broad factors will be discussed, followed by case material and discussion of a fusional attachment style referred to as desperate love.

Several psychoanalytic theorists (e.g., Giovacchini, 1976; Jacobson, 1964; Kernberg, 1975, 1976, 1980) have discussed the quality of the early maternal symbiotic relationship, and the importance of this dynamic to later love relations. Mahler (1952) introduced the notion of symbiosis between mother and infant, and later expanded on this: "The essential feature of symbiosis is hallucinatory or delusional, somatopsychic, omnipotent fusion with the representation of the mother and, in particular, delusion of a common boundary of the two actually and physically separate individuals" (Mahler, 1967, p. 742). Giovacchini (1976) emphasizes the normative and ascendant interconnections between symbiosis and intimacy, as well as creativity, intuitiveness and empathy. He believes that in order to achieve a positive interconnection, the infant must first have experienced a "smoothly balanced" symbiotic relationship. In such cases, "the infant fundamentally has the security that his needs will be met without having to recognize his dependency upon an external object for survival" (p. 420). This smoothly balanced relationship prevents the schizoidal need to turn inward for comfort and stability, or, similarly, the development of a sense of narcissistic omnipotence. Unlike the schizoid or severe narcissistic states, wherein very early, basic deficiencies in the quality of symbiotic attachment may be paramount, when fusional dynamics are later able to be enacted in intimate relations, the more likely it is that the early maternal relationship has allowed for introjection of a good symbiotic object. The next developmental task, however, comes in the face of separation and the rapprochement negotiation of the "optimal distance" (Mahler et al., 1975) from love objects. This also constitutes what I believe is the second mediating factor in differentiating healthy from pathologic fusion.

The ability to hold onto the internalized good symbiotic object image becomes increasingly taxed in the face of separation, at the same time as libido is being increasingly cathected onto a wider array of external objects. Altman (1977) comments that during this time "the love affair with someone and something other than oneself has begun. The libidinal investment in others, however, is a very precarious thing, ready, with any frustration, to turn about face to be reinvested in the self. Resolution of narcissism is never complete" (p. 40). Altman may be overestimating the immediate reactivity of the rapprochement child to frustrations and the resultant withdrawal of external cathexes, but I believe he does point to a critical process: When the separating child is not met with "good enough" mothering (Winnicott, 1960), a regressive pull for reinstatement of the earlier preambivalent symbiotic relation can gain prominence. To some extent this can be seen as a normal response to the frustrations of separation; to the degree that the child is inappropriately frustrated or overly gratified in his or her regressive attitude, fusional desires may strengthen.

Jacobson (1964) has discussed at length these early experiences of frustration and separation as awakening fantasies of incorporation of the gratifying object and reestablishment of the "lost unit," adding that such wishful fantasies of merging are the foundation for all later identifications and object relations. She offers the concept of refusion of self and object images to characterize this primitive type of identification which persists throughout one's lifetime, commenting: "Our subtle, empathic understanding of others, especially those we love, depends on such temporary—either short-lived or more lasting—identifications. However, such temporary fusions induced in the service of the ego do not normally weaken the boundaries between images of self and objects, whereas in the early infantile state, such firm boundaries have not yet been established" (pp. 40–41). From this description it is apparent that temporary refusions of self and object images can facilitate healthy connectedness with others. However, excessive frustration reinforces the normal disposition to regressive refusion, resulting in unneutralized fusional desires and potentially contributing to a borderline personality organization characterized by excessive aggression, attempts to retain or regain absolute gratification, object splitting and diffuse ego boundaries (Kernberg, 1975).

The third suggested factor that differentiates healthy versus pathologic fusion concerns the paths open to the child, and then adolescent, for enactment of relational imperatives. Overdetermined fusional desires resulting from preoedipal development may lead the oedipal child to experience intense incestuous guilt and masochistic tendencies in response to the first primitive sexual feelings toward the symbiotic mother. The task, then, for such a child in adolescence is twofold: to initiate adult-like intimate sexual relations without reawakening this incestuous guilt (Bergmann, 1980), while at the same time to sublimate considerable desires for fusional dependence. One possible avenue of negotiation is through idealization of the love object, who can be understood in part as a composite projection of the ego ideal and of the gratifying qualities of the symbiotic mother. In this regard, Chasseguet-Smirgel (1976) comments: "Love is probably one of the principal postoedipal manifestations of the ego's desire to be united with its ideal, a union which does not necessarily occur in a nonregressive way . . . in order to be again united with the ego it (the ego ideal) can choose either the shortest route, the most regressive one, or the evolutionary route which includes the integration of each stage of development" (pp. 355–356).

A fusional quality to intimacy is common in the relational testing grounds of adolescence. Fusion, as well as many other dynamics, is able to be experienced and explored during this period without serious long-term consequences. However, of interest to this discussion is the case where strong fusional desires persist and are regularly enacted in late adolescence and adulthood—when the shortest, more regressive route toward reunion of ego and ego ideal, or self and symbiotic object, is chosen.

I have previously referred to this style of adult love relations as *desperate love,* choosing this term because it highlights the urgency with which reciprocation is desired (Sperling, 1985). I have specifically not used the label *fusional love* in order to reinforce the distinction between the perpetuation of fusional desires in love relations and the actual attainment of fusion, which is developmentally well past. Arlow (1980) captures this distinction well in saying, "When poets describe the ecstasy of love or orgasm by saying that they feel completely united and indissolubly fused with the beloved, there is nonetheless some concomitant awareness of the existence of the other person as an independent object" (p. 119). When a person experiences desperate love there are prevailing themes such as much idealization and diminished interpersonal reality testing in order to construe the relation and the love object as wholly gratifying, a seemingly insatiable need for reciprocal affection, anxiety at separations, a sense of urgency, and diffuse ego boundaries.

The broad range of behaviors and dynamics characterized as desperate love bridge several diagnostic categories, as well as normative functioning. In this sense desperate love can be understood as falling within the third and fourth, or borderline and neurotic, positions on Kernberg's (1976) continuum regarding the capacity for falling in love and remaining in love, with pathological relations clustered in the third and more normative but maladaptive (to integrated adult functioning) relations clustered in the fourth. Kernberg suggests that the primitive idealization of the love object and clinging infantile dependency characteristic of the third position presuppose a lack of libidinal object constancy. They are typical of the chaotic love relations of individuals with borderline pathology who employ much splitting, projection and projective identification in dyadic contexts. This unintegrated, preambivalent attitude can regard the loved person as savior, source of all that is good in the object world. The idealization which facilitates such a response is primitive and fluid; hence, when reality-mediated interpersonal frustration impinges upon the relationship, it is likely to become stressed, requiring stronger defensive measures or an ending. The once-loved object (or idealized internal representation of the object) may be cast aside, and the same pattern repeated—quite frequently in the case of borderline love relations. The type of conflictual desperate love relation which bridges into the fourth position on Kernberg's continuum is marked by relative temporal stability, as there is some capacity for stable, internalized object constancy. Yet derivatives of earlier unresolved fusional dynamics with parents still persist and may dominate one's adult love relations, inhibiting fuller movement toward triadic, oedipally based "neurotic" relational conflicts.

Handley (1989) and Hull and Lane (1989) offer illustrations of fusional dynamics as expressed through aggressive and self-destructive acting out in patients with severe narcissistic and borderline character pathology. I will now present a case example of a dependent and masochistic patient with a less severe borderline personality organization who has frequently experienced desperate love, in order to further discuss the maladaptive and adaptive possibilities for enactment of fusional desires in intimate relations.

Case Example

The patient is a 35-year-old, single, white male I will refer to as Daniel. He was a fairly tall, bearded, sturdy-looking man at first glance, but in sessions his affect and body conveyed a sense of childlike helplessness and defeat, with occasional bursts of agitated strength, as if trying to prove that he was not burdened by his intrapsychic process. Daniel presented for evaluation at the outpatient clinic of a New York City hospital with complaints of depression, lethargy, poor sleep and appetite, poor concentration and suicidal ideation, claiming "I have been conflicted over whether I want to live or die. . . It seems I don't want to take care of myself." Over the past 18 years he had been in psychotherapy intermittently, with one brief hospitalization. He had worked at several jobs, mostly as a taxi driver or chauffeur, and was currently trying to complete a bachelor's degree in music performance. His intimate relational experiences were similarly inconsistent, with a pattern of involvement in either dependent, needy relationships, or distant, quasi-sadistic ones. Additionally, there was a history of symptoms and character traits which supported the diagnosis of a borderline personality organization, including: impulsivity, as marked by occasional displays of intense anger and excessive alcohol use; grandiosity; idealization, manipulation and devaluation in relationships; chronic, diffuse anxiety; poor identity integration; primitive defenses of splitting, projective identification and denial; and feelings of emptiness and meaninglessness.

His presenting difficulties began nine months earlier, when his girlfriend, Jean, ended a two-year relationship between them. The following day, during a session with his former therapist, he suffered a mild heart attack. He then believed erroneously that Jean would take him back. As Daniel expressed it, "The woman I thought would be there forever really abandoned me." After recovering from the acute effects of his medical condition, he became increasingly depressed and obsessed with Jean, phoning her numerous times each day, following her to work and fantasizing about killing her. Eventually she initiated a restraining order against him to prevent contact. During these months, he was hospitalized twice, briefly, for depression and suicidal ideation and treated with antidepressant medication. After the second hospitalization he was referred to day treatment, where he remained for two months before beginning outpatient psychotherapy.

The process of the 10-month psychotherapy falls generally into four phases: 1) an initial period characterized by Daniel's coexisting wishes to dominate and control relations with myself and others, yet also to be dominated and cared for, to find a new "mommy"; 2) a period of reunion fantasies during which, on several occasions, he became excited and grandiose prior to an anticipated social contact with Jean, followed by renewed suicidal ideation after the contact; 3) a period dominated by increased expression of transferential and external feelings of helpless dependency and sadistic rage, with a concurrent sense of "growing up," as well as initiation of a new intimate relationship; and 4) a final termination period during which he demonstrated increased ambivalence of feelings and improved reality testing in his intimate relationship and in the therapeutic relationship.

While the course of treatment was relatively brief, and Daniel's character pathology was by no means fully resolved, the flow of the process loosely parallels the developmental sequence of fusional dynamics, as discussed earlier in this paper. Specifically, the most salient dynamics in the first of the four phases outlined above correspond to a symbiotic, narcissistic position in early development, the second phase to a renewal of regressive refusion fantasies in the face of differentiation, the third to a rapprochement position of searching for the optimal distance, and the fourth phase to consolidation of more adaptive sublimatory channels for enactment of fusional desires. The necessary brevity of this presentation precludes a fuller elaboration of these sequential correspondences, but I would like to illustrate some of these dynamics as manifested in the transference.

For a person like Daniel, who repeatedly enacts fusional desires in desperate love relations, the central transferential theme of psychotherapy revolves around the question of how the patient can give up the illusory pursuit of refusion and, with some sense of safety and security, move toward a less idealized and controlling relational position. It can be said that this position is relevant to any patient with character difficulties (Giovacchini, 1976); however, I believe it to be a strikingly apparent transference theme in those who experience desperate love. For example, in one session during the second phase of reunion fantasies, Daniel arrived late and described his state as "devastated" after having recently seen Jean at a party. He was very angry and wanted to phone her to say that she "manipulated him into being babied," that "I want to be a man for you, to take care of you," and that "I can live without you." This tripartite message carries with it the contrasting communications that I want to care for you from a position of strength, that I don't need to be with you, presumably also a position of strength, and the blameful accusation that you caused me to act like a baby and lose my strength. For a few subsequent sessions he continued to focus on his anger at Jean, trying to defend against his fusional desires by reaffirming his strength and ability to care for himself. Gradually, then, as gratification was not forthcoming from Jean, he brought these feelings into the therapeutic relationship, saying that he wanted "answers" from me. He described me as withholding, and grew increasingly angry and "hateful" toward me, frequently arriving late for sessions. With interpretation of his hateful feelings and acting out as related to Jean's withholding, which, given the relationship's history, was an inevitable and predictable response to his demands for dependency, Daniel's anger faded and was replaced by awareness of his insatiability: "I can't take care of that part of me that feels lonely, neglected, needs constant attention, needs to be loved every minute otherwise he's gonna to die." He then offered a genetic explanation, claiming that his mother never let him grow up, but rather taught him how to be helpless, and that his father never intervened to teach him how to be older and stronger.

In the next session I asked Daniel what he would like most from me. He again gave me a tripartite message, saying that he wanted to be "left alone," wanted "caring," and was angry at me. Although contradictory, this message directly conveys the struggle of the rapprochement child to achieve an optimal distance, a struggle which is always reenacted in love relations and, in Daniel's case, also became the dominant dynamic in the therapeutic relation. He wants to be simultaneously fusionally attached and allowed to feel autonomous; yet, in the face of the inevitable frustration of these two desires in adulthood, he grows rageful. Then, in an attempt to compensate for this anger toward his love objects, he idealizes them and tries to enact the dependent side of the split by regressively refusing, as his early maternal relation has rendered the illusion that this is the safest path.

Although the reification of fusional desires can become problematic, the ability to enact them in the transference, as in external relationships, can also be seen as a good prognostic sign in psychotherapy, as the relational pathology is achieving its most direct manifestation. The cases presented by Handley and Hull and Lane illustrate indirect manifestations of fusional desires, which become more difficult to ameliorate. In Daniel's case, the relational pathology was directly enacted in the therapeutic relationship and, to some extent, worked through during the course of treatment. Moreover, as Kernberg (1980) has suggested, being able to reexperience through passion some of the bliss associated with fusion is not only gratifying and desirable, but is a healthy sign of an integrated love relation.

Summary

When, in adult life, the regressive pull toward refusion of self and object images takes on a quality of desperation for psychic survival, it becomes unhealthy in the sense of inhibiting growthfulness—it tends to lock a love relation into a fixed, recapitulative pattern. However, when temporary fusional identifications exist on a selective basis, they can become, as Jacobson (1984) has suggested, a normative and growthful dynamic in love relations. In this regard, the therapeutic relationship with Daniel became less symbiotic near the end of treatment, as he seemed to depend less on me to sustain a sense of wholeness—what Searles (1979) refers to as the ego defense of pathologic symbiosis. At the same time, the passion and intensity of his new intimate relationship deepened, albeit fraught with ambivalence, and the quality of our relation felt less coercive. He spoke of being "on the edge of becoming competent" as a musician, and then extended this to therapy, feeling as if he were about to be launched. The move in the dominant transference from symbiosis to identification was a significant development, which indicated his readiness to begin relinquishing persistent fantasies of regressive refusion, and instead to internalize the therapist as a differentiated object. This process was encapsulated in a benign acting out of his positive, yet differentiated, identification with me. He came to one of our last sessions having shaved off his beard, an action which I too had taken earlier during the treatment. He commented that every year he shaved the beard off, but each time grew it back the next day. He then added that this time was different, it had been six days and "I like my face."

Forms of Fusion

Charles R. Swenson, M.D.
(1986)

This symposium (see Handley, 1989; Hull & Lane, 1989; Sperling, 1989) has addressed a wide variety of loosely related issues: archaic ego states, boundary disruptions, primitive body imagery, and intimacy, to name but a few. At first the natural relationships and intersecting concerns may not appear so obvious. As I hope to draw out in this discussion, there is one central organizing construct to which the others refer. It is the one Sperling began with: *fusion,* or as he said, "the ubiquitous desire for symbiotic fusion (whether internal or acted out)." The concerns of the symposium are: What is fusion in intrapsychic and interpersonal life? Where does it come from? What are its various manifestations? What is healthy fusion? What is pathological fusion? And what does fusion have to do with love? Or with hate? It is my intention here to define the essential features of fusion, then to propose a typology of different manifestations of fusion as mediated through different levels of personality organization.

Definition

Jacobson (1964) has provided the central idea by referring to the "lost unit" of symbiosis "which never ceases to play a part in our emotional life" (p. 39). She claims that all object relations are built on the earliest wishful fantasies of merging on and being one with the mother. Searles (1979), referring to the same idea, claims that

---

Presented at the annual convention of the American Psychological Association, August 22–26, 1986, Washington, DC.

symbiosis is ever-present at a subterranean level of human relations. So, fusion refers to a relationship at the symbiotic phase of infantile development, to a longed for "lost unit," to a maternal-child relationship and its precipitates in psychic structure. Once the symbiotic phase is passed, the "lost unit" is thought to be represented in a deep layer of internalized object relations. Fusion refers to the joined relationship between the self and the object representations in the internal object world. There is a tendency toward reestablishing fusion, especially in the face of stress. But notice: Fusion is a concept referring to intrapsychic structuring, not relational behavior. Attachment, on the other hand, refers to seeking proximity and involvement relationally, in the real world. This gives "fusional attachment," frequently referred to in the symposium, an inherent tension. I understand it to mean the superimposition of a fused internal self-object representation upon a real relationship, coercing the latter to approximate the fusion of the former.

Having briefly discussed fusion, let me move on to a proposed typology of fusional manifestations, in order to provide a scheme for the integration of the various ideas brought out in the symposium. After proposing this typology, I will spend the rest of my time remarking on the individual presentations, with the scheme and definition of fusion in the background.

Typology

Fusion, then, is a concept referring to an internal object situation. It does not refer to subjective experience, to body imagery, or to actual interpersonal relations, but is intimately related to them all. In fact, in thinking about the interrelationships, it might help to refer to a grid, or chart (see Figure 1). Down the left side are the following categories: nature of self-object fusion, corresponding subjective experiences, corresponding body imagery, and implications for love relationships. Along the top are three categories: psychotic, borderline, neurotic, referring to three levels of personality organization (Kernberg, 1975). In other words, I am proposing that, depending upon the nature of the mediating personality organization, self-object fusion will have certain qualities, as will corresponding body imagery, subjective experiences, and attachment relationships.

	Psychotic Organization	Borderline Organization	Neurotic Organization
Nature of Self-Object Fusion	Merger of self and object images. Dissolution of boundaries. self ⟨⟩ object	Merger of part-self with part-object images. (+) or (−). Boundaries between self and object intact. self (+) (+) object self (−) (−) object	Closeness between integrated self-images and integrated object-images. self (+)(−) (+)(−) object
Corresponding Subjective Experiences	Global, extreme, fluctuating states. Confusion. Ecstasy, annihilation.	Heightened gratification when (+) fusion active. Heightened fear, rage, persecution when (−) fusion active.	Intimacy, empathy and anxiety about closeness.
Corresponding Body Imagery	Fragmented body images. Images of leaky, porous body surfaces.	Body boundaries intact. Themes of seduction, vulnerability, and control permeate imagery of body and body parts.	Intact body imagery with parts clearly related to whole body.
Features of Attachment Relationships	Minimal "real relatedness," contaminated and disrupted by delusional features.	Coercion. Persecution. Idealization.	Relative stability, wholeness, integration.

Figure 1. Forms of Fusion

Beginning with the psychotic: The self and object images, in fusion, lack a differentiating boundary. They merge into one another, and contents are mixed. The corresponding subjective experience is one of chaos, confusion, and flux. Depending on whether, at the moment, it is a libidinally or aggressively invested fusion, it leads to states of ecstasy or of annihilation. Corresponding body imagery has some of the hallmarks discussed by Hull and Lane regarding transient psychotic experiences: porous boundaries, leakage of contents, fragmented autoerotic and autosadistic sensational experiences, dismemberment, and so on. Implications for love relations follow: There is a near inability to have them with an-*other* person, since the other person and the self are seen as mixed with each other in ecstatic unions, or completely persecuted and contaminated by each other, or totally separate from each other. The internal situation of merger in a psychotic state is more commonly accompanied by an entire lack of relatedness to real objects: It precipitates a withdrawal of such investments, and a heightened internal investment, leading to a delusional or autistic situation.

Let's turn to fusion in the borderline. The unreconciled existence of different and opposing self-representations and different and opposing object-representations leads to an internal world of possible fusions between various different part-selfs and part-objects. A demanding, deprived self-representation can be fused with a persecutory part-object representation. A gratified part-self representation can be fused, in primitive idealization, with a totally nurturant and protective part-object representation. These can flip back and forth. Differing from the psychotic fusion, there is a boundary that, for most of the time, remains intact between self and object. In states of fusion in the borderline organization, parts are exchanged between self and object, and designations of what is the self and what is the object switch around. So, the fusion is not the boundariless *delusional* situation of the psychotic; it is an *illusory* state of fusion, with a coexisting awareness of a boundary except at those points, discussed by Hull and Lane, when boundaries temporarily dissolve. Corresponding subjective experiences include some confusion about who is who, and what belongs to whom, but more particular to the borderline organization is the experience of controlling or being controlled, idealizing or being idealized—that is, the imposition of an internal illusion of fusion, in a positive or negative state, upon the real relationship. Sperling's "desperate love," in this context, is the attempt, with insistence, to keep the illusion corresponding to positive fusion imposed upon the actually frustrating relationship, to keep from flipping to the emergence of a negative form of fusion.

Body imagery corresponding to borderline organization is vividly described by Handley's patient: the control, by the self or the object, over the body parts of the other one, usually by violent means such as taking possession, hitting, raping. The body boundaries, as described, remain overall intact, but parts are in fantasy dismemberable and interchangeable. The implications for attachment relations have been referred to: One sees primitive idealizations on the positive side, persecution and control on the negative side. And I would suggest that "desperate love" is a relationship on the cusp between idealization and persecution, with a failing attempt to keep the positive from shifting to negative in the face of frustration or separation.

Let's turn to the neurotic situation. Here fusion between self and object representations is profoundly different: Not only is there an established and maintained self-object boundary, but also the various part-selfs and part-objects have been reconciled into an integrated self and an integrated object. Whole object relations prevail. The boundary and the integrated structure remain intact, and fusion amounts to an adjacency and fantasied exchanges of contents on temporary bases and without such disruptive consequences. The corresponding feeling states are toned down by comparison to the annihilations, persecutions, ecstasies, and idealizations of the other organizations. There are positive feelings of intimacy, union, empathy, sharing, or, on the negative side, anxieties about closeness. Images of bodies remain on the whole intact, with temporary fantasied exchanges of body parts. Not too different from the polymorphously perverse body imagery of borderline, here the overall context is one of intactness, integration, whole-bodiness, and the body parts are more likely to be seen as related to a whole body and a whole person. Love relations among neurotics have the quality of more integration, more stability, more wholeness.

To summarize: In an archaic layer, lying deep within *each* person, regardless of level of personality organization, is the lost unit of symbiosis. It can itself have a positive or negative valence, or both. It exerts a kind of binding influence on relations between self and object representations experienced as a desire for positive or negative closeness. Its influence is qualitatively different depending on whether it is mediated through a psychotic, borderline or neurotic organization. And qualitatively different types of body imagery are characteristic of fusion in the three different organizations.

Remarks on Individual Presentations

At this point, I will review and comment on the individual presentations, with the definition and a typology of fusion in the background. Proceeding as I have been, from psychotic to borderline to neurotic, I will begin with the paper of Hull and Lane, who address the forms and contents of preverbal experience, particularly of the presymbiotic and symbiotic infant. It is their impression that the borderline patient undergoing a transient psychotic episode is reexperiencing and reenacting aspects of those phases. More specifically, they understand depersonalization, derealization, blurring of inner and outer, and withdrawal of investment from the outer world to be akin to forms of symbiotic experience. They understand the heightened awareness of tongue, mouth, skin and stomach to parallel the heightened investment of those body parts during the actual symbiotic phase. And they understand the vomiting, cutting and fantasies of skin mutilation to represent the attempted resolution of conflicts about merging with, versus differentiating from, the maternal object of symbiosis. That is, the psychotically regressed borderline patient is attempting to contact the maternal symbiotic object through the experience and enactment of these primitive, mostly bodily-experiential modes. In this interpretation, the vomiting, cutting, torturous and voluptuous skin experiences, and so on, are fragmentery outer signs of an inner attempt to regress to reestablish, in fantasy, the lost symbiotic unit. It is in this idea, the pursuit of fusion at a primitive level and with psychotic mechanisms, that this paper joins the symposium theme. This very creative and interesting way of thinking leads Hull and Lane to emphasize the importance in psychotherapy of exploring the meanings of these regressive phenomena.

The second case presented by Hull and Lane is of special interest here, as this patient, the man whose girlfriend left him suddenly and unexpectedly, functioned for a while on a borderline level and then regressed to a psychotic level. When borderline, he was pursuing the woman with ferocious intensity, trying to reestablish the lost unit intrapsychically and relationally, trying to ward off growing wishes to murder himself as her victim and shove it in her face. This represented desperate love as discussed by Sperling. At a certain point, the man suddenly regressed to a psychotic level, with various manifestations of depersonalization, derealization, boundary blurring, withdrawal, and self-inflicted violence to his body surface. He was, in their formulation, attempting to recontact the lost symbiotic mother and to reestablish the lost unit. This patient shifted from a controlling borderline interpersonal pursuit of the re-union to a frantic more internally directed psychotic pursuit of re-union.

Handley's paper is a dramatic demonstration of the relational and intrapsychic dynamics of a borderline patient desperately seeking a negatively charged fusion between her part-self and part-object worlds. He studied, with behavioral observational data about her external adjustment and psychotherapy-derived data about her internal adjustment, her reactions to a separation from him. He used the long-term inpatient unit in an inspiring way as a developmental laboratory for the microscopic study of a regressive episode. Of special interest, in view of infant studies, was his finding of a dramatically heightened aggressive reaction around reunion by comparison with the periods before and during the separation. We can speculate, in light of today's symposium, that this is due to a heightened conflict about reestablishing the lost unit with the now reavailable lost object.

Let us retrace Handley's findings. Immediately following his announcement of the vacation, he wondered if the patient would leave the inpatient unit when he did. She then announced her wish to rip off a piece of him, his head, to possess. This would help her to avoid her most feared experience: that Dr. Handley, by separating from her, would wipe her out, leaving her utterly alone, deserted. So, disruption in her real relationship with him led to a disruption in the internal self-object relations, and with a background terror of utter aloneness, galvanized her into action and fantasy to establish a negatively charged symbiotic unit, mostly with a persecutory or persecuted object. In dreams, fantasies and actions, she evidenced fears of being controlled, attacked and destroyed, and wishes to destroy and attack, and to force people to pursue her, grab her, and hold her tight. She experienced threats to the body image as manifested in dreams of cutting, bleeding, losing teeth, being raped, and in her fantasy that the nursing staff caused her menstrual period to come one week early. A composite verbal statement of the variety of messages being delivered by this patient might read:

> You have begun to be someone I depend on and need. I can't bear that you are leaving me at all. I can feel that this is going to push me toward a position of aloneness, utter emptiness, a wiped-out condition of near nonexistence. I won't let you do this. I want to rip something off of yours,

to take it inside me and hang on to it. Forget that. I want to
hurt you badly; you have hurt me. In fact, the entire place
here seems to be out to get me, to grab me, to restrict me,
to persecute me, and to punish me. Thank God you will
not let me go.

There is, in other words, a persecutory situation that she is
fighting with, which is better than a situation of total aloneness. She
activates and projects and struggles in the environment with the so-
called bad or persecutory internalized object. These projections
shift around from patients as recipients to staff as recipients, and the
self and object designation alternates rapidly. This leads to a focus
on action rather than thought, on outside rather than inside, on
contact rather than desertion, and on blurring of the real situation
and its accompanying emptiness. It provides an experience of
blurred, exciting and frightening content.

For the purposes of the symposium, and the typology of fusional
phenomena, this patient is, in reaction to object loss, attempting to
reestablish the fused unit: a fusional attachment, negatively endowed, to a hostile and persecutory object world. In this context, I
would underline Handley's quotation from Blum (1986): "The
constant, hostile persecution is the reciprocal of libidinal object
constancy as a desperate effort to preserve an illusory contact with
an object while constantly fearing betrayal and loss."

Sperling's patient presents a glimpse of a positive fused state in
a borderline patient, and its transformation, triggered by rejection,
to a negative fused state. "The woman I thought would be there
forever really abandoned me." This moment represented, for Daniel,
the devastating impingement of reality upon his illusion of symbiotic
oneness. His illusion was that she would be there for him forever, in
isolation from limitations and loss. She would live for him and he
would live for her. Her unbelievable refusal to take him back after his
heart attack finally sank in. She did not play her part, and this
disrupted the internal self-object fusion. He grew depressed, then
obsessed with pursuit, "phoning her numerous times each day,
following her to work and fantasizing about killing her." His fusional
bliss coldly undone, he set out aggressively to reinstate it in a new
form. If he couldn't have her, no one would have her, and she would
have no one, and in that sense he would possess her, even if dead, all
for himself. If he could not have her in fusional bliss, he would have
her in fusional destruction. Such is the underlying power of
desperate love.

I would like to close with Edgar Allan Poe's poem "Annabel Lee," a tribute to the persistence of the idealized symbiotic lost unit. I looked it up the other day when a reference was made to it in the Clint Eastwood movie, "Play Misty for Me," an exquisite and tragic depiction of desperate love.

Annabel Lee

It was many and many a year ago,
    In a kingdom by the sea,
That a maiden there lived whom you may know
    By the name of Annabel Lee;
And this maiden she lived with no other thought
    Than to love and be loved by me.

I was a child and she was a child,
    In this kingdom by the sea,
But we loved with a love that was more than love—
    I and my Annabel Lee—
With a love that the winged seraphs of heaven
    Coveted her and me.

And this was the reason that, long ago,
    In this kingdom by the sea,
A wind blew out of a cloud, chilling
    My beautiful Annabel Lee;
So that her highborn kinsmen came
    And bore her away from me,
To shut her up in a sepulchre
    In this kingdom by the sea.

The angels, not half so happy in heaven,
    Went envying her and me—
Yes!—that was the reason (as all men know,
    In this kingdom by the sea)
That the wind came out of the cloud by night,
    Chilling and killing my Annabel Lee.

But our love it was stronger by far than the love
    Of those who were older than we—
    Of many far wiser than we—
And neither the angels in heaven above,

Nor the demons down under the sea,
Can ever dissever my soul from the soul
    Of the beautiful Annabel Lee.

For the moon never beams, without bringing me dreams
    Of the beautiful Annabel Lee;
And the stars never rise, but I feel the bright eyes
    Of the beautiful Annabel Lee:
And so, all the night-tide, I lie down by the side
Of my darling—my darling—my life and my bride,
    In the sepulchre there by the sea—
    In her tomb by the sounding sea.

Some Comments on the Treatment of Borderline Children

Saralea Chazan, Ph.D.
(1987)

The symptoms of borderline children vary from a multiplicity of neurotic complaints to marked disturbances in interpersonal relationships to a variety of management problems, including temper tantrums, poor judgment, impulsivity, unevenness in development. However, as observed by Marcus (1963), many of these symptoms, especially the neurotic ones, may appear and disappear suddenly, or be interchangeable. Clearly, the manifold symptoms are only the manifest signs of a deeper, more pervasive disturbance. The purpose of this paper is to illustrate the prominence of a core conflict involving issues of living versus nonliving, or death, in the lives of borderline children through the description of an individual case. What made this case significant was the poignancy with which the child patient was able to pinpoint the essence of her problem and the therapeutic course which ensued. Far from being unique, I view this child's struggle as prototypical, illustrative of the kinds of children I am meeting in my work, and particularly eloquent in evoking a dilemma which seems in our times to be an almost ubiquitous source of maladjustment.

General Observations Regarding Treatment

It is the assumption of this writer that borderline conditions refer to difficulties which arise during pregenital stages of development. Although at times pinpointed at the rapprochement phase (Pine, 1974; Mahler et al., 1975), they can also be traced to earlier disturbances in the symbiotic and practicing phases. What distinguishes borderline children from more disturbed psychotic children is not the exact point of genesis, but rather the extent to which a measure of adaptability remains, enabling them to come to terms with their individual reality (P. Kernberg, 1983). Reality testing, degree of tolerance for frustration, control of impulses, level of anxiety are the major processes which are assessed in making a differential diagnosis. These functions belong to the domain of the ego. In terms of object relations, these children experience severe separation anxiety, intense ambivalence, and a marked deficit in sustaining the concept of an object as permanent. So marked is this deficit that it is at times pessimistically referred to as a defect, something that is irreversible and can only be modified through lifelong intervention. Defenses vary with degree of pathology. Denial and splitting are used extensively, resulting in a tuning out to people and events or a jagged, unpredictable pattern of response. As the trauma becomes less intense, more compulsive obsessive mechanisms come to the fore, including doing and undoing, rituals and perfectionism. As the condition modifies to become an internalized neurotic conflict, repression begins to function as a more advanced level of defense.

The essence of childhood borderline conditions is that they have their origins in early infancy. They often have roots in intergenerational dynamics and frequently reflect modifiable maladaptive patterns of accommodation to life circumstances. These patients' life experience is not that of a single trauma. Rather their birth and the meaning of its occurrence are traumatic to the family system, producing continuous trauma and struggle for parents and child. Repetitive reliving of the core conflict, which imposes continuous strain, is seen most clearly in the rapprochement period but can occur earlier. Strengths prevent psychosis from developing, but stress precludes neurotic solution. Difficulties flow not only from the nurturing environment, but from its particular fit with the temperamental characteristics of a given child. Treatment occurs not in discrete stages, but rather within a continuous flow between regression and progression, splitting off of feelings, and integration of self. The most regressed diffuse themes remain, but are gradually less dominant and become interwoven with more differentiated themes, which allow for the development of stability and a sense of permanence.

Although the degree of emotional intensity is high and the resultant behaviors often destructive in nature, the child's dependency upon his/her environment is the key to fostering change. It is precisely because the child is still enmeshed with family that change is possible. Through altering the external family atmosphere which fostered the pathology, and with intensive individual psychotherapy for the child, the pathology need not be a continuous one.

What we are describing, then, is a treatment process which enables the child through monitored regression to return to the point of disintegration and reexperience the feeling of helplessness and repair within a therapeutic relationship. The assumption is that the core conflict around which the pathology becomes organized is the issue of living versus not living, or death. This conflict may have an initial point of origin, discrete memory traces for mother and child, but nonetheless reflects an ongoing series of events which is constantly being rehearsed within the inner life of the child. Thus, the symptoms reported are reenactments of this core conflict and its reverberating trauma of rejection and annihilation. Due to its original intensity and early point of origin the conflict is retained in an action-oriented sphere and not processed cognitively to enable further modification to occur. Primitive defense mechanisms of denial and splitting preserve the rigidity of these patterns.

In order for these traumatic feelings to be modified they need to be reenacted in treatment either directly in the transference relationship or indirectly in play and fantasy. At first the action-oriented impulses are expressed physically through direct assault upon the therapist, concrete surroundings, or inanimate play objects. Gradually the child is able to use play as an intermediate stage to gain entrance to a representational mode of expression. The use of language, through interpretive statements which enhance communication and understanding, enables symbolic process to emerge in the linking of words with feelings.

Despite the availability of enhanced levels of cognition, the essence of the core conflict remains the same. The crucial issue is one of maintaining continuity in personal existence, shared experience, and attunement with others. This core conflict, which forms a repetitive theme in treatment, is itself a reflection of unresolved dynamics between immediate and extended family members. Thus, the child patient has become tied to an ascribed meaning within the life history of the family. Frequently the child is a container for the split-off fragments of parental personality, the embodiment of one or more unconscious characteristics of the parents. Because the child is not simply representative of these traits, but embodies them in a way that they become central to his/her unique identity, there is little opportunity for variability. The child's sense of self emerges with a rigidity predetermined by temperament and the constraints placed by caregivers, narrowing the range of options available in the resolution of conflict. The child's efforts at contact with others occur within these narrow constraints and appear both alien and unfathomable to others. The therapeutic task for the child is to be reborn, to establish for him/herself a new identity separate from the prescribed unconscious role of the past. The child is the active creator, while the therapist provides the holding environment which makes possible the child's exploration.

Why this particular child? Why not a different family member? Is it a question of timing? Is it the outcome of a poor fit between caregiver and child? Is it largely predetermined by temperamental and constitutional characteristics? Is it the product of exposure to a chaotic environment? Is it reactive to a sibling position, or the experience of loss? Certainly all of these factors impinge to a greater or lesser extent in any single case. Etiology being uncertain, the one shared characteristic is the centrality of the issue of developing a sense of permanence about oneself, an identity.

As the child patient becomes less driven by compulsive activity, a fantasy life emerges. Prior to each new development in therapy, it is common that the crescendo of feeling is so intense that it is accompanied by a new wave of attack or vulnerability. These regressions are not true reversals; rather, they mark a peak of emotion which is experienced as painful and heralds the emergence of the child's true sense of self. The helplessness of the child must be met with calm and understanding by the therapist. By functioning as an empathic self-object, the therapist allows the child to experience his/her true feelings, while setting protective limits. If both child and therapist feel helpless in the face of these onslaughts of impulsivity, the child cannot experience him/herself as a separate being. At these points, the therapist often feels increasingly inadequate and overwhelmed by the pain endured by the child. As tension mounts, the therapist may feel, along with frustration and pain, his or her own inability to turn the tide alone. It is at this juncture that the child takes hold, follows a new course and gives some sign of his/her recognition of humanity in the other, and a new sense of self is born.

What is the nature of this original intense trauma, which is repeated over and over again in search of resolution? An assumption is that the early injury occurred during a shared moment of terror. When merging with the significant other, instead of being experienced as alive and active, the caregiver is experienced as dead or absent. For many complicated reasons, the caregiver is unable to relate in an alive, empathic way to the child. The reality evokes in the child a horror, or terror, which the child seeks to defend against through the use of splitting, denial and shifting levels of ego functioning. Use of these defenses further impedes accessibility to the caregiver, acting to prolong and intensify the original trauma. The visual gestalt of the face and auditory patterning of the voice, as well as kinesthetic cues and context, are crucial to the original pathological interaction. Sensitivities to these cues are acute and lasting. The child takes in as part of him/herself aspects of the persecuting, traumatizing, or abandoning caregiver. Although the child may lose contact with the external object through splitting and avoidance, the internal introject can continue to exist without undergoing modification of its primitive intense state. With further development these rigidly preserved feelings can lead to an experience of inner disharmony and fragmentation. The loss of control on the part of the child can be understood as an attempt to restore contact with the caregiver by repeating, or causing to come about, the circumstance of the original injury.

By making contact with the therapist, who responds empathically, the child can then be freed to restore him/herself. Although the child's actions may be experienced by the caregiver as destructive, attacking and persecuting, it is essential that the nonthreatening stance of accessibility, dependability, calmness and realness be maintained. It is the therapist's capacity for empathy, for meeting the child where the child is in his/her trauma and enduring it along with the child, that is therapeutic. The encounter between therapist and child occurs at different levels. The most primitive engagement occurs on the symbiotic level and permits a joining or merger to occur. Loss of boundaries, poor reality testing and projective identification are characteristic of the therapeutic relationship at this level. With increasing space, the therapist becomes an observer as the child reenacts the drama in play and fantasy. Later, the use of verbal interventions permits confrontation, reflection, clarification and finally interpretation of events. It is only at this stage that the conflict can be worked through. To the extent that development is free to progress onward, resolution of the conflict can be claimed to have been achieved. In treatment the core trauma undergoes progressive change in a sequential manner, with much movement back and forth between levels. As mentioned above, it is when ready to move forward that the child often experiences the most profound emotion, anxiety and pain. At this point the child is free to experience feelings with a new degree of accessibility; to that extent the child is also experiencing the event more fully. This new capacity for feeling accounts for what appear to be regressive shifts before the child can take significant steps forward.

Is consolidation of gains possible given the open state of childhood and ongoing development? Consolidation is a relative term and must be applied within the limits of any particular state of development. The issues of permanence are subject to intensified reexamination at puberty and again in late adolescence. Perhaps these children are always particularly vulnerable to the stress of change. However, treatment gains can be considered consolidated within the expectations for a given age group. It is in terms of these proximate goals that effective therapeutic amelioration can be measured and attained.

Case Vignettes

Relevant Family and Developmental History

Anna, the younger of two siblings living in an intact urban middle-class family, was six years old at the time of referral for treatment. Presenting problems included extreme negativism and fears, uncontrolled outbursts of aggression, and interpersonal difficulties with family, teachers and peers. Anna met all six summary criteria for the borderline child described by Vela, Gottlieb and Gottlieb (1983).

Review of family relationships revealed an unsettled environment, partially in response to Anna and her difficulties, partially reflecting marital disharmonies and partially in response to external extended family and financial pressures. Developmental history revealed that, although a second child was planned for sometime in the future, Anna's conception was unanticipated and occurred at a time when Mrs. A was still recovering from the birth of her first child and feeling overwhelmed by the demands of mothering. Despite these pressures, pregnancy and labor were normal. Anna was breastfed for four months, after which time Mrs. A felt she no longer seemed interested and she was weaned. Mrs. A did not recall Anna's temperament or moods as a child. Sometime during the first year she began to reject her mother, turning her head away from an offered kiss or embrace. Anna slept normally as an infant, giving up her nap early. Although an active child, she had problems with her feet, which required casts on both feet when she was a month old, followed by a bar and special shoes. Motor and language milestones were within normal limits. Toilet training was spontaneous at about two years of age. There was no history of bedwetting or daytime accidents. Anna was generally healthy, suffering the usual childhood illnesses. At two and a half years she developed a vaginal infection. For sometime after this, she complained of vaginal burning, requiring several return trips to the doctor. No further infection was found. Anna attended a two-day nursery program for two hours daily beginning at age three, then proceeded on to a five-day program for half-day at age four. Separation problems did not appear until later in kindergarten and began insidiously as dawdling getting ready for school. By first grade departure from the home was a source of ongoing stress and hostility between mother and child, reverberating as disagreements as to child management between husband and wife.

General Impressions at Beginning of Treatment

At her initial visit Anna came willingly into the therapist's office. She was unable to share an understanding of why she was there, but responded spontaneously saying, "I like this house." She separated from her mother without difficulty. Anna was a slender and lithe child of average build for her age. She had long, dark black hair, large black eyes with a somber, intense alertness, and a friendly smile which broke through at odd moments as contact was established. In total, her carriage was graceful and she had the capacity of generating almost a fairytale quality of beauty. She was curious about her surroundings, investigated the playroom, and quickly noticed the therapist's dog. At the first meeting, she enjoyed curling up in a chair in different positions and made a small boat of paper "to carry a little mouse." The therapist responded, "Like a mommy carries a baby," to which Anna responded, "I knew a dog who had babies in its womb and it died. The babies died too." With great sadness she continued, "It happened over two years ago and I still remember.

At the next two meetings, the Children's Apperception Test was administered. Anna enjoyed making up stories, until finishing card six, at which time she refused to continue until the following session. The remaining cards were either rejected at second administration, or responded to briefly. Card six depicts two large bears and a smaller bear curled together in a cave, with their eyes closed. Anna responded: "Once upon a time there were three bears. They were very mean bears. The baby bear goes hunting everyday, and he catches a lot of food. The three bears all went out one day to look for food. An animal came to their cave—a deer. The deer had babies there. Then, it went down the mountain to look for food. Then the bears came back from hunting animals and saw deers lying there. There were six. The bears were surprised, They killed the six babies and ate them. Then, the mother deer came back and peeked in and saw the bears eating her children. She went away very sad."

The theme of babies being killed was to emerge as a dominant one during treatment. Anna's terror of being destroyed made her extremely fearful of closeness with others. If one became a baby again (her regressive wish), then one could be killed. "To be a baby is to die." This intense belief dominated Anna's existence. Despite her exaggerated need for safety, to be close was dangerous. Incorporation by the other was a source of terror and brought with it the certainty of loss of integration. As a defense against annihilation, Anna utilized a variety of modes of relating. These attempts at making contact with others included merging, distancing, shadowing/coercing, and attacking. In each instance, the patterns of relating were initially used protectively as a defense against the awareness of a sense of inner deadness. Anna's interpersonal functioning was characterized by slippage and fluidity, as levels of relating fluctuated in an unpredictable, often chaotic manner in response to her inner states of alarm and upset. The immediate access to regression and feelings of annihilation resulted in chaotic interaction, which seemed at first a frantic attempt to incorporate and control the other ("I am everything, everything is me"). For Anna to repair, it was necessary for her to return to the point of disintegration, which in her case was also the point of earliest integration. She needed to reexperience earliest states of helplessness within a "good enough" holding environment. Her discovery of various aspects of herself through establishing a connectedness with the therapist was expressed in recurring play themes of creation and rebirth. Several of these vignettes will be described below.

Creation of the Therapeutic Baby

Following a brief honeymoon period of cooperativeness, Anna became increasingly oppositional and attacking. She would insist to her mother that she hated the therapist and would not go to therapy. Direct physical attacks alternated with wild mean looks and periods of puppet play depicting sadistic patterns between a king and queen. This was an intense period of confusion as Anna tried to fend me off by perceiving me as frightening. In one session during this period, as we worked with watercolors, there was good control, with only a hint of spills. On the paper she drew a hill with a circle on top and covered the painting with water, making the picture fade away. On another sheet she muddled the colors all together; I interpreted that these were her confused feelings and that this is why she came to therapy. Each time she would make a mess of the colors in the box, she would ask my assistance in wiping them clean. Anna: "Where did the yellow go?" I linked the colors with feelings and suggested that, when we worked together, feelings became clearer and less confused, for example, happiness (yellow), grey (sadness). She needed a larger piece of paper. I supplied it. She tore it up with a malicious smile. I asked her if she could use parts. At this point she checked her watch against mine and commented that mine was fast by three minutes. I agreed to follow hers. Anna replied the parts were "too small" and started to tear progressively smaller bits, saying in a baby voice, "Too small, too small." I joined in the refrain and added, "A little, little baby sometimes feels the world is a confusing place—everything seems to run together. It's good to have a place to bring these baby feelings." Anna responded with a twinkle in her eye. She wanted to spell a word. I suggested she use the blackboard. With my assistance, she wrote the word "humorous" over and over again on the blackboard. I responded that it was very, very humorous, adding a "very" for each new word. She added that my name, "Saralea is humorous." "Yes, I am pretty funny, but maybe even a bit scary, too. Who else do you know who is humorous on the outside?" Anna: "Nobody." Therapist: "This then is the place to bring all of your humorous feelings." Anna drew my face clearly. Then, she erased the features and made them jagged, like lightning flashes. Therapist: "Sometimes I am humorous and it feels comfortable with me; sometimes I am humorous and I have a lightning face. It can be very confusing here."

These were sessions marked by fluctuating ambivalence toward the therapist. During periods of harmonious work, confusion would suddenly surface, particularly if a "mistake" occurred. I wondered aloud how it must feel when good feelings get confused so quickly. Responding with a malicious smile, she threw a ball directly at me. I said this hurt me and directed her to a doll instead. She immediately accepted the surrogate object and created a game of throwing balls at the doll and keeping score. I commented on her angry feelings and the hitting of the doll, how the doll becomes angry when she cannot do what she wants to do. Playing the game is the way she, Anna, can tell me how she feels. She can't hit me, but she can show me how she feels. I commented that the doll did not have its own feelings or otherwise it would be hurt. Anna responded: "The doll is humorous; it likes getting hurt." Therapist: "No one likes getting hurt; that's why we have toys to play with." Anna examined the anus of the doll and pulled its legs apart. Anna: "The vagina would be here—this kind of doll takes water from a bottle. The water comes out the back, but the bottle is lost. We could put the water in its mouth." As the session ended Anna maintained control, despite some anxious clinging, at separation.

Another session the following week began with messy pasting play. Anna used up a small bottle of glue pasting all the tissues in a box into a large wad. Therapist: "It's fun to bring all your messy feelings into therapy—somehow they are all holding together—but, we've run out of supplies." Anna began kicking me and I directed her to the doll. She threw down the doll and stood on top of it. Therapist: "Do you think she likes being thrown down and getting hurt?" Anna wrote on a sheet of paper, "You are humorous." Therapist: "That means you think I like getting hurt. No one likes getting hurt. These feelings come on so suddenly. At first you enjoy messy feelings, and then they become frightening—suddenly you felt attacked." Anna began a game of catch with the doll. Anna: "Who is that? Really me." I responded, "Who is that? Really Anna." Anna hit the baby on the head four times, counting 1, 2, 3, 4. Therapist: "Big girl Anna and baby Anna. When big girl Anna hits baby Anna, does big girl Anna hurt baby Anna? It seems like big girl Anna is confused. She thinks that, if her baby is hit, it will feel better; I think it just hurts. Has anyone ever hit you this way?" Anna denied ever being hit. At the close of the session Anna drew a whole figure, a snowman with parts that came together.

Two sessions later Anna came in very upset. She made reference to a statue covered with paint on mischief night and proceeded to paint off the paper, staring at me as if not seeing the mess. She would not accept limits and physically attacked me. I had to hold her. Therapist: "Nobody likes to get hurt. I don't like to get hurt. You don't like to get hurt. These are angry feelings that come when you don't get what you want. I think you were angry when you saw the statue all covered with paint." I explained mischief night. Anna: "No, I was happy. They threw eggs on my car. I threw apples out the window." Therapist: "You were protecting your car. Maybe someone should have protected the statue. It bothers you when these things happen. Can you tell me about it?" Anna took the doll and repeatedly let it fall. She painted bruises on the doll. I commented, "Poor doll is getting hurt. She keeps falling down. You are pushing her down. She doesn't like it. It hurts. This is a very, very precious baby. She is humorous. She has a high spirit and many, many needs. She needs lots of care. Maybe she'd rather get a hug than a hit. Maybe the baby is getting hit because she can't get a hug. A humorous baby is one you can hug." Anna stopped throwing the baby and held her. She fed her until she had "had enough."

At the next session Anna began by searching for the doll. She found her with some measure of relief and declared, "She is dead." Anna worked on cleaning the doll's bruises, fed her, made her go wee-wee, and made a heart for the baby so she could live. I commented that baby Anna has been treated with love and can now feel loved. Anna continued over the next few weeks to fluctuate between loving and hating baby Anna. These ambivalent feelings were also clear in the transference, as Anna was often overwhelmed by the intensity of her bad feelings for me. At times she was terrified. At one of these moments she drew my face going though gradual transformations of becoming increasingly scary. As we worked together, she suggested that we play a make-believe game "that part of me is part of you." She talked about a kitty she used for masturbation and how rubbing made her feel good and forget the bad feelings.

First Sustained Play Fantasy Not Interrupted by Thrusts of Aggression

The play objects are dinosaurs. The meat eaters fight each other to "dead" the bird who teases: "Come and get me." The plant eaters take over the world, thanks to the bird. The meat eaters eat each other up and become extinct. "They are not only dead, they are gone forever." The dinosaurs are bigger and stronger, but the bird can make them chase him and get a lot of attention by teasing and being bad. The little bad bird wants the dinosaurs to chase him. Anna played at being the bird, jumping up and down on the couch. She laid eggs.

At this juncture the transference took a decidedly positive turn. Anna wanted to know, "Does Taffy [the therapist's dog] like you when you have to say no?" Anna still resisted separation from me and repeatedly wanted to take toys home from the playroom. I interpreted her feelings; tantrums usually ensued. Anna found a new hiding place under my desk where she kept her secrets. She played she was a jellyfish that stings and hurts while hiding in the ocean, then she became an octopus which continues to eat even after it is dead.

In the next session, from her secret place Anna told a story about a desert dog who lived in a tent left by explorers. They didn't know they had left her since she was so very, very tiny—a baby. "I don't want to talk about it." Anna made a drawing. She crossed out the dogs and put in eggs instead. The drawing she didn't like she gave to me (but didn't tear up); the drawing she liked she gave to her mother. The change in feeling that occurred within the transference seemed to generalize to her mother. In play she was welcoming, inviting me to a tea party, feeding babies and being gratified by play. There were less violent fantasies concerning her mother, whom she began to see as nurturing. Mrs. A brought afterschool snacks to session for Anna, who often looked out to check on her presence for reassurance during a difficult play period. Anna began practicing her gymnastics and jump rope skills. She often entertained me by having me watch her perform.

Rebirth of the Therapeutic Baby

Anna began playing with a baby doll with hair she named David. "We'll cut his hair and make him a penis." She cut the penis off and he cried; she pasted it on again. Anna spoke for David: "I feel weird, I don't have a penis. I don't have a vagina. I don't know what I am." Anna: "Be still or I'll cut off your arm." She turned to me, "Tell him I'm not serious. My Dad told me when I was very, very little, he cut my hair like this. He saved it, but I never saw it." We collected the doll's hair and put it in an envelope. Anna turned to the Anna doll; she hurt the doll. Anna: "I don't know if it is a boy or a girl." Therapist: "This doll hurt itself because it felt different. Its scars are better now." Anna looked at the sores on the eyes and decided that they are better too. She decided it was a boy and hurt its head so it was bleeding; she also drew on new bruises.

At the next session she went immediately to the baby Anna doll and decided that it was a girl. She drew a vagina on it, with a clitoris and a place to pee. I commented that some kids think that, if they do not have a penis, something is wrong—it fell off or got lost. Anna: "It didn't. She's a girl and has a vagina. She knows she doesn't have a penis." She continued putting sores on the doll because she is "bad." She made a red rear end and put multiple hurts on her stomach. I commented, "Some kids feel so bad they do not have a penis—they feel they have to hurt themselves—they are so different." Anna volunteered, "Let's clean her up." She made a diaper. I asked, "How did she get so hurt?" Anna replied, "Her parents got shot. She jumped off the Empire State Building. She couldn't find her mommy and daddy. They went to the Museum of Natural History and are with the dinosaurs." I reflected with Anna how terrible it is when parents argue—you feel like they cannot take care of themselves, like something terrible might happen. Anna might lose them and worry it was her fault. Anna took the doll and immersed her totally in water. She cleaned her completely and she "came out like new." Anna wanted her mother to see.

On Mother's Day Anna drew a face, my face as she first saw me. Then she drew a succession of three faces: a composite face of myself and her mother, a frenzied face, and a clown's face. She was intent on showing me the changes in her mother's face and how she was different from me. She was particularly concerned with the mouth and used a mirror to search for her own uvula. We talked about changes which occur from day to day, differences between people, such as eye color, etc. Anna drew a precious little girl. She continued to hide in her tiny space and asked not to be laughed at because she wished to be small. "This little girl walks and talks at one second old." Anna acknowledged that this is unreal. She remembered that, when she was little, she slept in her parents' room and ate potatoes and applesauce and from her mommy's breast. When I inquired how her brother felt about that, she responded, "He did not see me. I was in the crib in mommy's room." On the blackboard Anna wrote the words: "I am." This was the first session to end with no manifest separation anxiety.

Thematic Continuities in Later Phases of Treatment

The previous vignettes are brief selections from the first year of treatment, which was to continue for three years. The course of therapy was marked by recurrent regressions and the resurgence of hostility as Anna would claim again and again that I was humorous and wanted to destroy and devour everything. The beginning of the second year brought the creation of a fantasy world of birds, which was to involve us in sustained play for a three-month period. The activity followed a visit to a medieval museum where Anna viewed the tapestries of the unicorn, which terrified her with its depiction of blood and battle, and the collection of church treasures. Each bird was made of a different metal which formed a hierarchy of treasures. Subsequently, a lineage of different colored birds emerged, each with its distinctive characteristics. In this fantasy world, there were also a pair of turtles, a snake, and a vulture. The gold jay would nest and have babies. This play depicted inner conflict within a framework which made mastery possible. From this play and its themes, Anna was able to begin to talk directly about her relationships at home. Sibling rivalry and her brother's wish that she were dead were central themes in the middle period of treatment.

Work with the parents was an essential part of this therapeutic process. Anna's parents were seen together for weekly counseling sessions, in addition to Anna's bi-weekly sessions. They were encouraged to bring in concrete descriptions of events that occurred at home, and we would problem-solve together. Mrs. A was able to identify closely with the therapist. Considerable gains in self-esteem followed gains in management at home for both parents. Mr. A's resistance to therapy was considerable but diminished following events surrounding the death of Anna's pet bird. Anna wanted to caress and hold the dead animal. Her father was frightened by these feelings, called the therapist for suggestion and responded to reassurance. A funeral was performed and Anna was permitted to grieve. In therapy she was able to relate the entire episode and her sadness. Her fantasy was of rebirth, like a "jack-in-the-box." She was angry at Bluebird for leaving. She took out the doll and began caring for it. "When I grow up, I will be a big girl, and then a teenager, then a woman, then a mother." "I will not be able to care for twins or triplets by myself, with just the help of mother; I will need a grandmother and grandmother will need a great-grandmother." "Do I have a great-grandmother?" We talked about her awareness of death. Anna talked to me more about Bluebird: "I feel completely good about her." It was a moving experience for her parents as well, who took pride in their management of the loss.

Termination concerns were first expressed at the time of the death of Anna's bird. She began to become aware that there might be a time when she would no longer need to come to treatment. Coincidental with these concerns were some definite signs of progress, both within her inner world and with those in the world around her. Anna's fantasy world became a less tyrannical and punitive place. Her characters became playful, and events that before seemed scary now at times could be perceived as amusing. Anna was no longer a passive agent in her play, but willfully imposed outcomes and suggested alternative versions of scripts. She became very involved with the case of Baby Fae, an infant who was given an artificial heart. In the therapy room, Baby Susan was born. She suffered from a congenital defect of a split heart, which needed to be healed. Baby Susan survived, even in the face of the death of Baby

Fae, and was nurtured well by parents and doctors. Within the transference, sadistic projections decreased and there was increased pleasure in being together. Anna remained a strong-willed individual and was able to assert herself positively with peers. Along with increased social competence came gains in physical prowess and capacity to care for herself, including self-regulation of moods. Particularly significant was Anna's newfound ability to make reparation: "I want to apologize. Sometimes when I get angry, that's how I act."

These forward steps alternated with regressive periods, recalling the earlier days of treatment. Outbursts of aggression, extreme fearfulness, and physical attacks would indicate the resurgence of old issues. The therapist would indicate to Anna that these frightening concerns had come back again, and we would work on them as long as was necessary. Anna created two games which pointed toward a comprehension of the treatment process. One was called "looking forward and looking backward," the other involved discerning the ending and beginning of a maze. These games would recur spontaneously at different points during the last half of treatment.

A new bird to replace the lost bird brought a resurgence of concerns regarding separation. Anna talked about the loss of her old bird who had eggs; the new one was a male. Anna would sit in my rocking chair with her "baby" alongside her and ask if she could always visit me and if I would visit her. We talked about her wish to be my baby and always be with me. With increased acceptance of the treatment relationship, the bond between us became stronger. The unicorn became the gold jay's best friend. Anna often used the couch and associated freely. She talked about metamorphosis, which she defined as "something transformed, that undergoes change, like a butterfly, or a frog." The room was her cocoon and I reflected how comfortable she seemed to feel now in the cocoon while undergoing change. Anna welcomed the new school year, and in early fall sessions were decreased to once a week.

Decisions to decrease sessions and to terminate were undertaken through a three-part process: 1) between Anna and myself; 2) between Anna and her parents; 3) between her parents and myself. It was understood that, although Anna and I would recommend, the final decision lay with her parents. The termination process was extremely gradual and, until the present, some occasional contact is maintained with the family. It was her choice to see me the following year on her birthday. Counseling sessions were continued on a once-a-month basis for her parents for nine months following cessation of patient contact, at their request.

As Anna and I reached the end of our work together, a new game was created. She would fall off the couch and roll further and further away, playing at being the baby delivered by the doctor. She asked if, when she grew up, she could bring her child to me. She looked at my bookshelves and observed, "At first I hated them, now I love them." I remarked that it seemed that the butterfly had reached its final stage of growth within the cocoon. There had been so many changes. Anna replied, "But it's the same body, the same blood, the same caterpillar." The strong positive attachment was described by Anna: "The first year we were only friends; the second year we were good friends; now we are the greatest of friends." She drew a picture of a flower with a part missing. A bird was coming to the flower for nectar. "I so much like coming here."

Summary

This brief case vignette supports the suggestion by Paulina Kernberg (1983) that borderline conditions in childhood may stem not only from the rapproachment crisis, but also from fixations or regressions to earlier differentiation or practicing phases of the separation-individuation process. In Anna's case, part-objects and self-representations were not integrated. As Kernberg observes, in these instances, the external object is usually utilized by the patient as a prop for projections, so that at times the patient experiences him/herself as the therapist, while simultaneously the therapist is induced to reenact an aspect of the personality of the patient. The shifting ego states in Anna's case clearly corresponded to organized self-object representations utilized for defensive purposes. Coercion, shadowing, withdrawal, and temper outbursts were all activated in correspondence to a different level of subject-object representation. Through extended play therapy these themes were stabilized, clarified, linked to real life circumstances, and finally underwent modification. Hopefully, these experiences with difficult child patients will encourage other child therapists to invest in them and the long, arduous process which can lead to their recovery.

The Fairy Godmother and the Wicked Witch of the West

Simone Sternberg, Ed.D.
(1987)

Fairy tales help children to make some sense and give order to the world around them—the confusing and gargantuan world of adults. They also appeal to the child's wish to simplify, to see things as black or white, and they enable the child to project his or her own internal drama onto the characters of the tale, the better to see them, to own or disown them. Borrowing from Joyce McDougall's (1985) theatrical metaphor in the understanding of internal psychic drama, I am proposing two characters to personify the play of opposite forces, taken from the original film version of *The Wizard of Oz*. The Fairy Godmother, or good fairy character, was played in this version by the blonde-haired, blue-eyed Billie Burke, as Belinda, the Good Witch of the North. In the opposite corner we have the Wicked Witch of the West, dark-haired and darker complexioned, sharp featured, dressed in black (another version is the Wicked Stepmother of fairy tales), played unforgettably by Margaret Hamilton. Through them I wish to demonstrate some aspects of more "primitive" defenses, characteristically used by our more fragile patients.

To return for a minute to our film classic. Images are often more powerful than words, and a brief scene from *The Wizard of Oz* offers us, very succinctly and dramatically, a version of the concept of splitting. Dorothy (Judy Garland), looking into the Magic Ball of the Wicked Witch of the West, first sees Auntie Em expressing concern

---

The author extends special thanks to those persons in supervision who provided some of the clinical examples used in this paper.

and offering comfort and love. This image is soon obliterated and replaced by that of the cackling, murderous Wicked Witch. The ball, as screen for the internal projection, cannot tolerate both images at once, and the one image literally wipes out the other.

The borderline patient has been written about extensively in recent years. A wide range of patients has been included under this designation, as well as a gamut of treatment modalities from traditional psychoanalysis and variants thereof (Abend et al., 1983) through expressive psychoanalytic psychotherapy (Kernberg, 1975) to more supportive modalities.

In this paper I am not concerned with "borderline" patients per se, but with some of the more fragile aspects of patients I have either worked with directly or have learned about from supervisees.

Fenichel (1945), presenting the traditional psychoanalytic view, speaks of "perversions" in the adult as a return to childhood sexuality. Those zones and practices which gave pleasure and reduced anxiety when we were young children are never abandoned or are reactivated later on. Similarly, the defenses of the fragile patient can be seen as a return to those ways of being and perceiving that seemed to work in childhood. The fact that they didn't work that well or are no longer appropriate for an adult functioning in an adult world is ignored by the psyche. Some of the more "primitive" defenses, often used by "borderline" patients (Kernberg, 1975) and at times by all of us under sufficient stress, are denial, projection, projective identification, splitting, and concretization. These are by no means discrete defensive maneuvers; rather, they overlap and support each other. Their utilization by the fragile person is an attempt to reduce suffering and make some childlike sense of the world. According to McDougall (1985), they can be seen as creations, which allow the person to live as best he or she can, the alternative being psychic chaos, perhaps psychic death.

Following are brief examples of the use of concretization by adults: A young male patient has to cross a long bridge to get to his therapist's office. One morning there was an extensive traffic tieup and the patient arrived late for his appointment. He proceeded to relate at length the vicissitudes of his journey—the poor road conditions, thousands of cars, the condition of his car and of the bridge, all described in infinite detail. (One recognizes here a favorite pastime of obsessive-compulsive patients.) The journey as symbolic, the bridge as a metaphor of his tie to his therapist (still tenuous at present), and his lateness as an aspect of this were all very obscure notions to him.

Another example of the use of the concrete is found in an adult male patient's dream and his associations to the dream. This patient, often flooded with sexual thoughts, had a dream of a trumpet flying around the room. In the dream, the patient receives admiration for playing the trumpet and subsequently joins a band. While the dream might have served as a sublimation of his sexual feelings (a cleaned up wet-dream of sorts), all the patient could think of was that he wants to buy a trumpet and that they are fun to play.

Had this been a child and not an adult, his response would be considered appropriate and expectable. Even in latency and early adolescence, such a response could be considered normal. However, when concrete thinking is used exclusively, predominantly and/or inappropriately by an adult, one is led to speculate about the fragility (including the possibility of organicity and brain damage) of the person in question.

Children, especially young children, cling to the literal meanings of words; physical attributes and exterior presentation, or packaging, are accepted as representative of what the package (or person) contains. Black can mean the color black, but also that which is dark, fearful, mysterious, sexual, evil. These aspects of concretization are considered normal in childhood thinking. As an example, a seven-year-old was recently asked by an adult how many times he had driven to Pennsylvania. "Never," said the child, "but I'll be able to drive there in 10 years." This child wasn't joking, but the adult meant how many times had the child driven in the car with his parents to Pennsylvania. As children become older and more secure, they can abandon "literal" meanings, play with words and concepts, and increasingly feel comfortable with metaphor.

Following is an example of the use of the concrete combined with splitting. Linda, age 5, came to therapy with two stuffed animals, Good Mousie and Bad Mousie. The two animals were small, grey and looked identical. To Linda, however, they were clearly distinguishable and had to be kept apart, on different sides of the room. The way she could tell which was which was by smelling them. Bad Mousie had a fecal smell. Earlier, Linda described her good mother as smelling of cotton candy and her bad mother of poo-poo. In a collateral session her mother had reported that Linda was constantly smelling things, at a time when most children have largely relinquished smell as a primary source of information. Also, the cathexis to the anal stage is clearly evident.

Much of the conflict was worked through in therapy and eventually Linda came to sessions with a teddy bear which represented the therapist, a kind of Hegelian synthesis of the thesis and antithesis. Interestingly, Teddy, according to Linda, had no smell.

In the discussion of Linda, I mentioned her splitting of the Mousies into Good Mousie and Bad Mousie. The concept of splitting lends itself to a certain amount of confusion, as it has been used somewhat differently by various theoreticians, described at length by some authors (notably Kernberg, 1975), ignored by others, and mentioned very briefly by still others. Fine (1986), discussing the history of theories of narcissism, speaks of the basic emotional split in the infant between love and hate (p. 311). He describes the etiology of the concepts of splitting, projection and projective identification, usually linked together, primarily as used by Melanie Klein and her followers. Fine makes the point that, historically, insufficient reference has been made "to the overwhelming anxieties that set these defenses off" (p. 47).

Webster's English Dictionary (1962) defines splitting in the practical sense: "To divide lengthwise: To tear asunder violently: Cleave: Disunite." This pithy definition is the one to which I find myself returning when trying to sort out the uses made of the term in the psychoanalytic literature.

Laplanche and Pontalis (1973) tell us that the term *Spaltung* has very old and varied uses. In Freud's early papers on hysteria, some written with Breuer, he talked about alternating states of consciousness, a kind of dual personality, such as found in certain hysterias and as a result of hypnosis. The mind is split and only part of it is accessible to conscious thought and reality. In his 1940 paper on the splitting of the ego Freud describes it as a defensive process in the context of his work on fetishism and psychoses. Two attitudes toward external reality coexist in the ego. The first takes account of reality while the second "disavows it and replaces it by a product of desire. The two attitudes persist side by side without influencing each other" (Laplanche & Pontalis, 1973, p. 427). Due to conflict there is an intrasystemic split in the ego, in order to obtain instinctual gratification.*

---

* Stoller, in his excellent book *Splitting/A Case of Female Masculinity* (1973), goes back to Freud in describing splitting as a process in which the ego is altered as it attempts to defend itself. One current in mental life disavows another, both acting as if independent of each other, i.e., split off (p. xvi). His use of "splitting" simply as a descriptive term to describe a process used to preserve the self and identity is both sobering and a great relief. He describes theorizing as "a process of endlessly palpating and stroking one's words and thoughts" (p. xvi).

Klein (1975) described the dependent position of the infant as intolerable as early as the first half year of existence. In rage, the infant uses the defenses of splitting, introjection and projection in an attempt to deal with mother (the need satisfier), against whom both erotic and destructive instincts are directed. The object is split into "good" and "bad." This splitting of the object was viewed by Klein as the most primitive defense against anxiety.

This splitting transpires in the "paranoid schizoid" position, wherein the mother is treated as a part object, but splitting also affects the mother as whole object later on in the "depressive" position. The child's ego is concomitantly split into "good" and "bad" as it is constituted essentially through the introjection of objects (Klein, 1975, p. 430).

Most definitions of splitting in the current literature overlap with that of projective identification. The *Harvard Guide to Modern Psychiatry* (Nicholi, 1978) describes splitting as part of projective identification, a secondary defense used to alleviate anxiety:

> The patient splits off painful parts of the self relating to the people he has lost and projects them onto the available person. The split-off state of his ego and projection of these aspects onto others then leads to alterations in his ego boundaries; this process increases anxiety, which fosters regressive dependence and counteractive aggression. (p. 232)

Grotstein (1981), in his book *Splitting and Projective Identification,* also discusses the concepts similarly as "both a benign defense which simply wishes to postpone confrontation with some experience that cannot yet be tolerated," but can also "negate, destroy, and literally obliterate the sense of reality" (p. 131).

We see, then, that splitting can be viewed as normal when age appropriate, a benign defense; and also as a pretty serious matter, smacking of gross pathology.

Kernberg, following Klein, points to the primitive idealization of the all-good mother and the need to protect this image against the all-bad object image of the frustrating and/or engulfing mother. Another object can become the receptacle of the "bad" mother, for example, the stranger in Spitz's (1965) concept of eight-month stranger anxiety. Later, splitting is used defensively by the emerging ego to prevent spreading and generalization of anxiety. "This defensive division of the ego, in what was at first a simple defect in integration is then used actively for other purposes" (Kernberg,

1975, p. 427). Ordinarily it is used in very early stages of ego development (during the first year) and is then replaced by the higher level defenses of isolation and undoing. For Kernberg (1975), there is an intensification and pathological fixation of splitting processes in the borderline. He considers these mechanisms as diagnostic indicators of "lower level character disorders" (p. 13).

Anna Freud (Sandler et al., 1980), in talking about child therapy, said that the therapist might be used "for the externalization of an introject on which the patient depends for self-esteem or other narcissistic supplies" (p. 107). The therapist may also be used for the splitting of ambivalence and can become the "good" mother in contradistinction to the "bad" mommy at home. In what is to follow I embroider variations on this theme, often with the positive feelings directed not toward the therapist, but some other external figure or object, another therapist or supervisor. The "good" mommy/"bad" mommy battle has been largely displaced from the person of the mother herself onto two other "actors" whom the patient has cast in the roles of Good Fairy and Wicked Witch. (The same actor can be cast in both roles, in oscillating fashion, during the same session, while the patient briefly assumes the opposite role. Kernberg, 1975, discusses this phenomenon in detail.)

Fred, a patient in his mid-twenties, is very intelligent and has a shy, elfin smile. In the winter he came to sessions wearing two or three jackets and a woolen cap on his head, most of which usually stayed on throughout the session. In the old days, we would have characterized him as "schizoid." Fred had few relationships and spoke to few people. He quickly developed intense and painful feelings of love for me. His falling "head over heels in love" can be viewed as a transference phenomenon, a transference "psychosis," or simply as resistance to treatment. His feelings were so strong that they effectively negated his view of me as his therapist, thereby thwarting our therapeutic dialogue and my ability to do my job.

Freud (1915) warned of the dangers of women patients falling in love with their male analysts and the destructive effects on the analysis. Wanting real gratification from the analyst, they were unable to tolerate the frustrations imposed by the analytic contract and usually left treatment. With Fred and his female therapist, only the gender was changed. Fred had split me off as a "real love object" and was unable to hold onto the idea of me as therapist at the same time.

Fred also couldn't tolerate the idea of paying me. If he paid me, I was further split off as the prostitute to whom he was giving money for love. The confusion was such that he left therapy for several months. The distance enabled him to feel less anxious and more in control and, finally, to return to treatment. Thus the splitting of the therapist into the idealized, beloved woman and the degraded, servile, greedy prostitute can gradually be played out and worked through in therapy.

Abraham (1924) wrote about the case of a male patient who, when depressed, would look for mother-of-pearl buttons in the street. No other buttons would do. The patient was obsessed with mother-of-pearl buttons. Mother-of-pearl was associated with the idea of brightness and cleanliness and was therefore of special worth. This patient, as a child, was greatly disappointed in his "wicked" mother and sought solace in the shop of the widowed mother of a playmate who would give him Johannis bread to eat. Abraham tells us that the elongated shape and brown color of the bread were associated with patient's desire to eat excrement (an anal/oral fantasy of some depressives) melded with his desire for maternal love and care. Another association of this patient, also from childhood, was the unearthing of some shells by workmen constructing a road in his hometown. One side of the shells, covered with earth and dirt, contrasted sharply with the other side, which glistened like mother-of-pearl. These shells were the forebears of the mother-of-pearl buttons, which in the analysis represented the patient's ambivalence toward his mother. The very name, mother-of-pearl, seemed to indicate his high esteem for his mother, the pearl. But the smooth, shining surface was deceptive. The other side was not so beautiful. In likening this other side, covered with dirt (excrement), to his "wicked" mother, from whom he had to withdraw his love, he was abusing her and holding her up to scorn. Only one side could be seen at a time.

Fred offers another version of this good/bad, idealization/denigration dichotomy. I returned from a week's vacation to find a letter from him, after seeing him intermittently in therapy for almost a year. During that time, Fred never openly expressed negative thoughts or feelings about me. The letter displays intelligence, insight, as well as a fair amount of aggression, which until that point he was unable to discharge in sessions.

> Although I can possibly grasp the notion I may not be such a terrible person, oftentimes I do not feel these things. I am too wrapped up in my own self to be concerned with others. . . . There are some thoughts I sometimes have of

you which I don't like to admit. Today, when you
mentioned the word "bitch" . . . I could have mentioned
that I think I have occasionally, if not often, engendered
this term when thinking of you. . . Finally, and this is even
worse, I sometimes, when thinking of you, think of you as
Dr. Shitbag. Almost comical.

In talking about the letter, Fred said that he really likes me quite
a bit, but these thoughts are hard to control, obsessional thoughts
which force themselves on him. Although the scatalogical nature of
these thoughts gets intertwined with sexual images, the regression
to the anal level is clear. This is an example of his ambivalent feelings
about me and reminiscent of Abraham's depressive patient. Fred is
still using higher order cognitive function, however, and playing
around with words, distorting my name, etc. Whether he might be
considered borderline or an obsessive-compulsive with borderline
features could be a point of discussion but is not the subject of this
paper.

Some degree of splitting is inherent in any situation where the
patient is seen by more than one therapist. Splitting of the
transference can be done not only with another therapist but with a
supervisor, instructor, friend, spouse, parent, ad infinitum. In its
more benign form it weakens the transference, but if persistent and
severe, it can inhibit or stop treatment altogether. While this division
of attention (and libido) is not necessarily pathological, it must be
analyzed. A benign example is that of a female patient who went with
her husband to another therapist for marital counseling at his
request, after having already left the conjugal domicile. Her rationale
was that she could ease her husband into therapy for himself (she
also felt guilty about having been the one to leave). In this case, the
marital therapist was split off as the receptacle of the patient's
negative feelings. She was seen as too intrusive, too loose (her dog
was in the office during the session), and too frightening, as though
the therapist could somehow coerce my patient to return to her
husband. I, on the other hand, remained the "good mother." By
unloading all the negatives on the couple's therapist, she could
preserve me as the kind, maternal figure she so much wanted as an
ally during her time of need.

A less benign example is shown by Nola, who, when I first saw
her in therapy, was concomitantly in a group for agoraphobics. She
also had an adult lifetime history of therapy, mainly with males. The
leader of this group, a woman, was immensely liked and admired by

themselves, although one had specifically requested it. Neither wanted to return to her former male therapist and each wanted to work with a woman.

The first, Gwen, felt a special kinship with her supervisor, having had her previously as an instructor. In addition, two of Gwen's friends were in therapy with her supervisor. In early sessions with me she denied her desire to have her supervisor as her therapist, but displaced this wish onto the male therapist of a third friend, for whom Gwen kept threatening to leave me. Her initial denial of wanting her supervisor as therapist was in the service of giving me a chance, maintaining a more "professional" supervisory relationship (all seemingly positive), but also of not allowing herself to feel the full fury of her jealousy toward her friends, who did indeed get the full benefit of her supervisor as their therapist.

Some months after beginning treatment, Gwen, via a phone message, requested the name of a child therapist in an outlying area for a friend.

During my absence Gwen made the same request of her supervisor, from whom she obtained the name of a child therapist personally known to and highly recommended by her. Gwen, in addition to wanting the information (which she could have also obtained from other sources), was testing us both and let me know that her supervisor had better information. This was related with obvious glee (there was a playful element as well) and led to the unearthing of Gwen's feelings of jealousy and that her friends, patients of the supervisor, were getting the better deal.

Gwen's supervisor was described by her as blonde and blue-eyed, feminine and soft in manner, dress and voice. I, on the contrary, was seen as efficient, successful, well-dressed in a somewhat masculine way, with a sharp-edged voice. Gwen herself has dark hair, as did her mother. A version of her idealized self, or ego ideal, had been projected onto her supervisor, while I for the time represented aspects of her more tarnished self as well as her unattuned, narcissistic mother. There was another dichotomy as well. When the supervisor was described as warm, feminine and maternal and I was felt to be the more masculine, I was the receptacle of a father transference in addition to being the "phallic mother."

Another, more dramatic example of a split in the transference is in the work with Harriet, a psychiatric nurse. Like Gwen's mother, Harriet's mother also had dark hair. That and the fact that I am female might be slim straws on which to hang a maternal transference. We know that a blonde, male analyst could have equally been the receptacle of the maternal transference. However, I am particularly stressing the concrete elements of the resemblance in the transference.

Harriet had carefully and lovingly chosen her supervisor of six years, part of the time overlapping her treatment with a male therapist she eventually stopped seeing. After terminating her therapy she began using her supervisory sessions more and more as quasi-therapy sessions. In discussing countertransference issues, Harriet would talk increasingly about herself, to the point where she became the major and sometimes the sole focus of sessions. When it became clear that Harriet needed further treatment, she requested therapy with her supervisor. After reflection the supervisor demurred, citing their long supervisory relationship and the difficulty, at that point, of switching gears.

Harriet was referred to me and initially welcomed the referral, as I basked in the glow as the choice of her idealized and loved supervisor. Her disappointment and feelings of rejection by the supervisor were initially not readily available to her. However, Harriet soon split supervisor and therapist into an idealized, beloved mother figure, who happened to be light-haired, and the de-idealized, dark-haired mother in the transference, as I was cast in the role of her own mother and her bad, unlovable self. Harriet's mother was a narcissistic woman, ill prepared for motherhood and viewed by the patient as never providing the warm, maternal love and care she needed. Nonetheless, Harriet loved her mother very much, was "in love with her" until age seven. Adjectives she has used to describe me, such as slim, dark, beautiful, fashionable, youthful, are similar to or the same as those used to paint a picture of her early mother. At age seven she longed for, fell in love with her father, at which point her mother was transformed into a bad, ugly witch. Psychically this is what her mother has remained for many decades, and the role in which I am intermittently cast.

The split in the two transference "mothers" in which Harriet is currently immobilized is a reenactment of a childhood schism between her pre-seven and post-seven, beloved and hated mother, and that between her mother and her father. She felt that she couldn't have them both, and the price of loving one was renunciation of the other.

Some atypical features of this "oedipal triangulation" are the relative lateness at which it occurs, her inability to have ever reached and felt loved by her "pre-oedipal" mother, and that there is no real triangulation. Harriet is involved in two dyads and is still unable to tolerate the triangle.

As a child, Harriet also enacted this drama with her two teddies, not unlike Linda's use of her two mousies, described earlier. Harriet had two teddies, a black one and a white one. She always felt torn between the two, as she did between her parents. To love one was to be disloyal to the other. As Harriet had great difficulty relating to the two teddies at the same time (one had to be physically removed from the presence of the other), she now feels guilty toward her supervisor when feeling positive about me and vice-versa. Consequently she abandons one of us and then the other alternately, fearing our anger as well as her own.

In a recent session Harriet expressed her deep ambivalence about being in therapy; she wants double sessions with me and has simultaneously been thinking of stopping both therapy and supervision. She is angry with both of us. When her supervisor asks her if she has discussed some issue with me that she had raised in supervision, Harriet draws a blank. She can't remember what she talks about in therapy when in supervision, nor does she remember the content of discussion about her own psyche in supervisory sessions when she reaches my door. In fact, the forgetting probably took place when she left her supervisor's door, and has a hysterical quality to it. Not only must she keep us apart, but the memory of what transpires in each "home" must be split off as well.

Harriet, who selected her supervisor after long scrutiny, feels a deep trust in her presence (as mentioned earlier, the supervisory relationship has lasted many years), expresses much affect in supervision and cries easily. By saving the tears for her supervisory session and keeping them out of therapy, she reinforces the split between the supervisor as the recipient of her emotions and the therapist as the receptacle of her intellectual formulations. She, in fact, splits the work of therapy between the two of us. Combined, if she could put us together and the two parts could communicate with each other, we would make one good therapist.

Margaret Mahler (1971), in her discussion of the understanding of borderline phenomena, writes of "the importance of reconciliation and thus of integration of the image of the erstwhile 'good' symbiotic mother, whom we long for 'from the cradle on to the grave,' this image to become blended with the representation of the ambivalently loved—dangerous because potentially re-engulfing—mother after separation" (p. 416). This is also a good characterization of Harriet's formulation of her pre-seven and post-seven mothers. Part of the task, then, is to help her to establish a dialectical relationship between all of her dichotomies—intellectual and emotional, pregenital and postgenital mothers, mother and father, supervisor and therapist, good self and bad self, loved self and hated self, supervisor and therapist, black teddy and white teddy.

Sandler, Kennedy and Tyson (1980), in their book on child analysis in collaboration with Anna Freud, speak eloquently about the resolution of the transference. Their remarks, while applicable to the work with any patient, have a particular relevance for the case just discussed. While we are still far from resolutions, these are goals to keep in mind:

> The question of resolution of the transference, or the myth of the resolution of the transference, is relevant to transference development. Resolution of the transference implies that an active conflict involving the person of the therapist—one that represents the externalization of an internal conflict of some sort—should have receded as a consequence of the analytic work. The patient should also have a more realistic assessment of the therapist as a person, and the ties that remain to the therapist should ideally be less emotion laden and conflictual. (p. 103)

Just as children simplify and tend to see things in absolutes, in black and white, they are also capable of living happily with ambiguity. We even see this as a sign of growth and maturation. (While to accept blatant contradictions simultaneously might have much to do with isolation and denial, I am referring more to the acceptance of gradations of good and bad, black and white, in the same person.) An example is the concept, evolved independently when he was four years old, that my child called the Good Wicked Witch. This is an important part of the work we hope to accomplish with patients (especially the fragile ones): the ability to play with words, to use metaphor freely, and to accept the idea that good fairies may be tarnished and wicked witches might also be good.

Summary

Reuben Fine, Ph.D.

In the past two decades the borderline patient has occupied an increasing amount of attention in the professional journals; yet, in spite of intensive study, the essential problems regarding the borderline remain unresolved. The papers in this volume are designed to give the reader both the background of the controversies and a variety of contemporary positions on them.

"Borderline" obviously means "on the border"; historically it has meant the border between neurosis and psychosis, although in recent years the meaning has shifted somewhat from that to the border between normality and neurosis. This immediately raises the question of schizophrenia (psychosis); therefore, the first part of the monograph centers on the background of thinking about schizophrenia.

The classical view of schizophrenia is best represented by Emil Kraepelin, whose views as of 1917 are reprinted here. Kraepelin saw the schizophrenic (whom he called *dementia praecox*) as hereditarily tainted, organically impaired, and essentially inaccessible to any kind of rational therapy. In spite of his dismal view of 70% incurable, he claims that "we have discovered the approach to be followed henceforth in psychiatry."

Although Eugen Bleuler was somewhat more optimistic in his 1911 textbook, the opinion that schizophrenia is essentially hopeless prevailed until World War II. In spite of the dramatic changes in outcome, this position is still the usual one held by psychiatrists today.

Many somatic treatments developed during the present century; virtually all have been discarded, except for the neuroleptics. Here some optimism is found, although the outcome for the schizophrenic is seen as gloomy at best (Tissot et al., 1977). Many psychiatrists,

407

especially those with a psychoanalytic background, have been sharply critical of the Kraepelinian theories. Warner (1986), for example, claims that "schizophrenia is an illness that is shaped, to a large extent, by political economy." Robards (1980) maintains that psychiatry seeks power more than it seeks to understand or cure. Breggin (1983) claims that when drug therapy does work, its effect is to cause brain damage; the same claim is made by him for all somatic treatments. Bellak (1979) writes that "most recently pharmacotherapy has been a source of disappointment even to its most enthusiastic adherents" (p. 5).

The first break in Kraepelin's dreary attitude was provided by the American Harry Stack Sullivan in the 1920s. After extensive treatment of young male schizophrenic patients at Shepard and Enoch Pratt Hospital near Baltimore, he summed up his experiences in the two papers that are reproduced here. In contrast to Kraepelinian hopelessness, he found that in cases with acute onset, somewhat over 61% showed marked improvement, "in a considerable number, the change has amounted to a recovery from the mental disorder" (1931b, p. 238). He presented a modified psychoanalytic treatment of the disorder which he had practiced with much success over a period of some 10 years.

In spite of the startling nature of his claims, it took several generations to catch up with him. The vast majority of psychiatrists continued for many years to incarcerate the majority of their patients for a long time, often for life, and ridiculed the notion that any psychological treatment was feasible.

The conviction that schizophrenia is an organic disorder has persisted, and is probably the majority view among psychiatrists today. With the discovery of the neuroleptics in the 1950s, this position seemed strongly reinforced. Nevertheless, there are many dissenting voices, among them persons of considerable prominence. For example, Manfred Bleuler, son of Eugen, stated flatly that the "overwhelming majority of schizophrenics are physiologically, and particularly endocrinologically, healthy" (1979, p. viii). The issue of the etiology of schizophrenia remains controversial, although with the combined approaches common today, in 20-year follow-up studies, 60–85% of schizophrenic patients, depending on the criteria used, had achieved good social recoveries (Mosher, 1987). Karon and VandenBos (1981) regard psychotherapy as the treatment of choice in schizophrenia.

The major issue relates to the degree of regression present in the schizophrenic. All studies indicate that some 10% are untreatable by any means; but this leaves 90% who are amenable to treatment. No one really questions the fact that the outcome of treatment depends more on social and psychological factors than on anything else. Thus, most would agree that the schizophrenic, if seen early enough, can get better, in varying measure, but what this "early point" is remains a matter of dispute.

It was after World War II that the concept of the "borderline" patient began to take hold. Although used earlier, it was first given explicit formulation by Knight in 1953. He stated: "The term 'borderline state' has achieved almost no official status in psychiatric nomenclature, and conveys no diagnostic illumination other than the implication that the patient is quite sick but not frankly psychotic." Although by now the term has crept into the official psychiatric diagnostic system (DSM-III), Knight's statement is still valid: "The patient is quite sick but not frankly psychotic." The DSM-III, although it lists the disorder, states: "No single feature is invariably present" (APA, 1980, p. 321).

What the work of analysts and analytically oriented psychiatrists accomplished was to puncture the old myth that psychosis is on one side, neurosis on the other, and never the twain shall meet. It became quite clear that there are many borderline conditions, though what is meant by borderline is a matter for investigation. A long series of studies began on what the borderline really is, studies which are still going on, apparently at an increased pace.

Once psychoanalysis entered the psychiatric picture, after World War I, analytic explanations of the various disorders began to dominate the field. This was especially true in America. In 1929, at the opening of the Psychiatric Institute of Columbia University, Ernest Jones expressed the opinion that America had actually created a new profession; he went on to say, even, that the profession of psychiatry does not exist in any other country in the world. The change, he thought, was brought about by a developing attitude on the part of society in general quite as much as by the influence of a few outstanding personalities.

In this paper Jones also, in effect, rejected the traditional psychiatric diagnostic entities: "All mental morbidity . . . is a state of schizophrenia." Mental disorder represents the endless variety of ways in which the threatened ego struggles for its preservation. With these observations, Jones made a considerable advance on Freud's (1924) formula, that in neurosis there is a conflict between the ego and the id, in psychosis, between the ego and reality. Psychosis, neurosis and normality all required more careful examination, which became one of the goals of psychoanalytic research. The common-sense notions that psychosis represents an inability to live in society, while the normal is the one who can "get along," were both turned on their heads by psychoanalytic thought. As Jones had said, an entirely new science was created, even though the terms remained in many cases the same.

In the meantime, psychoanalytic theory made considerable strides after Freud. There was first of all the exploration of the oral stage, which began around 1940, after Freud had died. The close examination of the pathology of parent-child relationships, first with the mother, more recently with the father, came to light. Then came the awareness of the significance of hostility. This was ushered in with Freud's death instinct theory, but while his death instinct was almost universally rejected, the importance of hostility was univer-sally recognized. The defense mechanisms, first described by Freud, were later codified and presented in clear form by his daughter Anna in *The Ego and the Mechanisms of Defense* (1936). World War I and World War II even more so facilitated the recognition of the cultural factors in mental and emotional disturbance. They had been recognized much earlier, but for political reasons, together with the reluctance to seem too grandiose, had not been stressed. Yet as early as 1932 Roheim could write that every culture has its own neurosis. When Rennie and his colleagues (1962) found that more than 80% of the New Yorkers they investigated were emotionally disturbed, some 25% so seriously that they could not function, new questions were raised about the nature of normality in our or any culture. To all of this must be added ongoing research in child development, anthropology, sociology, ethology, neurology and numerous allied sciences. The early formulas remained true but had to be filled out with the newer information.

Space does not permit a full discussion of all these factors (cf. Fine, 1979); our concern is with the borderline. Since the war and subsequent developments had made all too plain the emotional disturbances of the human being, the very definitions of psychotic, neurotic and normal required extensive restatements. One line of investigation concerned the borderline.

The first extensive study of the traits of the borderline was conducted by Grinker and his associates in Chicago (1968). Their main finding was that the borderline syndrome includes anger as the main or only affect, defect in affectional relationships, absence of indications of self-identity, and depressive loneliness.

The theoretician who has played the greatest role in the attempts to define the borderline is, of course, Otto Kernberg. In a long series of papers and a book he has tried to define as minutely as possible how the borderline differs from the psychotic and the normal. The essentials of his theory have been given in the introduction to this volume. Since his papers in the 1970s, most other writings about the borderline have focused on his theories. Yet in spite of this enormous literature pro and con Kernberg, neither clarity nor consensus has emerged.

Gunderson and Kolb (1978) enumerated seven criteria: 1) low achievement; 2) impulsivity; 3) manipulative suicide; 4) heightened affectivity; 5) mild psychotic experiences; 6) high socialization; and 7) disturbed close relationships. Although their work, like that of Grinker et al.'s, is based on careful statistical comparisons, they do not seem to say much beyond what Knight had said a quarter of a century earlier, and Jones a quarter of a century before him: The borderline is a patient who is seriously disturbed but not frankly psychotic.

In a more recent paper (1985) Gunderson and Elliott found an interface between borderline and affective disorder. George and Soloff (1986) noted a high percentage of borderline patients with schizotypal disorders, which is scarcely surprising since schizotypal symptoms are included in Kernberg's overall description, and borderline is often just a new word for what used to be called "schizoid."

Criticism of the Kernbergian formulations is common. Perhaps the most trenchant critique came from Calef and Weinshel (1979), who pointed out that if Kernberg's criteria were adhered to faithfully, it would be hard to find a patient who could not in some respect be called borderline. Reiser and Levenson (1984) went further and identified six ways in which the term "borderline" is commonly abused: 1) as an expression of countertransference hate; 2) to mask sloppy and imprecise diagnostic thinking; 3) to rationalize mistakes in the treatment or treatment failure; 4) as a justification for acting out in the countertransference; 5) to defend against sexual material, including oedipal material, in clinical work; and 6) as a rationale for avoiding medical and pharmacologic treatment interventions.

In a similar vein, the New York group of Abend, Porder and Willick (1983) expressed sharp disagreement with Kernberg:

> Our conclusion that the term "borderline" does not refer to a specific diagnostic entity but to a diffuse and heterogeneous group of patients who are sicker than the more typical neurotic but not as severely disturbed as patients with psychosis is consistent with our view that

there is no specific etiological determinant in the development of borderline pathology. (p. 241)

Numerous other contradictory findings have been reported in
the literature. Palombo (1982) reviewed the concept of the borderline child. He raised questions about the generally held assumption
that a similarity exists between the dynamics of borderline children
and those of borderline adults, suggesting that no data are currently
available to substantiate such a view. Stone (1985) summarized the
borderline's plight by stating that among borderlines, one often sees
sex without love, or love without sex, or both sex and love with an
unsuitable partner. In other words sex and love remain unintegrated.
But Stone does not explain how this differs from the average
individual in our culture, whose inability to integrate sex and love
was described by Freud almost 100 years ago. McGlashan (1985),
comparing borderlines with schizophrenics, found that the borderlines had a somewhat better prognosis, but that outcome was highly
unpredictable, and premorbid functioning had little to do with their
illness. Greene, Rosenkrantz and Muth (1986) suggest that psychotherapy research should shift from signs and symptoms (such as
those of Kernberg and Gunderson) to direct studies of the therapeutic relationship, with a particular focus on countertransferential
dynamics. Finally mention may be made of the study by Zubenko,
George, Soloff and Schulz (1987), in which they found homosexuality
was 10 times more common among the men and six times more
common among the women with borderline personality disorder
than in the general population or in a depressed control group.

In the final section, a number of case presentations are included.
In a symposium held at the American Psychological Association in
1986 with Swenson, Handley, Hull, Lane and Sperling the emphasis
was on fusion with the early mother, which in transference became
fusion with the therapist. When this wish for fusion was satisfactorily
analyzed, the patient could enter into a more normal kind of life. The
last two papers highlight case material with children. While the same
dynamics are operative, they appear in different ways with different
children.

What is one to make of this voluminous body of literature on the
borderline? While many dynamic mechanisms are described, the
notion of a distinct entity that should be labeled "borderline" is not
borne out. All the papers point to persons who are seriously
disturbed, but not frankly psychotic, or who, if they are at times
psychotic, recover quickly.

Diagnosis has been anathema to many analysts. Anna Freud once wrote, "The descriptive nature of many current diagnostic categories runs counter to the essence of psychoanalytic thinking" (1965, p. 110). Menninger (1963) has shown how the conventional psychiatric nomenclature has changed but little over the centuries. And Laplanche and Pontalis (1973, p. 269) note that the attempt to define neurosis tends to become indistinguishable from psychoanalytic theory itself.

The innumerable attempts to define borderline all end up with the same conclusion: seriously disturbed, but not frankly psychotic, full of a variety of infantile mechanisms, harder to treat than the "more typical" neurotic, yet not as hard to treat as the overtly psychotic. Inevitably further research will have to take these findings as a point of departure for more careful investigation.

References

Abend, S. M., Porder, M. S., & Willick, M. S. (1983). *Borderline patients: Psychoanalytic perspectives.* New York: International Universities Press.

Abraham, K. (1924). A short study of the development of the libido, viewed in the light of mental disorders. In *Selected papers on psychoanalysis* (pp. 418–501). London: Hogarth, 1965.

Ackerman, N. (1958). *The psychodynamics of family life.* New York: Basic Books.

Adler, G. (1970). Valuing and devaluing in the psychotherapeutic process. *Archives of General Psychiatry, 22,* 454–461.

Adler, G. (1973). Hospital treatment of borderline patients. *American Journal of Psychiatry, 130,* 32–35.

Adler, G. (1974). Regression in psychotherapy: Disruptive or therapeutic? *International Journal of Psycho-Analytic Psychotherapy, 3,* 252–264.

Adler, G. (1975). The usefulness of the "borderline" concept in psychotherapy. In J. E. Mack (Ed.), *Borderline states in psychiatry* (pp. 29–40). New York: Grune & Stratton.

Ainsworth, M. D. S., Blehar, M. C., Waters, E., & Wall, S. (1978). *Patterns of attachment.* Hillsdale, NJ: Lawrence Erlbaum.

Akiskal, H. S. (1981). Subaffective disorders; dysthymic, cyclothymic and bipolar II disorders in the "borderline" realm. *Psychiatric Clinics of North America, 4,* 25–46.

Altman, L. L. (1977). Some vicissitudes of love. *Journal of the American Psychoanalytic Association, 25,* 35–52.

American Psychiatric Association. (1980). *Diagnostic and statistical manual of mental disorders* (3rd ed.). Washington, DC: APA.

Andrulonis, P. A., Glueck, B. C., Stroebel, C. F., et al. (1980). Organic brain dysfunction and the borderline syndrome. *Psychiatric Clinics of North America, 4,* 47–66.

Andrulonis, P. A., Vogel, N. G. (1984). Comparison of borderline subcategories to schizophrenic and affective disorders. *British Journal of Psychiatry, 144,* 358–363.

Apfelbaum, B. (1966). Ego psychology: A critique of the structural approach to psychoanalytic theory. *International Journal of Psycho-Analysis, 47,* 451–475.

Arlow, J. A. (1980). Object concept and object choice. *Psychoanalytic Quarterly, 49,* 109–133.

Aronson, T. H. (1985). Historical perspectives on the borderline concept: A review and critique. *Psychiatry, 48,* 209–222.

Atkin, S. (1974). A borderline case: Ego synthesis and cognition. *International Journal of Psycho-Analysis, 55,* 13–19.

Atkin, S. (1975). Ego synthesis and cognition in a borderline case. *Psychoanalytic Quarterly, 44,* 29–61.

Baldessarini, R. J. (1983). *Biomedical aspects of depression and its treatment.* Washington, DC: American Psychiatric Press.

Bannister, D. (1965). The rationale and clinical relevance of the repertory grid technique. *British Journal of Psychiatry, 111,* 977–982.

Barasch, A., Frances, A., Hurt, S., et al. (1985). Stability and distinctness of borderline personality disorder. *American Journal of Psychiatry, 142,* 1484–1486.

Baron, M. (1981). A diagnostic interview for schizotypal features. *Psychiatry Research, 4,* 213–228.

Barrash, J., Kroll, J., Carey, K., et al. (1983). Discriminating borderline disorder from other personality disorders: Cluster analysis of the Diagnostic Interview for Borderlines. *Archives of General Psychiatry, 40,* 1297–1302.

Basaglia, F. (1987). *Psychiatry inside out.* New York: Columbia University Press.

Beck, S. J. (1964). Symptom and trait in schizophrenia, *American Journal of Orthopsychiatry, 34,* 517–526.

Beckett, P. G. S., Robinson, D. B., Frazier, S. H., Steinhilber, R. M., Duncan, G. M., Estes, H. R., Litin, E. M., Gratton, R. T., Lorton, W. L., Williams, G. E., & Johnson, A. M. (1956). The significance of exogenous traumata in the genesis of schizophrenia. *Psychiatry, 19,* 137–142.

Behrends, R. S., & Blatt, S. J. (1985). Internalization and psychological development throughout the life cycle. *Psychoanalytic Study of the Child, 40,* 11–39.

Bell, J., Lycaki, H., Jones, D., et al. (1983). Effect of preexisting borderline personality disorder on clinical and EEG sleep correlates of depression. *Psychiatry Research, 9,* 115-123.

Bellak, L. (Ed.) (1979). *Disorders of the schizophrenic syndrome.* New York: Basic Books.

Bellak, L., & Hurvich, M. (1969). A systematic study of ego functions. *Journal of Nervous and Mental Disease, 148,* 569–585.

Bergeret, J. (1970). Les états limites. *Revue Française de Psychoanalyse, 34,* 605–633.

Bergeret, J. (1972). *Abrege de psychologie pathologique.* Paris: Masson & Cie.

Bergeret, J. (1975). *La dépression et les états limites.* Paris: Payot.

Bergmann, M. S. (1980). On the intrapsychic function of falling in love. *Psychoanalytic Quarterly, 49,* 56–77.

Bion, W. (1959). *Experiences in groups.* New York: Basic Books.

Birdwhistell, R. L. (1966). The American family. *Psychiatry, 29,* 204–212.

Bishop, E. R., & Holt, A. R. (1980). Pseudopsychosis: A re-examination of the concept of hysterical psychosis. *Comprehensive Psychiatry, 21,* 150–161.

Blatt, S. J., & Shichman, S. (1983). Two primary configurations of psychopathology. *Psychoanalysis and Contemporary Thought, 6,* 187–254.

Blum, H. (1972). Psychoanalytic understanding and psychotherapy of borderline regression. *International Journal of Psychoanalytic Psychotherapy, 1,* 46–60.

Blum, H. (1974). The borderline childhood of the Wolf-Man. *Journal of the American Psychoanalytic Association, 22,* 721–742.

Blum, H. (1986). Object inconstancy and paranoid conspiracy. In R. F. Lax, S. Bach, & J. A. Burland (Eds.), *Self and object constancy: Clinical and theoretical perspectives* (pp. 253–270). New York: Guildford Press.

Boisen, A. T. (1936). *The exploration of the inner world: A study of mental disorder and religious experience.* New York: Harpers.

Book, H. E., Sadavoy, J., & Silver, D. (1978). Staff countertransference to borderline patients on an inpatient unit. *American Journal of Psychotherapy, 32,* 521–532.

Boyer, L. (1971). Psychoanalytic technique in the treatment of certain characterological and schizophrenic disorders. *International Journal of Psycho-Analysis, 52,* 67–85.

Boyer, L., & Giovacchini, P. (1967). *Psychoanalytic treatment of characterological and schizophrenic disorders.* New York: Science House.

Bradley, S. J. (1979). The relationship of early maternal separation to borderline personality in children and adolescents: A pilot study. *American Journal of Psychiatry, 136,* 424–426.

Breggin, P. R. (1983). *Psychiatric drugs: Hazards to the brain.* New York: Springer.

Brinkley, J. R., Beitman, B. D., & Friedel, R. O. (1979). Low dose neuroleptic regimes in the treatment of borderline patients. *Archives of General Psychiatry, 36,* 319–326.

Brody, E. B. (1960). Borderline state, character disorder, and psychotic manifestations—Some conceptual formulations. *Psychiatry, 23,* 75–80.

Brown, L. J. (1980). Staff countertransference reactions in the hospital treatment of borderline patients. *Psychiatry, 43,* 333–345.

Buie, D., & Adler, G. (1972). The uses of confrontation with borderline patients. *International Journal of Psychoanalytic Psychotherapy, 1,* 90–108.

Buie, D., & Adler, G. (1982). Definitive treatment of the borderline personality. *International Journal of Psychoanalytic Psychotherapy, 9,* 51–87.

Burke, W. F., & Tansey, M. J. (1985). Projective identification and countertransference turmoil: Disruptions in the empathic process. *Contemporary Psychoanalysis, 21,* 372–402.

Calef, V., & Weinshel, E. M. (1979). The new psychoanalysis and psychoanalytic revisionism. *Psychoanalytic Quarterly, 48,* 470–491.

Carpenter, W. T., Jr., & Gunderson, J. G. (1977). Five-year follow-up comparison of borderline and schizophrenic patients. *Comprehensive Psychiatry, 18,* 567–571.

Carpenter, W. T., Jr., Gunderson, J. G., & Strauss, J. S. (1977). Considerations of the borderline syndrome: A longitudinal comparative study of borderline and schizophrenic patients. In P. Hartocollis (Ed.), *Borderline personality disorders.* New York: International Universities Press.

Carroll, B. J., Greden, J. T., Feinberg, M., et al. (1981). Neuroendocrine evaluation of depression in borderline patients. *Psychiatric Clinics of North America, 4,* 89–99.

Cary, G. (1972). The borderline condition: A structural-dynamic viewpoint. *Psychoanalytic Review, 59,* 33–54.

Charney, D. S., Nelson, J. C., & Quinlan, D. M. (1981). Personality traits and disorder in depression. *American Journal of Psychiatry, 138,* 1601–1604.

Chasseguet-Smirgel, J. (1976). Some thoughts on the ego ideal—A contribution to the study of the "illness of ideality." *Psychoanalytic Quarterly, 46,* 345–373.

Chessick, R. D. (1966). The psychotherapy of borderline patients. *American Journal of Psychotherapy, 20,* 600–614.

Chessick, R. D. (1971). Use of the couch in the psychotherapy of borderline patients. *Archives of General Psychiatry, 25,* 306–313.

Chethic, M. (1979). The borderline child. In J. D. Noshpitz (Ed.), *Basic handbook of child psychiatry* (Vol. 2). New York: Basic Books.

Cole, J. O., Salomon, M., Gunderson, J. G., et al. (1984). Drug therapy in borderline patients. *Comprehensive Psychiatry, 25,* 249–262.

Cole, J. O., Sunderland, P., III. (1982). The drug treatment of borderline patients. In L. Grinspoon (Ed.), *Psychiatry 1982: The American Psychiatric Association annual review.* Washington, DC: American Psychiatric Press.

Collum, J. M. (1972). Identity diffusion and the borderline maneuver. *Comprehensive Psychiatry, 13,* 179–184.

Conte, H. R., Plutchik, R., Karasu, T. B., et al. (1980). A self-report borderline scale: Discriminative validity and preliminary norms. *Journal of Nervous and Mental Disease, 168,* 428–435.

Coppolillo, H. P. (1967). Maturational aspects of the transitional phenomenon. *International Journal of Psycho-Analysis, 48,* 237–246.

Dahl, H. (1974). Discussion of O. Kernberg's paper, "Instincts, affects, and objects relations," at the meeting of the New York Psychoanalytic Society, October 15.

Dahl, H., Teller, V., Moss, D., & Trujillo, M. (1978). Countertransference examples of the syntactic expression of warded-off contents. *Psychoanalytic Quarterly, 47,* 339–363.

Deutsch, H. (1942). Some forms of emotional disturbance and their relationship to schizophrenia. *Psychoanalytic Quarterly, 11,* 301–321.

Deutsch, H. (1949). *Applied psychoanalysis: Selected objectives of psychotherapy.* New York: Grune & Stratton.

Dickes, R. (1974). The concepts of borderline states: An alternative proposal. *International Journal of Psychoanalytic Psychotherapy, 3,* 1–27.

Doane, J. A., West, K. L., Goldstein, M. J., Rodnick, E. H., & Jones, J. E. (1980). *Parental affective style and communication deviance as predictors of subsequent schizophrenia spectrum disorders in vulnerable adolescents.* Los Angeles: Department of Psychology, UCLA.

Dorpat, I. L. (1979). Is splitting a defense? *International Review of Psycho-Analysis, 6,* 105–113.

Duvocelle, A. (1971). L'état limite ou borderline personality organization. These pour le doctorat en medecine, Lille.

Ekstein R., & Wallerstein, J. (1954). Observations on the psychotherapy of borderline and psychotic children. *Psychoanalytic Study of the Child, 9,* 344–369.

Ekstein, R., & Wallerstein, J. (1956). Observations on the psychology of borderline and psychotic children. *Psychoanalytic Study of the Child, 11,* 303–311.

Emslie, G. J., & Rosenfeld, A. (1983). Incest reported by children and adolescents hospitalized for severe psychiatric problems. *American Journal of Psychiatry, 140,* 708–711.

Erikson, E. H. (1956). The problem of ego identity. *Journal of the American Psychoanalytic Association, 4,* 56–121.

Evans, A. L. (1976). Personality characteristics of child-abusing mothers. Unpublished PhD dissertation, Michigan State University.

Fast, I. (1974). Multiple identities in the borderline personality organization. *British Journal of Medical Psychology, 47,* 291–300.

Fast, I. (1975). Aspects of work style and work difficulty in borderline personalities. *International Journal of Psycho-Analysis, 56,* 397–403.

Fast, I., & Chethik, M. (1972). Some aspects of object relationships in borderline children. *International Journal of Psycho-Analysis, 53,* 479–485.

Federn, P. (1934). *Ego psychology and the psychoses.* New York: Basic Books, 1952.

Fenichel, O. (1945). *The psychoanalytic theory of neurosis.* New York: Norton.

Fine, R. (1979). *A history of psychoanalysis.* New York: Columbia University Press.

Fine, R. (1981). *The psychoanalytic vision.* New York: Free Press.

Fine, R. (1986). *Narcissism, the self and society.* New York: Columbia University Press.

Finkelhor, D. (1979). *Sexually victimized children.* New York: Free Press.

Fintzy, R. T. (1971). Vicissitudes of the transitional object in borderline children. *International Journal of Psycho-Analysis, 52,* 107–114.

Fisher, C. (1965). Psychoanalytic implications of recent research on sleep and dreaming. *Journal of the American Psychoanalytic Association, 13,* 197–303.

Fleck, S. (1966). An approach to family pathology. *Comprehensive Psychiatry, 7,* 307–320.

Freud, A. (1936). *The ego and the mechanisms of defense.* New York: International Universities Press.

Freud, A. (1963). The concept of developmental lines. *Psychoanalytic Study of the Child, 18,* 245–265.

Freud, A. (1965). *Normality and pathology in childhood.* New York: International Universities Press.

Freud, S. (1913). Further recommendations in the technique of psycho-analysis. On beginning the treatment. The question of the first communication. The dynamics of the cure. *Collected Papers, 2,* 342–365. London: Hogarth Press, 1946.

Freud, S. (1914). From the history of an infantile neurosis. *Standard Edition, 18,* 1–122.

Freud, S. (1915). Papers on Technique. Observations on transference love. *Standard Edition, 12,* 157–176. London: Hogarth.

Freud, S. (1922). Some neurotic mechanisms in jealousy, paranoia, and homosexuality. *Standard Edition, 18,* 223–232.

Freud, S. (1924). Neurosis and psychosis. *Standard Edition, 19,* 149–156.

Freud, S. (1924). The loss of reality in neurosis and psychosis. *Collected Papers, 2,* 277–282. London: Hogarth Press, 1946.

Freud, S. (1930). Civilization and its discontents. *Standard Edition, 21,* 59–148.

Freud, S. (1937). Analysis terminable and interminable. *Standard Edition, 23,* 209–254.

Freud, S. (1940). Splitting of the ego in the process of defense. *Standard*

Edition, 23, 275–278.

Friedman, H. J. (1970). Dr. Friedman replies (Correspondence). *American Journal of Psychiatry, 126,* 1677.

Friedman, H. J. (1975). Psychotherapy of borderline patients: The influence of theory on technique. *American Journal of Psychiatry, 132,* 1048–1052.

Friedman, R. C. (1983). Review of "Homosexuality" by C. W. Socarides. *Journal of the American Psychoanalytic Association, 31,* 316–323.

Friedman, R. C., Aronoff, M. S., Clarkin, J. F., et al. (1983). History of suicidal behavior in depressed borderline patients. *American Journal of Psychiatry, 140,* 1023–1026.

Frieswyk, S. H., Allen, J. G., Colson, D. B., et al. (1986). Therapeutic alliance: Its place as a process and outcome variable in dynamic psychotherapy research. *Journal of Consulting and Clinical Psychology, 54,* 32–38.

Frijling-Schreuder, E. C. (1969). Borderline states in children. *Psychoanalytic Study of the Child, 24,* 307–327.

Frosch, J. (1964). The psychotic character: Clinical psychiatric considerations. *Psychoanalytic Quarterly, 38,* 81–96.

Frosch, J. (1967). Severe regressive states during analysis: Introduction. *Journal of the American Psychoanalytic Association, 15,* 491–507.

Frosch, J. (1967). Severe regressive states during analysis: Summary. *Journal of the American Psychoanalytic Association, 15,* 606–625.

Frosch, J. (1970). Psychoanalytic considerations of the psychotic character. *Journal of the American Psychoanalytic Association, 18,* 24–50.

Frosch, J. (1971). Technique in regard to some specific ego defects in the treatment of borderline patients. *Psychoanalytic Quarterly, 45,* 216–220.

Frosch, J. (1983). *The psychotic process.* New York: International Universities Press.

Garbutt, J. C., Loosen, P. T., Tipermas, A., et al. (1983). The TRH test in patients with borderline personality disorder. *Psychiatry Research, 9,* 107–113.

Gardiner, M. (Ed.) (1971). *The Wolf-Man.* New York: Basic Books.

Gaviria, M., Flaherty, J., & Val, E. (1982). A comparison of bipolar patients with and without a borderline personality disorder. *Psychiatric Journal of the University of Ottawa, 7,* 190–195.

Gedo, J. E., & Goldberg, A. (1973). *Models of the mind: A psychoanalytic theory.* Chicago: University of Chicago Press.

Geleerd, E. (1958). Borderline states in childhood and adolescence. *Psychoanalytic Study of the Child, 13,* 279–295.

Geleerd, E. (1958). Borderline states. *Psychoanalytic Study of the Child, 15,* 19–41.

Gershon, E. S., Bunney, W. E., Leckman, J. F., et al. (1976). The inheritance of affective disorders: A review of data and hypotheses. *Behavior and Genetics, 6,* 227–261.

Gill, M. M. (1963). *Topography and systems in psychoanalytic theory.* New York: International Universities Press.

Giovacchini, P. L. (1965). Transference, incorporation and synthesis. *International Journal of Psychoanalysis, 46,* 287–296.

Giovacchini, P. L. (1973). Character disorders: with special reference to the borderline state. *International Journal of Psychoanalytic Psychotherapy, 2,* 7–36.

Giovacchini, P. L. (1976). Symbiosis and intimacy. *International Journal of Psychoanalytic Psychotherapy, 5,* 413–436.

Glover, E. (1932). A psycho-analytical approach to the classification of mental disorders. *Journal of Mental Science, 78,* 819–842.

Glover, E. (1955). *The technique of psychoanalysis.* New York: Basic Books.

Goldfarb, W. (1955). Emotional and intellectual consequences of psychological deprivation in infancy. In P. H. Hoch & J. Zubin (Eds.), *Psychopathology of childhood.* New York: Grune & Stratton.

Gossett, J. T., Lewis, J. M., & Barnhard, F. D. (1983). *To find a way: The outcome of hospital treatment of disturbed adolescents.* New York: Brunner/Mazel.

Green, A. (1972). The borderline concept. In P. Hartocollis (Ed.), *Borderline personality disorders.* New York: International Universities Press.

Greene, L. R. (1983). The patient-staff community meeting as therapeutic agent for borderline personality disorders. In L. Wolberg & M. Aronson (Eds.), *Group and family therapy 1982.* New York: Brunner/Mazel.

Greene, L. R., Rosenkrantz, J., & Muth, D. Y. (1985). Splitting dynamics, self-representations and boundary phenomena in the group psychotherapy of borderline personality disorders. *Psychiatry, 48,* 234–245.

Greenson, R. (1970). The unique patient-therapist relationship in borderline patients. Presented at the annual meeting of the American Psychiatric Association.

Grinberg, L. (1979). Countertransference and projective counter-identification. *Contemporary Psychoanalysis, 15,* 226–247.

Grinker, R. R. (1979). Diagnosis of borderlines: A discussion. *Schizophrenia Bulletin, 5,* 47–52.

Grinker, R. R., & Holzman, P. S. (1973). Schizophrenic pathology in young adults. *Archives of General Psychiatry, 28,* 168–175.

Grinker, R. R., & Werble, B. (1977). *The borderline patient.* New York: Jason Aronson.

Grinker, R., Sr., Werble, B., & Drye, R. (1968). *The borderline syndrome.* New York: Basic Books.

Grotstein, J. (1981). *Splitting and projective identification.* New York: Jason Aronson.

Gunderson, J. G. (1974). The influence of theoretical model of schizophrenia on treatment practice. *Journal of the American Psychoanalytic Association, 22,* 182–199.

Gunderson, J. G. (1977). Characteristics of borderlines. In P. Hartocollis (Ed.), *Borderline personality disorders.* New York: International Universities Press.

Gunderson, J. G. (1982). Empirical studies of the borderline diagnosis. In L. Grinspoon (Ed.), *Psychiatry 1982: The American Psychiatric Association annual review.* Washington, DC: American Psychiatric Press.

Gunderson, J. G. (1984). *Borderline personality disorder.* Washington, DC: American Psychiatric Press.

Gunderson, J. G., Carpenter, W. T., Jr., & Strauss, J. S. (1975). Borderline and schizophrenic patients: A comparative study. *American Journal of Psychiatry, 132,* 1259–1264.

Gunderson, J. G., & Kolb, J. E. (1976). Diagnosing borderlines: A semi-structured interview. Presented at the 129th annual meeting of the American Psychiatric Association, Miami Beach, FL, May 10–14.

Gunderson, J. G., & Kolb, J. E. (1978). Discriminating features of borderline patients. *American Journal of Psychiatry, 135,* 792–796.

Gunderson, J. G., Kolb, J. E., & Austin, V. (1981). The diagnostic interview for borderline patients. *American Journal of Psychiatry, 138,* 896–903.

Gunderson, J. G., Siever, L. J., & Spaulding, E. (1983). The search for a schizotype: Crossing the border again. *Archives of General Psychiatry, 40,* 15–22.

Gunderson, J. G., & Singer, M. T. (1975). Defining borderline patients: An overview. *American Journal of Psychiatry, 132,* 1–10.

Guze, S. B. (1975). Differential diagnosis of the borderline personality syndrome. In J. E. Mack (Ed.), *Borderline states in psychiatry* (pp. 69–74). New York: Grune & Stratton.

Hamburg, D., et al. (1967). Report of the ad hoc committee on central fact-gathering data of the American Psychoanalytic Association. *Journal of the American Psychoanalytic Association, 15,* 841–861.

Handley, R. B. (1989). Therapist-patient separations: Fusional attachment phenomena in a borderline personality. In R. Fine & J. S. Stroan (Eds.), *Current and historical perspectives on the borderline patient.* New York: Brunner/Mazel.

Hartley, D. E., & Strupp, H. H. (1983). The therapeutic alliance: Its relationship to outcome in brief psychotherapy. In J. Masling (Ed.), *Empirical studies of psychoanalytic theories.* New York: Analytic Press.

Hartmann, H. (1939). *Ego psychology and the problem of adaptation.* New York: International Universities Press.

Hartmann, H. (1964). *Essays on ego psychology.* New York: International Universities Press.

Hartocollis, P. (1977). Affects in borderline disorders. In P. Hartocollis (Ed.), *Borderline personality disorders.* New York: International Universities Press.

Hay, G. G. (1970). Dysmorphophobia. *British Journal of Psychiatry, 116,* 399–406.

Heimann, P. (1966). Comment on Dr. Kernberg's paper. *International Journal of Psychoanalysis, 47,* 254–260.

Hirschfeld, R. M. A., Klerman, G. L., Clayton, P. J., et al. (1983). Assessing personality: Effects of the depressive state on trait measurement. *American Journal of Psychiatry, 140,* 695–699.

Hoch, P. H., & Cattell, J. P. (1959). The diagnosis of pseudoneurotic schizophrenia. *Psychiatric Quarterly, 33,* 17–43.

Hoch, P. H., Cattell, J. P., Strahl, M. O., & Pennes, H. (1962). The course and outcome of pseudoneurotic schizophrenia. *American Journal of Psychiatry, 119,* 106–115.

Hoch, P. H., & Polatin, P. (1949). Pseudoneurotic forms of schizophrenia. *Psychiatric Quarterly, 23,* 248–276.

Hoffer, W. (1950). Development of the body ego. *Psychoanalytic Study of the Child, 5,* 18–23.

Holzman, P. S. (1976). The future of psychoanalysis and its institutes. *Psychoanalytic Quarterly, 45,* 250–273.

Horner, A. J. (1975). Stages and processes in the development of early object relations and their associated pathologies. *International Review of Psychoanalysis, 2,* 95–105.

Horwitz, L. (1983). Projective identification in dyads and groups. *Interna-*

tional Journal of Group Psychotherapy, 33, 259–79.

Horwitz, L. (1985). Divergent views on the treatment of borderline patients. *Bulletin of the Menninger Clinic, 49,* 525–545.

Hull, J. W., & Lane, R. C. (1989). Bodily representation of conflicts around fusion and individuation in borderlines. In R. Fine & H. S. Strean (Eds.), *Current and historical perspectives on the borderline patient.* New York: Brunner/Mazel.

Hurt, S., Hyler, S., Frances, A., et al. (1984). Assessing borderline personality disorder with self-report, clinical interview, or semistructured interview. *American Journal of Psychiatry, 141,* 1228–1231.

Hurvich, M. (1970). On the concept of reality testing. *International Journal of Psychoanalysis, 51,* 299–312.

Isakower, O. (1938) A contribution to the psychopathology of phenomena associated with falling asleep. *International Journal of Psychoanalysis, 19,* 331–345.

Jacobson, E. (1954). Psychotic identifications. In *Depression* (pp. 242–263). New York: International Universities Press, 1971.

Jacobson, E. (1964). *The self and object world.* New York: International Universities Press.

Jacobson, E. (1975). Comment in the issue of *Psychotherapy and Social Science Review* (*9,* 4, March 14), announcing the publication of O. Kernberg's *Borderline conditions and pathological narcissism.*

Jones, E. (1929). Psychoanalysis and psychiatry. In *Collected papers* (5th ed.). London: Baillière, Tindall and Cox, 1948.

Kafka, E. (1971) On the development of the experience of mental self, the bodily self, and self consciousness. *Psychoanalytic Study of the Child, 26,* 217–237.

Karon, B., & VandenBos, G. (1981). *Psychotherapy of schizophrenia: The treatment of choice.* New York: Jason Aronson.

Kasl, S. V., & Mahl, G. F. (1965). Disturbance and hesitation in speech. *Journal of Personality and Social Psychology, 1,* 425–433.

Keiser, S. (1958). Disturbances in abstract thinking and body-image formation. *Journal of the American Psychoanalytic Association, 6,* 628–652.

Kernberg, O. F. (1966). Structural derivatives of object relationships. *International Journal of Psychoanalysis, 47,* 236–253.

Kernberg, O. F. (1967). Borderline personality organization. *Journal of the American Psychoanalytic Association, 15,* 641–685.

Kernberg, O. F. (1968). The treatment of patients with borderline personality organization. *International Journal of Psychoanalysis, 49,* 600–619.

Kernberg, O. F. (1970). Factors in the psychoanalytic treatment of narcissistic personalities. *Journal of the American Psychoanalytic Association, 18,* 51–85.

Kernberg, O. F. (1970). A psychoanalytic classification of character pathology. *Journal of the American Psychoanalytic Association, 18,* 800–802.

Kernberg, O. F. (1971). Prognostic considerations regarding borderline personality organization. *Journal of the American Psychoanalytic Association, 19,* 595–635.

Kernberg, O. F. (1974). Further contributions to the treatment of narcissistic personalities. *International Journal of Psychoanalysis, 55,* 215–240.

Kernberg, O. F. (1975). *Borderline conditions and pathological narcissism.* New York: Jason Aronson.

Kernberg, O. F. (1976). *Object relations theory and clinical psychoanalysis.* New York: Jason Aronson.

Kernberg, O. F. (1976). Technical considerations in the treatment of borderline personality organization. *Journal of the American Psychoanalytic Association, 24,* 795–829.

Kernberg, O. F. (1977). The structural diagnosis of borderline personality organization. In P. Hartocollis (Ed.), *Borderline personality disorders.* New York: International Universities Press.

Kernberg, O. F. (1979). Two reviews of the literature on borderlines: An assessment. *Schizophrenia Bulletin, 5,* 53–58.

Kernberg, O. F. (1980). *Internal world and external reality.* New York: Jason Aronson.

Kernberg, O. F. (1984). *The severe personality disorders.* New Haven, CT: Yale University Press.

Kernberg, O. F. (1986). Institutional problems of psychoanalytic education. *Journal of the American Psychoanalytic Association, 34,* 799–834.

Kernberg, O. F., Burstein, E., Coyne, L., Appelbaum, A., Horwitz, L., & Voth, H. (1972). Psychotherapy and psychoanalysis: Final report of the Menninger Foundation's psychotherapy research project. *Bulletin of the Menninger Clinic, 36,* 1/2.

Kernberg, P. (1983). Borderline conditions: Childhood and adolescent aspects. In K. Robson (Ed.), *The borderline child.* New York: McGraw-Hill.

Kernberg, P. (1983). Issues in the psychotherapy of borderline conditions in children. In K. Robson (Ed.), *The borderline child.* New York: McGraw-Hill.

Kety, S. S. (1978). The biological bases of mental illness. In Bernstein (Ed.), *Clinical psychopharmacology.* Littleton, MA: PSG.

Kety, S. S., Rosenthal, D. Wender, P. H., et al. (1968). The types and prevalence of mental illness in the biological and adoptive families of adopted schizophrenics. In D. Rosenthal & S. S. Kety (Eds.), *The transmission of schizophrenia.* New York: Pergamon Press.

Khan, M., & Masud, R. (1964). Ego distortion, cumulative trauma, and the role of reconstruction in the analytic situation. *International Journal of Psycho-Analysis, 45,* 272–279.

Khan, M., & Masud, R. (1969). On symbiotic omnipotence. In J. A. Lindon (Ed.), *The psychoanalytic forum.* New York: Science House.

Khouri, P., Haier, R., Rieder, R. O., et al. (1980). A symptom schedule for the diagnosis of borderline schizophrenia: A first report. *British Journal of Psychiatry, 137,* 140–147.

Klein, D. F. (1975). Psychopharmacology and the borderline patient. In J. E. Mack (Ed.), *Borderline states in psychiatry* (pp. 75-91). New York: Grune & Stratton.

Klein, D. F. (1977). Psychopharmacological treatment and delineation of borderline disorders. In P. Hartocollis (Ed.), *Borderline personality disorders.* New York: International Universities Press.

Klein, M. (1946). Notes on some schizoid mechanisms. *International Journal of Psychoanalysis, 27,* 99–100.

Klein, M. (1946–1963). *Envy and gratitude and other works.* New York: Delacorte Press/Seymour Lawrence, 1975.

Knight R. P. (1953). Borderline states. *Bulletin of the Menninger Clinic, 17,* 1–12.

Knight, R. P. (1953). Borderline states. In *Psychoanalytic psychiatry and psychology* (pp. 97–109). New York: International Universities Press.

Koenigsberg, H. W., Kernberg, O. F., Haas, G., et al. (1985). Development of a scale for measuring techniques in the psychotherapy of borderline patients. *Journal of Nervous and Mental Disease, 173,* 424–431.

Koenigsberg, H. W., Kernberg, O. F., & Schomer, J. (1982). Diagnosing borderline conditions in an outpatient setting. *Archives of General Psychiatry, 40,* 49–53.

Kohut, H. (1971). *The analysis of the self.* New York: International Universities Press.

Kolb, J. E., & Gunderson, J. G. (1978). Diagnosing borderlines with a semi-standard interview. Presented at the 131st annual meeting of the American Psychiatric Association, Atlanta, GA, May 8–12.

Kolb, J. E., & Gunderson, J. G. (1980). Diagnosing borderline patients with a semistructured interview. *Archives of General Psychiatry, 37,* 37–41.

Kolb, L. C., & Brodie, H. K. H. (1982). *Modern clinical psychiatry.* Philadelphia: W. B. Saunders.

Koupernik, C. (1982). Psychopathologie de l'adolescence. In C. Koupernik, H. Loo, & E. Zarifian (Eds.), *Précis de psychiatrie.* Paris: Flammarion.

Kraepelin, E. (1917). *One hundred years of psychiatry.* New York: Citadel Press.

Kraepelin, E. (1921). *Manic-depressive insanity and paranoia.* Edinburgh: E. & S. Livingstone.

Kroll, J., Carley, K., Sines, L., et al. (1982). Are there borderlines in Britain? A cross-validation of US findings. *Archives of General Psychiatry, 39,* 60–63.

Kroll, J., Sines, L., Martin, K., et al. (1981). Borderline personality disorder. *Archives of General Psychiatry, 38,* 1021–1026.

Laplanche, J., & Pontalis, J. B. (1973). *The language of psychoanalysis.* New York: Norton.

Laufer, M. (1976). The central masturbation fantasy, the final sexual organization, and adolescence. *Psychoanalytic Study of the Child, 31,* 297–316.

Lehmann, H. E. (1975). Psychopharmacological treatment of schizophrenia. In A. M. Freedman, H. I. Kaplan & B. J. Saddock (Eds.), *Comprehensive textbook of psychiatry* (pp. 890–923). Baltimore: Williams & Wilkins.

Leone, N. F. (1982). Response of borderline patients to loxapine and chlorpromazine. *Journal of Clinical Psychiatry, 43,* 148–150.

Lerner, H. D., & St. Peter, S. (1984). Patterns of object relations in neurotic, borderline and schizophrenic patients. *Psychiatry, 47,* 77–92.

Lerner, H. D., Sugarman, A., & Barbour, C. (1985). Patterns of ego boundary disturbance in neurotic, borderline and schizophrenic patients. *Psychoanalytic Psychology, 2,* 47–66.

Levy, D. M. (1943). *Maternal overprotection.* New York: Columbia University Press.

Lichtenstein, H. (1964). The role of narcissism in the emergence and maintenance of a primary identity. *International Journal of Psychoanalysis, 45,* 49–56.

Lichtenstein, H. (1965). Towards a metapsychological definition of the concept of self. *International Journal of Psychoanalysis, 46,* 117–128.

Lidz, T. (1973). *The origin and treatment of schizophrenic disorders.* New York: Basic Books.

Lidz, T., Fleck, S., & Cornelison, A. R. (1965). *Schizophrenia and the family.* New York: International Universities Press.

Liebowitz, M. R., & Klein, D. G. (1981). Interrelationship of hysteroid dysphoria and borderline personality disorder. *Psychiatric Clinics of North America, 4,* 67–87.

Loewald, H. W. (1960). On the therapeutic action of psychoanalysis. *International Journal of Psycho-Analysis, 41,* 16–33.

Loewald, H. W. (1971). On motivation and instinct theory. *Psychoanalytic Study of the Child, 26,* 91–128.

Loosen, P. T., & Prange, A. J., Jr. (1982). Serum thyrotropin response to thyrotropin-releasing hormone in psychiatric patients: A review. *American Journal of Psychiatry, 139,* 405–414.

Loranger, A. W., Oldham, J. M., Russakoff, L. M., et al. (1984). Structured interviews and borderline personality disorder. *Archives of General Psychiatry, 41,* 565–568.

Loranger, A. W., Oldham, J. M., & Tulis, E. (1982). Familial transmission of DSM-III borderline personality disorder. *Archives of General Psychiatry, 39,* 795–799.

Mahler, M. S. (1952). On child psychoses and schizophrenia. *Psychoanalytic Study of the Child, 7,* 286–305.

Mahler, M. S. (1967). On human symbiosis and the vicissitudes of individuation. *Journal of the American Psychoanalytic Association, 15,* 740–763.

Mahler, M. S. (1968). *On human symbiosis and the vicissitudes of individuation.* New York: International Universities Press.

Mahler, M. S. (1971). A study of separation-individuation process and its possible applications to borderline phenomena. *Psychoanalytic Study of the Child, 26,* 403–424.

Mahler, M. S. (1972). The rapprochement subphase of the separation-individuation process. *Psychoanalytic Quarterly, 41,* 487–506.

Mahler, M. S., & Kaplan, D. W. (1977). *Developmental aspects in the assessment of narcissistic and so-called borderline personalities.* New York: International Universities Press.

Mahler, M. S., Pine, F., & Bergman, A. (1975). *The psychological birth of the human infant.* New York: Basic Books.

Main, T. F. (1957). The ailment. *British Journal of Medical Psychology, 30,* 129–145.

Malitz, S., Wilkins, B., & Esecover, H. (1962). A comparison of drug-induced hallucinations with those seen in spontaneously occurring psychosis. In L. J. West (Ed.), *Hallucinations.* New York: Grune & Stratton.

Maltsberger, J. T., & Buie, D. H. (1974). Countertransference hate in the treatment of suicidal patients. *Archives of General Psychiatry, 30,* 625–633.

Marcus, J. (1963). Borderline states in childhood. *Journal of Childhood Psychology and Psychiatry, 4,* 207–218.

Masterson, J. F. (1972). *Treatment of the borderline adolescent: A developmental approach.* New York: Wiley.

Masterson, J. F. (1976). *Psychotherapy of the borderline adult.* New York: Brunner/Mazel.

Masterson, J. F. (1978). The borderline adult: Therapeutic alliance and transference. *American Journal of Psychiatry, 135,* 437–441.

Masterson, J. F. (1978). *New perspectives on the psychotherapy of the borderline adult.* New York: Brunner/Mazel.

Masterson, J. F. (1980). *From borderline adolescent to functioning adult: The test of time.* New York: Brunner/Mazel.

Masterson, J. F. (1981). *The narcissistic and borderline disorders.* New York: Brunner/Mazel.

Masterson, J. F., & Rinsley, D. B. (1975). The borderline syndrome: The role of the mother in the genesis and psychic structure of the borderline personality. *International Journal of Psycho-Analysis, 56,* 163–177.

McDougall, J. (1985). *Theaters of the mind.* New York: Basic Books.

McGinniss, J. (1983). *Fatal vision.* New York: G. P. Putnam's Sons.

McGlashan, T. H. (1983). The borderline syndrome, I: Testing three diagnostic systems for borderline. *Archives of General Psychiatry, 40,* 1311–1318.

McGlashan, T. H. (1983). The borderline syndrome, II: Is it a variant of schizophrenia or affective disorder? *Archives of General Psychiatry, 40,* 1319–1323.

McGlashan, T. H. (1984). The Chestnut Lodge follow-up study, II: Long-term outcome of schizophrenia and the affective disorders. *Archives of General Psychiatry, 41,* 586–601.

McGlashan, T. H. (1985). The prediction of outcome in chronic schizophrenia: Part IV of the Chestnut Lodge follow-up study. *Archives of General Psychiatry, 43,* 167–176.

McGlashan, T. H. (Ed.) (1985). *The borderline: Current empirical research.* Washington, DC: American Psychiatric Press.

McGlashan, T. H. (1985). The prediction of outcome in borderline personality disorder: Part V of the Chestnut Lodge follow-up study. In T. H. McGlashan (Ed.), *The borderline: Current empirical research.* Washington, DC: American Psychiatric Press.

McGlashan, T. H. (1986). The Chestnut Lodge follow-up study: III. Long-term outcome of borderline personalities. *Archives of General Psychiatry, 43,* 20–30.

McNamara, E., Reynolds, D. F., III, Soloff, P. H., et al. (1984). EEG sleep evaluation of depression in borderline patients. *American Journal of Psychiatry, 141,* 182–186.

Meissner, W. W. (1971). Notes on identification. II. Clarification of related concepts. *Psychoanalytic Quarterly, 40,* 277–302.

Meissner, W. W. (1976). New horizons in metapsychology: View and review (panel report). *Journal of the American Psychoanalytic Association, 24,* 161–180.

Meissner, W. W. (1978). *The paranoid process.* New York: Jason Aronson.

Meehl, P. E. (1964). *Manual for use with checklist of schizotypic signs.* Minneapolis: Psychiatric Research Unit, University of Minnesota Medical School.

Melnick, B., & Hurley, J. R. (1969). Distinctive personality attributes of child-abusing mothers. *Journal of Consulting Clinical Psychology, 33,* 746–749.

Menninger, K. (1963). *The vital balance.* New York: Viking.

Meyer, R. G., & Karon, B. P. (1967). The schizophrenogenic mother concept and the TAT. *Psychiatry, 30,*173–179.

Meza, C. (1970). Anger—A key to the borderline patient (Correspondence). *American Journal of Psychiatry, 126,* 1676–1677.

Meza, C. (1970) *El colérico* (borderline). Mexico: Editorial Joaquín Mortiz.

Mezzich, J. E., Coffman, G. A., & Goodpastor, S. M. (1982). A format for DSM-III diagnostic formulation: Experience with 1,111 consecutive patients. *American Journal of Psychiatry, 139,* 591–596.

Miller, W. R. (1940). The relationship between early schizophrenia and the neuroses. *American Journal of Psychiatry, 96,* 889–896.

Mischler, E., & Waxler, N. (1966). Family interaction processes and schizophrenia. *International Journal of Psychiatry, 2,* 375–428.

Mitchell, K. M. (1968). An analysis of the schizophrenic mother concept by means of the TAT. *Journal of Abnormal Psychology, 73,* 571–574.

Mitchell, K. M. (1969). Concept of "pathogenesis" in parents of schizophrenic and normal children. *Journal of Abnormal Psychology, 74,* 423–424.

Modell, A. H. (1961). Denial and the sense of separateness. *Journal of the American Psychoanalytic Association, 9,* 533–547.

Modell, A. H. (1963). Primitive object-relationships and the predisposition to schizophrenia. *International Journal of Psychoanalysis, 44,* 282–292.

Modell, A. H. (1968). *Object love and reality.* New York: International Universities Press.

Modell, A. H. (1975). A narcissistic defense against affects and the illusion of self-sufficiency. *International Journal of Psycho-Analysis, 56,* 275–282.

Moore, B. E. (1975). Toward a clarification of the concept of narcissism. *Psychoanalytic Study of the Child, 30,* 243–276.

Moore, T. V. (1929–30). The empirical determination of certain syndromes underlying praecox and manic-depressive psychoses. *American Journal of Psychiatry, 86,* 719–738.

Morselli, E. (1866). Sulla dismorfofobia e sulla tafefobia. *Boll. Acad. della Scienze Med. di Genova, 6,* 110.

Mosher, L. R. (1982). Italy's revolutionary mental health law: Assessment. *American Journal of Psychiatry, 38,* 199–203.

Mosher, L. R. (1987). Review of Warner: Recovery from schizophrenia. *American journal of Psychiatry, 144,* 956–957.

Mosher, L. R., & Gunderson, J. G. (1973). Special report on schizophrenia: 1972. *Schizophrenia Bulletin, 1,* 10–52.

Murray, J. M. (1964). Narcissism and the ego ideal. *Journal of the American Psychoanalytic Association, 12,* 477–528.

Nameche, G., & Ricks, D. (1966). Life patterns of children who became adult schizophrenics. Presented at the annual meeting of the American Orthopsychiatric Association, San Francisco, April 16.

Nelson, H., Tennen, H., Tasman, A., et al. (1985). Comparison of three systems for diagnosing borderline personality disorder. *American Journal of Psychiatry, 142,* 855–858.

Nemetz, S. J. (1979) Panel on Conceptualizing the Nature of the Therapeutic Action of Psychoanalytic Psychotherapy. *Journal of the American Psychiatric Association, 27,* 127–144.

Nuetzel, E. J. (1985). DSM-III and the use of the term borderline. *Bulletin of the*

Menninger Clinic, 49, 124–134.

Nicholi, A. M. (Ed.) (1978). *Harvard guide to modern psychiatry.* Boston: Harvard University Press.

Nichols, N. (1970). The relationship between degree of maternal pathogenicity and severity of ego impairment in schizophrenic offspring. PhD dissertation, University of Michigan.

Ornstein, P. (1974). On narcissism: Beyond the introduction, highlights of Heinz Kohut's contributions to the psychoanalytic treatment of narcissistic personality disorders. *Annual of Psychoanalysis, 2,* 127–149.

Osgood, C. E., Suci, G. J., & Tannenbaum, P. H. (1957). *The measurement of meaning.* Urbana: University of Illinois Press.

Palombo, J. (1979). Perceptual deficits and self-esteem in adolescence. *Clinical Social Work Journal, 7,* 34–61.

Paz, C. (1969). Reflexiones técnicas sobre el proceso analítico en los psicóticos fronterizos. *Revista de Psicoanálisis, 26,* 571–630.

Perry, H. S. (1982). *Psychiatrists of America.* Cambridge, MA: Belknap Press.

Perry, J. C., & Klerman, G. L. (1978). The borderline patient: A comparative analysis of four sets of diagnostic criteria. *Archives of General Psychiatry, 35,* 141–150.

Perry, J. C., & Klerman, G. L. (1980). Clinical features of the borderline personality disorder. *American Journal of Psychiatry, 137,* 165–173.

Pfister, O. (1931). Donjuanismus und Dirnetum. *Die Liebe vor der Ehe und ihre Fehlentwicklung, Almanach, 13,* 190–200.

Pine, F. (1974). The concept of "borderline" in children: A clinical essay. *Psychoanalytic Study of the Child, 29,* 241–368.

Pines, M. (1978). Group analytic psychotherapy of the borderline patient. *Group Analysis, 11,* 115–126.

Pious, W. L. (1950). Obsessive-compulsive symptoms in an incipient schizophrenic. *Psychoanalytic Quarterly, 19,* 327–351.

Pope, H. G., Jonas, J. M., Hudson, J. I., et al (1983). The validity of DSM-III borderline personality disorder. *Archives of General Psychiatry, 40,* 23–30.

Porder, M. S., Abend, S. M., & Willick, M. S. (1983). *Borderline patients.* New York: International Universities Press.

Pruyser, P. W. (1975). What splits in "splitting"? *Bulletin of the Menninger Clinic, 39,* 1–46.

Racker, H. (1968). *Transference and countertransference.* New York: International Universities Press.

Raifman, I. (1984). Diagnostic issues in borderline disorders. *Psychoanalytic Psychology, 1,* 301–318.

Rangell, L. (1955). The borderline case (panel report). *Journal of the American Psychoanalytic Association, 3,* 285–298.

Rapaport, D. (1958). *The structure of psychoanalytic theory: A systematizing attempt.* New York: International Universities Press.

Rapaport, D. (1967). *The collected papers of David Rapaport.* New York: Basic Books.

Rapaport, D., Gill, M., & Schafer, R. (1945 & 1946). *Diagnostic psychological testing* (2 Vols.). Chicago: Yearbook Publishers.

Reich, A. (1953). Narcissistic object choice in women. *Journal of the American Psychoanalytic Association, 1,* 22–44.

Reiser, D. E., & Levenson, H. (1984). Abuses of the borderline diagnosis: A clinical problem with teaching opportunities. *American Journal of Psychiatry, 141,* 1528–1532.

Rennie, T. A. C., et al. (1962). *Mental health in the metropolis: The midtown study.* New York: McGraw-Hill.

Rickman, J. (1928). *The development of the psycho-analytical theory of the psychoses, 1893–1926.* London: Baillière, Tindall & Cox.

Ricoeur, P. (1970). *Freud and philosophy: An essay on interpretation.* New Haven, CT: Yale University Press.

Rinsley, D. B. (1982). *Borderline and other self disorders.* New York: Jason Aronson.

Robards, J. (1980). *The powers of psychiatry.* Boston: Houghton-Mifflin.

Robbins, L. L. (1956). A contribution to the psychological understanding of the character of Don Juan. *Bulletin of the Menninger Clinic, 20,* 166–180.

Robbins, L. L. (1956). The borderline case (panel report). *Journal of the American Psychoanalytic Association, 4,* 550–562.

Robbins, M. D. (1976). Borderline personality organization: The need for a new theory. *Journal of the American Psychoanalytic Association, 24,* 831–853.

Rochlin, G. (1973). *Man's aggression: The defense of the self.* Boston: Gambit.

Roheim, H. (1932). Psychoanalysis of primitive cultural types. *International Journal of Psycho-Analysis, 13,* 1–224.

Roiphe, H., & Galenson, E. (1986). Maternal depression, separation, and a failure in the development of object constancy. In R. F. Lax, S. Bach & J. A. Burland (Eds.), *Self and object constancy: Clinical and theoretical perspectives* (pp. 304–323). New York: Guildford Press.

Rosenfeld, D. (1984). Hypochondrias, somatic delusion and body scheme in psychoanalytic practice. *International Journal of Psycho-Analysis, 65,* 377–387.

Rosenfeld, H. (1965). *Psychotic states.* London: Hogarth Press.

Rosenfeld, S. K. (1965). Some thoughts on the technical handling of borderline children. *Psychoanalytic Study of the Child, 20,* 495–517.

Rosenfeld, S. K. (1975). Some reflections arising from the treatment of a traumatized borderline child. *Studies in child analysis.*

Rosenfeld, S. K., & Sprince, M. P. (1963). An attempt to formulate the meaning of the concept "borderline." *Psychoanalytic Study of the Child, 18,* 603–635.

Rosenfeld, S. K., & Sprince, M. P. (1965). Some thoughts on the technical handling of borderline children. *Psychoanalytic Study of the Child, 20,* 495–517.

Rubin, J. (1965). *Optimal taxonomy program (7090-IBM-0026).* International Business Machines Corp., Program Information Dept., Hawthorne, New York.

Sandler, J. (1976). Countertransference and role-responsiveness. *International Review of Psychoanalysis, 3,* 43–47.

Sandler, J. Kennedy, H., & Tyson, R. L. (1980). *The technique of child analysis. Discussions with Anna Freud.* Cambridge, MA: Harvard University Press.

Schafer, R. (1948). *The clinical application of psychological tests.* New York: International Universities Press.

Schafer, R. (1968). *Aspects of internalization.* New York: International

Universities Press.

Schilder, P. (1931–32). Scope of psychotherapy in schizophrenia. *American Journal of Psychiatry, 88,* 1181–1182.

Schmideberg, M. (1947). the treatment of psychopaths and borderline patients. *American Journal of Psychotherapy, 1,* 45–70.

Searles, H. F. (1965). *Collected papers on schizophrenia and related subjects.* New York: International Universities Press.

Searles, H. F. (1979). *Countertransference and related subjects.* New York: International Universities Press.

Searles, H. F. (1979). Pathologic symbiosis and autism. In *Countertransference and Related Subjects* (pp. 132–148). New York: International Universities Press.

Segal, H. (1964). *Introduction to the works of Melanie Klein.* New York: Basic Books.

Shapiro, E. R. (1978). The psychodynamics and developmental psychology of the borderline patient: A review. *American Journal of Psychiatry, 135,* 305–1315.

Siever, L. J. & Gunderson, J. G. (1979). Genetic determinants of borderline conditions. *Schizophrenia Bulletin, 5,* 59–86.

Singer, B. A., & Luborsky, L. (1977). Countertransference: The status of clinical versus quantitative research. In A. Gurman & A. Razin (Eds.), *Effective Psychotherapy.* New York: Pergamon.

Singer, J. L. (1985). Transference and the human condition: A cognitive-affective perspective. *Psychoanalytic Psychology, 2,* 189–220.

Singer, M., & Wynne, L. (1965). Thought disorder and family relations of schizophrenics: III. Methodology using projective techniques. *Archives of General Psychiatry, 12,* 187–200.

Singer, M. & Wynne, L. (1965). Thought disorder and family relations of schizophrenics: IV. Results and implications. *Archives of General Psychiatry, 12,* 201–212.

Singer, M. T., & Wynne, L. C. (1966). Communication styles in parents of normals, neurotics and schizophrenics. *American Psychiatric Research Report, 20,* 25–38.

Skodal, A. E., Buckley, P., & Charles, E. (1983). Is there a characteristic pattern to the treatment history of clinic outpatients with borderline personality? *Journal of Nervous and Mental Disease, 171,* 405–410.

Small, I. F. Small, J. G., & Anderson, J. M. (1966) Clinical characteristics of hallucinations of schizophrenia. *Diseases of the Nervous System, 27,* 349–353.

Snyder, S., Pitts, W. M., Goodpaster, W. A., et al. (1982). MMPI profile of DSM-III borderline personality disorder. *American Journal of Psychiatry, 139,* 1046–1048.

Soloff, P. H. (1981). Pharmacotherapy of borderline disorders. *Comprehensive Psychiatry, 22,* 535–543.

Soloff, P. H., George, A., & Nathan, R. S. (1982). The dexamethasone suppression test in patients with borderline personality disorder. *American Journal of Psychiatry, 139,* 1621–1623.

Soloff, P. H., & Millward, J. W. (1983). Psychiatric disorders in the families of borderline patients. *Archives of General Psychiatry, 40,* 37–44.

Soloff, P. H., & Millward, J. W. (1983). Developmental histories of borderline patients. *Comprehensive Psychiatry, 24,* 574–588.

Soloff, P. H., & Ulrich, R. F. (1981). The diagnostic interview for borderlines: A replication study. *Archives of General Psychiatry, 38,* 686–692.

Sperling, M. B. (1985). Discriminant measures for desperate love. *Journal of Personality Assessment, 49,* 324–328.

Sperling, M. (1989). Fusional relations in the borderline and normative realm: Desperate love. In R. Fine & H. S. Strean (Eds.), *Current and historical perspectives on the borderline patient.* New York: Brunner/Mazel.

Spiegel, J. (1966). Paradigms must be coordinated. *International Journal of Psychiatry, 2,* 422–431.

Spitz, R. (1955). The primal cavity: A contribution to the genesis of perception and its role for psychoanalytic theory. *Psychoanalytic Study of the Child, 10,* 215–240.

Spitz, R. (1965). *The first year of life.* New York: International Universities Press.

Spitzer, R. L., & Endicott, J. (1979). Justification for separating schizotypal and borderline personality disorders. *Schizophrenic Bulletin, 5,* 95–104.

Spitzer, R. L., Endicott, J., & Gibbon, M. (1979). Crossing the border into borderline personality and borderline schizophrenia: The development of criteria. *Archives of General Psychiatry, 36,* 17–24.

Spitzer, R. L., Endicott, J., & Robins, E. (1975). *Research diagnostic criteria (RDC) for a selected group of functional disorders* (2nd ed.). New York: New York State Psychiatric Institute, Biometrics Research.

Spitzer, R. L., Skodol, A. E., Williams, J. B., et al. (1982). Supervising intake diagnoses. *Archives of General Psychiatry, 39,* 1299–1305.

Spruiell, V. (1976). Paper presented at the December 1977 meeting of the American Psychoanalytic Association.

Staercke, A. (1921). Psychoanalysis and psychiatry. *International Journal of Psycho-Analysis, 2,* 361–415.

Stengel, E. (1945). A study of some clinical aspects of the relationship between obsessional neurosis and psychotic reaction types. *Journal of Mental Science, 91,* 166–187.

Stern, A. (1945). Psychoanalytic therapy in the borderline neuroses. *Psychoanalytic Quarterly, 14,* 190–198.

Sternbach, H. A., Fleming, J. Extein, E., et al. (1983). The dexamethasone suppression and thyrotropin-releasing hormone tests in depressed borderline patients. *Psychoneuroendocrinology, 8,* 459–462.

Stoller, R. J. (1973). *Splitting: A case of female masculinity.* New York: Quadrangle.

Stone, L. (1954). The widening scope of indications for psychoanalysis. *Journal of the American Psychoanalytic Association, 2,* 567–594.

Stone, M. H. (1973). Child psychiatry before the 20th century. *International Journal of Child Psychotherapy, 2,* 264–308.

Stone, M. H. (1977). The borderline syndrome: Evolution of the term, genetic aspects, and prognosis. *American Journal of Psychotherapy, 31,* 345–365.

Stone, M. H. (1979). Contemporary shift of the borderline concept from a subschizophrenic disorder to a subaffective disorder. *Psychiatric Clinics of North America, 2,* 577–594.

Stone, M. H. (1980). *The borderline syndromes: Constitution, personality and adaptation.* New York: McGraw-Hill.

Stone, M. H. (1981). Borderline syndromes: A consideration of subtypes and an overview, directions for research. *Psychiatric Clinics of North America, 4,* 3–24.

Stone, M. H. (1983). Premenstrual tension in borderline and related disorders. In R. C. Friedman (Ed.), *Behavior and the menstrual cycle.* New York: Marcel Dekker.

Stone, M. H. (1985). Disturbances in sex and love in borderline patients. In *Aspects of contemporary sexuality.* Westport, CT: Greenwood Press.

Stone, M. H., & Bernstein. (1980). Case management with borderline children: Theory and practice. *Clinical Social Work Journal, 8,* 147–166.

Stone, M. H., Kahn, E., & Flye, B. (1981). Psychiatrically ill relatives of borderline patients: A family study. *Psychiatric Quarterly, 53,* 71–84.

Strecker, E. A., & Wiley, G. F. (1925). Prognosis in schizophrenia. *Schizophrenia [Dementia Praecox], 5,* 403–431.

Strean, H. S. (1988). *Behind the couch: Revelations of a psychoanalyst.* New York: Wiley.

Sullivan, H. S. (1931). The modified psychoanalytic treatment of schizophrenia. *American Journal of Psychiatry, 11,* 519–540.

Sullivan, H. S. (1931). The relation of onset to outcome in schizophrenia. In *Schizophrenia as a human process* (pp. 233–255). New York: Norton, 1962.

Sullivan, H. S. (1962). *Schizophrenia as a human process.* New York: Norton.

Sutherland, J. (1983). The self and object relations: A challenge to psychoanalysis. *Bulletin of the Menninger Clinic, 47,* 525–541.

Tansey, M. J., & Burke, W. F. Projective identification and the empathic process: Interactional communications. *Contemporary Psychoanalysis, 21,* 42–69.

Tissot, R., et al. (1977). Long-term drug therapy in the psychoses. In C. Chiland (Ed.), *Long-term treatments of psychotic states.* New York: Human Sciences Press.

Tolpin, P. (1980). The borderline personality: Its makeup and analyzability. In Goldberg (Ed.), *Advances in self psychology,* New York: International Universities Press.

Tooley, K. (1973). Playing it right: A technique for the treatment of borderline children. *Journal of the American Academy of Child Psychiatry, 12,* 615–631.

Val, E., Flaherty, J. A., & Gaviria, F. (1982). *Psychological aspects in affective disorders: Psychopathology and treatment.* Chicago: Year Book Medical Publications.

Vallenstein, A. F. (1973). On attachment to painful feelings and the negative therapeutic reaction. *Psychoanalytic Study of the Child, 28,* 365–392.

Vanggaard, T. (1979). *Borderlands of sanity.* Copenhagen: Munksgaard.

Vaughn, C. E., & Leff, J. P. (1976). The influence of family and social factors on the course of psychiatric illness. *British Journal of Psychiatry, 129,* 125–137.

Vela, R., Gottlieb, E., & Gottlieb, H. (1983). Borderline syndromes in childhood: A critical review. In K. Robson (Ed.), *The borderline child.* New York: McGraw-Hill.

Voisin, F. (1826). *Des causes morales and physiques des maladies mentales.* Paris: J. B. Baillière.

Waelder, R. (1924). The psychoses: Their mechanism and accessibility to influence. *International Journal of Psycho-Analysis, 6,* 254–281.

Waldinger, R., & Gunderson, J. G. (1984). Completed psychotherapies with borderline patients. *American Journal of Psychotherapy, 38,* 190–202.

Wallerstein, R. S. (1986). *Forty-two lives in treatment.* New York: Guilford Press.

Walsh, F. (1977). Family study 1976: 14 new borderline cases. In R. R. Grinker, Sr., & B. Werble (Eds.), *Borderline patient.* New York: Jason Aronson.

Ward, H. (1926). *Thobbing.* New York: Bobbs-Merrill.

Warner, R. (1986). *Recovery from schizophrenia: Psychiatry and political economy.* New York: Methuen.

Watson, J. P. (1970). A repertory grid method of studying groups. *British Journal of Psychiatry, 117,* 309–318.

Webster's English Dictionary. New York: Holt, Rinehart & Winston, 1962.

Weil, A. P. (1973). Children with minimal brain dysfunction: Diagnostic and therapeutic considerations. In Sapir & Nitzburg (Eds.), *Children with learning problems.* New York: Brunner/Mazel.

Weil, A. P. (1978). Maturational variations and genetic dynamic issues. *Journal of the American Psychoanalytic Association, 26,* 461–492.

Weinshel, E. M. (1966). Panel on severe repressive states during analysis. *Journal of the American Psychoanalytic Association, 14,* 538–568.

Weinshel, E. M. (1976). Concluding comments on the congress topic. *International Journal of Psychiatry, 57,* 451–460.

Weisfogel, J., Dickes, R., & Simons, R. (1969). Diagnostic concepts concerning patients demonstrating both psychotic and neurotic symptoms. *Psychiatric Quarterly, 43,* 85–122.

Weissman, M. M., Myers, J. K., & Thompson, D. (1981). Depression and its treatment in a US urban community—1975–1976. *Archives of General Psychiatry, 38,* 417–421.

Werble, B. (1970). Second follow-up study of borderline patients. *Archives of General Psychiatry, 23,* 3–7.

Widiger, T. A. Psychological tests and borderline diagnosis. *Journal of Personality Assessment, 46,* 227–238.

Wilson, C. P. (1971). On the limits of the effectiveness of psychoanalysis: Early ego and somatic disturbances. *Journal of the American Psychoanalytic Association, 19,* 552–564.

Winnicott, D. W. (1953). Transitional objects and transitional phenomena. In *Playing and Reality* (pp. 1–25). New York: Basic Books, 1971.

Winnicott, D. W. (1960). Ego distortion in terms of true and false self. In *The maturational process and the facilitating environment* (pp. 140–152). New York: International Universities Press, 1965.

Winnicott, D. W. (1960). The theory of the parent-infant relationship. In *The maturational processes and the facilitating environment* (pp. 37–55). New York: International Universities Press, 1965.

Witenberg, E. G. (1976). To believe or not to believe. Presidential Address to the American Academy of Psychoanalysis. *Journal of the American Academy of Psychoanalysis, 4,* 433–445.

Wittman, P. (1941). A scale for measuring prognosis in schizophrenic patients. *Elgin State Hospital Papers, 4,* 20–33.

Wolberg, A. (1952). The borderline patient. *American Journal of Psychother-*

apy, 6, 694–701.

Wolberg, A. (1973). *The borderline patient.* New York: Intercontinental Medical Book Corporation.

Woodbury, M. (1966). Altered body-ego experiences: A contribution to the study of regression, perception and early development. *Journal of the American Psychoanalytic Association, 14,* 273–303.

Worden, F. G. (1955). A problem in psychoanalytic technique. *Journal of the American Psychoanalytic Association, 3,* 255–279.

World Health Organization. (1973). *Report of the International Pilot Study of Schizophrenia: Results of the initial evaluation phase.* Geneva: WHO.

Wynne, L. C., & Singer, M. T. (1963). Thought disorder and family relations of schizophrenics. *Archives of General Psychiatry, 9,* 199–206.

Wynne, L. C., & Singer, M. T. (1963). Thought disorders and family relations of schizophrenics. I. A research strategy, *Archives of General Psychiatry, 9,* 191–198.

Zetzel, E. (1971). A developmental approach to the borderline patient. *American Journal of Psychiatry, 127,* 867–871.

Zilboorg, G. (1941). Ambulatory schizophrenias. *Psychiatry, 4,* 149–155.

Zilboorg, G. (1956). The problem of ambulatory schizophrenias. *American Journal of Psychiatry, 113,* 519–525.

Zilboorg, G. (1957). Further observations on ambulatory schizophrenias. *American Journal of Orthopsychiatry, 27,* 677–682.

Zinner, J., & Shapiro, E. R. (1975). Splitting in families of borderline adolescents. In J. E. Mack (Ed.), *Borderline states in psychiatry* (pp. 103–122). New York: Grune & Stratton.

Zubenko, G. S., et al. (1987). Sexual practices among patients with borderline personality disorder. *American Journal of Psychiatry, 144,* 748–752.

Zuk, G. H., & Boszormenyi-Nagy, I. (1967). *Family therapy and disturbed families.* Palo Alto, CA: Science and Behavior Books.